Home Health Care

Home Health Care:
A Guide for Occupational
Therapy Practice

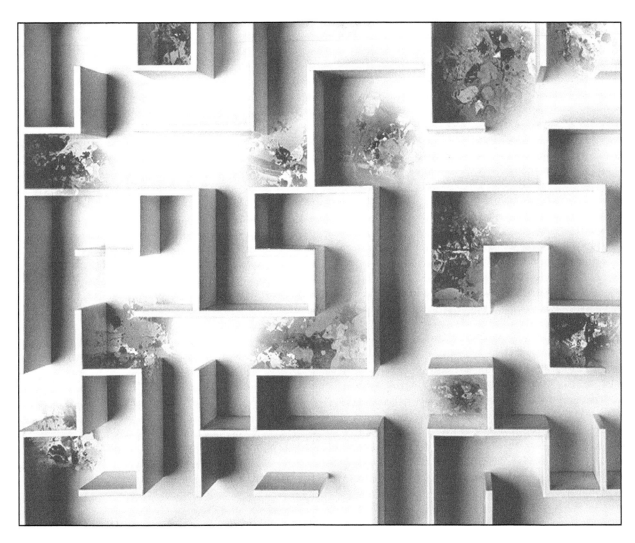

Edited by Karen Vance, BSOT

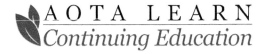

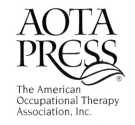

AOTA Centennial Vision

We envision that occupational therapy is a powerful, widely recognized, science-driven, and evidence-based profession with a globally connected and diverse workforce meeting society's occupational needs.

Mission Statement

The American Occupational Therapy Association advances the quality, availability, use, and support of occupational therapy through standard-setting, advocacy, education, and research on behalf of its members and the public.

AOTA Staff

Frederick P. Somers, *Executive Director*
Christopher M. Bluhm, *Chief Operating Officer*
Maureen Peterson, *Chief Professional Affairs Officer*

Chris Davis, *Director, AOTA Press*
Caroline Polk, *Digital Publishing Manager and* AJOT *Managing Editor*
Ashley Hofmann, *Development Editor*
Barbara Dickson, *Production Editor*

Debbie Amini, *Director, Professional Development*
Sarah Hertfelder, *Continuing Education Consultant*

Rebecca Rutberg, *Director, Marketing*
Amanda Goldman, *Marketing Manager*
Jennifer Folden, *Marketing Specialist*

American Occupational Therapy Association, Inc.
4720 Montgomery Lane
Bethesda, MD 20814
301-652-AOTA (2682)
TDD: 800-377-8555
Fax: 301-652-7711
www.aota.org
To order: 1-877-404-AOTA or store.aota.org

Disclaimers

This publication is designed to provide accurate and authoritative information in regard to the subject matter covered. It is sold or distributed with the understanding that the publisher is not engaged in rendering legal, accounting, or other professional service. If legal advice or other expert assistance is required, the services of a competent professional person should be sought.

—From the Declaration of Principles jointly adopted by the
American Bar Association and a Committee of Publishers and Associations

It is the objective of the American Occupational Therapy Association to be a forum for free expression and interchange of ideas. The opinions expressed by the contributors to this work are their own and not necessarily those of the American Occupational Therapy Association/AOTA Press.

ISBN: 978-1-56900-379-4

Library of Congress Control Number: 2016931358

Cover design by Debra Naylor, Naylor Design, Inc., Washington, DC
Composition and printing by Automated Graphic Systems, Inc., White Plains, MD
Publication management by Steve Pazdan, College Park, MD

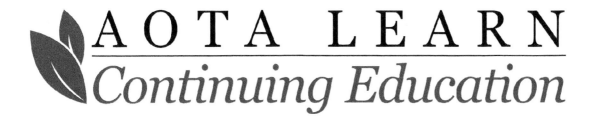

A O T A L E A R N
Continuing Education

Make Your Learning Count!

**Earn Continuing Education (CE) Credit (AOTA CEUs/Contact Hours/NBCOT® PDUs)
With This Publication.**

Publication Purchase: If you purchased the text non-CE publication version of *Home Health Care: A Guide for Occupational Therapy Practice,* you can purchase the CE exam and earn CE credits (20 contact hours; 2 AOTA CEUs; 25 NBCOT PDUs).

Ordering is easy! As a purchaser of this publication, order the Self-Paced Clinical Course (SPCC) exam only (price will reflect exam only):

- Enter **Order #3035CE** online at **http://store.aota.org,** or by phone at 877-404-AOTA (2682).
- Once you place an order, you will immediately receive an email with your CE exam access information.

SPCC Purchase: If you purchased *Home Health Care: A Guide for Occupational Therapy Practice* as an AOTA SPCC, you are enrolled in the CE activity (exam) for this publication. After placing your order, you will receive an email with instructions on how to access and complete the CE activity for this course at AOTA LEARN (**www.aota.org/learn**), AOTA's online center for professional development.

- The CE exam is available on AOTA LEARN to print and review as you read the SPCC.
- When you finish reading, complete the CE exam on AOTA LEARN.
- Successful completion of the exam requires a minimum passing score of 75%. You are provided with two attempts to pass the exam. If required, additional attempts to pass the exam can be purchased by calling 877-404-AOTA (2682).
- With successful course completion, you will instantly receive a certificate and transcript to download or print to verify your learning for state licensure, certification, employers, or your own professional development portfolio.

There are even more reasons to learn with an AOTA SPCC:

- Upon successful completion of the SPCC exam, for an additional cost, you can earn **nondegree graduate credits from Colorado State University.** Learn more on the next page.
- Learning with AOTA SPCCs provides a **depth of knowledge from experts** that can assist in achieving clinical excellence. Your colleagues and clients benefit when you apply your enhanced expertise.

Discontinuation: When an AOTA SPCC is discontinued, notification is provided at **aota.org/ce,** in AOTA periodicals, and via email to SPCC learners who have not yet completed the exam. SPCC learners have 1 year from first notification of discontinuation to complete the SPCC exam and receive CE credits.

Colorado State University (CSU) Nondegree Graduate Credit

To obtain nondegree graduate credit from CSU, do the following:

Contact CSU at the following address to obtain the most current registration form and tuition rate; refer to course number *OT 590 734 Workshop*: *Home Health Care: A Guide for Occupational Therapy Practice*.

Colorado State University Online
Division of Continuing Education
1040 Campus Delivery
Fort Collins, CO 80523-1040
Attn: Contract Courses

Phone: 970-491-5288
Email: onlineplus_questions@colostate.edu

You may obtain 2 CSU nondegree graduate credits for completing this course.

The following terms and conditions apply:

1. SPCC learners have 2 years from the time of purchase to complete the AOTA SPCC for optional, non-degree graduate credit from CSU, for an additional cost.
2. AOTA allows learners to retake the SPCC exam 2 times. After 2 attempts, learners can purchase additional attempts.
3. When learners pass an exam, AOTA issues them a continuing education certificate of completion. If you have registered for CSU nondegree graduate credits, CSU will contact AOTA at the end of each semester for grades of registered learners.
4. Learners who have not obtained a satisfactory grade on their exam and have applied for CSU non-degree graduate credit should contact CSU directly, at the address above, to discuss the timeline for keeping the CSU registration process active.
5. CSU tuition and fees are subject to change.

Contents

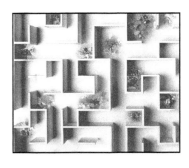

Boxes, Exhibits, Figures, and Tables

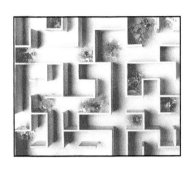

Boxes

Exhibits

Figures

Tables

Acknowledgments

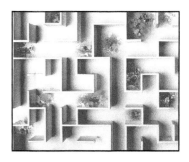

I would like to thank the authors who provided premier substance to this Self-Paced Clinical Course and publication, *Home Health Care: A Guide for Occupational Therapy Practice*. I appreciate their knowledge, expertise, passion, and patience for the time it took to complete this project. They persisted through the death of parents, personal health issues, and even retirement to see this through. I am also deeply grateful to Sarah Hertfelder, MEd, MOT, FAOTA, Continuing Education Consultant, whose ability to understand the blend of practice and policy important to this subject helped advocate for this publication to be the most accurate and comprehensive resource on this topic.

I would like to thank Christina Metzler, AOTA's Chief Public Affairs Officer, for supporting not only this publication but also all the practitioners working in home health care every day. I also want to thank my coworkers, Mark P. Sharp, CPA, Partner, and M. Aaron Little, CPA, Managing Director, at BKD LLP Health Care Group, for supporting me and helping me understand the home health industry in ways I could not have without them. Finally, thank you to Chris Davis, Director, AOTA Press, and the editorial and production staff, Ashley Hofmann, Hyde Loomis, Kathie Porta Baker, Steve Pazdan, and Barbara Dickson, for their editorial and production expertise, patience, and professionalism in finalizing this publication.

—Karen Vance, BSOT

The editor appreciates the time and thoughtful comments of our reviewers, who helped us reflect on and improve on our work:

- **Jennifer DeRosa, OTR/L, CAPS**
  Owner, AdaptABLE for Life
  Seattle

- **Mary St. Pierre, RN, BSN, MGA**
  Vice President for Regulatory Affairs
  National Association for Home Care & Hospice
  Washington, DC

- **Peggy Strecker Neufeld, PhD, OTR/L, FAOTA**
  Community Consultant and Advocate
  Research and Community Liaison
  St. Louis NORC (Naturally Occurring Retirement Community)
  Jewish Federation
  St. Louis

- **Pamela E. Toto, PhD, OTR/L, BCG, FAOTA**
  Assistant Professor of Occupational Therapy
  University of Pittsburgh
  Pittsburgh

- **Tracy Van Oss, DHSc, MPH, OTR/L, SCEM, CHES, CAPS**
  Associate Professor of Occupational Therapy
  Quinnipiac University
  Hamden, CT

About the Editor and Authors

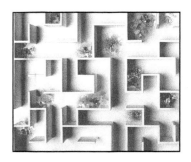

About the Editor

Karen Vance, BSOT, has been practicing in home care since 1981 in clinical, management, and consulting positions. She has served twice as chairperson of the American Occupational Therapy Association (AOTA) Home & Community Health Special Interest Section (HCHSIS) and was part of the original formation committee for HCHSIS. Karen has served on the National Association for Home 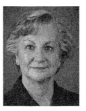 Care & Hospice Therapy Advisory Committee, the Technical Expert Panel for the Centers for Medicare & Medicaid's Home Health Quality Improvement Campaign, and the Agency for Healthcare Research and Quality's Consumer Assessment of Healthcare Providers and Systems and as liaison to the Joint Commission's Home Care Professional and Technical Advisory Committee. Karen has worked since 2003 as a consultant for BKD Health Care Group in Springfield, Missouri, providing clinical and operational consulting for home care and hospice agencies to establish and maintain quality management practices. Karen is a 1978 graduate of the University of Missouri, Columbia, with a bachelor of science degree in occupational therapy.

About the Authors

Ann O'Sullivan, OTR/L, LSW, FAOTA, has more than 38 years of experience working in adult rehabilitation, seating and positioning, home health, marketing, management, aging services, and education. She received her BS in occupational therapy from Tufts University in 1978 and her Maine social work license in 2002. In 2011, she was 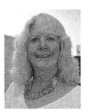 named an AOTA Fellow for tireless leadership in home care and family caregiving. She coordinates the Family Caregiver Support Program for the Southern Maine Agency on Aging and is past chair of the HCHSIS. She is a lead trainer for the evidence-based and evidence-informed A Matter of Balance: Lay Leader Model, the Savvy Caregiver Program, and the Savvy Caregiver Advanced Program, and she is a certified interventionist for the Rosalynn Carter Institute for Caregiving Resources' Enhancing Alzheimer's Caregiver Health program. Ann has authored or coauthored eight chapters in professional texts and 13 journal articles. She presents both locally and nationally on topics related to home health, dementia, and family caregivers.

Tina Shadley, OTR/L, received her degree in occupational therapy from the University of Puget Sound in 1976. Retired at the end of 2015, Tina worked as a therapy consultant for the South Carolina Department of Health and Environmental Control, Division of Home Health Services, in Columbia, South Carolina, in home health for a total of 27 years. She also served as a board member for the South Carolina Home Care and Hospice Association for 9 of those years.

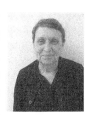

Carol Siebert, MS, OTR/L, FAOTA, has worked in home- and community-based practice since 1989. Her work in home health has been primarily as a staff occupational therapist. She has served as chairperson of the AOTA HCHSIS and as editor of the *HCHSIS Quarterly.* Carol served as a member of the Joint Commission Homecare Professional and Technical Advisory Committee from 2008 to 2011 and served as vice chair of that committee from 2012 to 2013. She served on the National Association for Home Care & Hospice Therapy Advisory Committee from 2009 to 2010 and was chair of that committee from 2011 to 2012. She has also established home health fieldwork experiences and served as a home health clinical educator at several agencies. In 2006, Carol was named an AOTA Fellow for her leadership in home health, empowering practitioners and educating the industry. Carol is currently the principal of Home Remedy, Chapel Hill, North Carolina, an occupational therapy practice providing direct and contracted services in community health and primary care in central North Carolina.

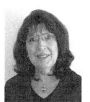

Missi Zahoransky, MSHS, OTR/L, owned a Medicare/Medicaid-certified home health agency with a zero-deficiency record for more than 14 years and is currently the owner of Total Rehabilitation Specialists, a therapy contract company that specializes in the provision of home care therapy services. Missi has presented at the national, state, and local levels both as an occupational therapist and as a home health care administrator and has written multiple articles and chapters on home health care and reimbursement issues. She is past chair of the AOTA HCHSIS; serves on the AOTA Advisory Council to the Special Interest Sections as an advisor on home health issues; and has served as the SIS Liaison to the AOTA Commission on Practice. Missi has received the Ohio Award of Merit, served on the steering committee for the Delta Therapy project, and was chair of the Visiting Committee for the College of Science at Cleveland State University, where she is a part-time faculty member and is currently on the development board. She received her bachelor's and master's degrees from Cleveland State University.

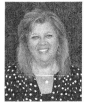

Abbreviations and Acronyms

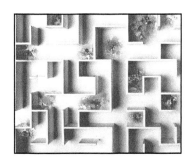

AAAs	Area Agencies on Aging
ACOTE	Accreditation Council for Occupational Therapy Education
ADLs	activities of daily living
ADRCs	Aging and Disability Resource Centers
AOTA	American Occupational Therapy Association
BADLs	basic activities of daily living
BRP	bathroom privileges
CAHPS	Consumer Assessment of Healthcare Providers and Systems
CDC	Centers for Disease Control and Prevention
CfCs	Conditions for Coverage
CFR	*Code of Federal Regulations*
CHAMP	Collaboration for Homecare Advances in Management and Practice
CHF	congestive heart failure
CMS	Centers for Medicare & Medicaid Services
CoP	Condition of Participation
CPE	continuing professional education
CPT®	*Current Procedural Terminology®*
DME	durable medical equipment
HCFA	Health Care Financing Administration
HCHSIS	Home & Community Health Special Interest Section [of AOTA]
HHA	home health agency
HHC	Home Health Compare

HHCAHPS	Home Health Consumer Assessment of Healthcare Providers and Systems
HHQI	Home Health Quality Initiative
HHRGs	home health resource groups
HI	health insurance
HIPAA	Health Insurance Portability and Accountability Act of 1996 (Pub. L. 104–191)
HIPPS	Health Insurance Prospective Payment System
IADLs	instrumental activities of daily living
ICD	International Statistical Classification of Diseases and Related Health Problems (aka International Classification of Diseases)
IOM	Institute of Medicine
LCDs	local coverage determinations
LUPA	low utilization payment adjustment
NBCOT®	National Board for Certification in Occupational Therapy®
NCHS	National Center for Health Statistics
OASIS	Outcome and Assessment Information Set
OBQI	Outcome-Based Quality Improvement
OBQM	Outcome-Based Quality Monitoring
PADLs	personal activities of daily living
PBQI	Process-Based Quality Improvement
PEO Model	Person–Environment–Occupation Model
PEP	partial episode payment
PHQ–2	Patient Health Questionnaire–2
POC	plan of care
POT	plan of treatment
PPS	prospective payment system
RAP	request for anticipated payment
RN	registered nurse
ROC	resumption of care
ROM	range of motion
SOC	start of care
SPCC	Self-Paced Clinical Course
UHF	United Hospital Fund
VA	U.S. Department of Veterans Affairs
WHO	World Health Organization

INTRODUCTION—

Home Health: The Perfect Context for Occupational Therapy

Karen Vance, BSOT

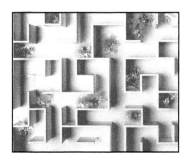

The practice of occupational therapy is an experience made very personal by the history, character, values, and talents of each occupational therapy practitioner. This personal context infuses meaning into practice for the practitioner as well as the client. The dictionary defines *context* as "the interrelated conditions in which something exists or occurs," including elements that "can throw light on its meaning" (Merriam-Webster, 2015). Practitioners exist within the fluid conditions that constitute their lives, and it is through the lens of context that they interpret their practice and see their clients.

The *Occupational Therapy Practice Framework: Domain and Process* (3rd ed.; American Occupational Therapy Association [AOTA], 2014b) focuses on the client in its definition of *context* as "elements within and surrounding a client that are often less tangible than physical and social environments but nonetheless exert a strong influence on performance" (p. S9). One of the conditions influencing clients' performance, of course, is the presence of an occupational therapy practitioner. The influence may be intentional, resulting from a planned intervention, or unintentional, resulting from the practitioner's own context interacting or sometimes colliding with the client's context. For example, the practitioner's subconsciously held cultural values may conflict with those of the client. Other interrelated conditions influencing the client's performance are the social and physical environments within which the client sits, both literally and figuratively.

Context is one of the fundamental concepts in the *Framework* and is integral to the framing of occupational therapy as a client-centered profession, regardless of the setting in which it is practiced. As the practitioner gathers information about a client during an evaluation, the client's context unfolds, helping the practitioner frame and define the optimal approach to successful occupational therapy interventions and client outcomes. In many settings, the practitioner must garner the entire client context through interviews and is dependent on the client's or caregiver's report of the client's context. In many other settings, the intervention is developed after an evaluation in a contrived environment in an attempt to re-create the client's context.

Evaluation in the home, however, allows the advantages inherent in the observation of spontaneous and habitual performance. The beauty of practicing in the client's own real environment is the natural display of the client's context, within which the occupational therapy practitioner can best support the client's health and participation in life through engagement in occupation: This context is home.

Home can be the house the client grew up in or moved into later in life, the residence of a family member, an assisted living facility, or even a homeless shelter. This practice setting envelops the client in his or her own rich social and environmental context, and practitioners are both challenged and benefited by the surroundings. Regardless of how the social or physical environment of the home helps or hinders health and participation in life, this is the context within which occupational therapy practitioners in home health practice must work to support engagement that is most meaningful to the client.

Historical Context: Influence of Medicare on Home Health Occupational Therapy Practice

Occupational therapy in the home may feel natural for a practitioner applying clinical reasoning one-on-one with a client. However, the practical application of occupational therapy in the home involves a much larger context than that of the practitioner and client alone. *Pragmatic reasoning,* the type of clinical reasoning that concerns the practice setting (Schell, 2008), elucidates the context of the home health practice setting as including not only the physical location of the client being served but also the reimbursement and regulatory requirements and population-driven considerations (e.g., diagnoses or conditions, demographics) specific to that setting. To begin comprehending how the larger context affects the day-to-day pragmatic reasoning of a home health occupational therapy practitioner, one must first understand the historical influence of Medicare on home health occupational therapy practice.

Medicare as payer and regulator has greatly affected occupational therapy in home health for many years. The financial incentives from past payment methodologies and regulations governing this setting shaped practice patterns that have had the unintended consequence of creating a perception in the home health industry that occupational therapy is a lesser or ancillary service. *Practice patterns* include the behaviors of health care practitioners, utilization of services, and results achieved or not achieved by the provision of services.

From the time Medicare began funding home health care in 1965 until late in 2000, home health agencies (HHAs) were reimbursed for the cost of each visit rendered to a beneficiary. This payment methodology created an incentive to make frequent visits or to provide services over long periods. The incentive to maximize visits influenced practice for 35 years. Indeed, many practice patterns established before 2000 persisted long after the change in payment methodology. Simply put, before 2000, it was not in HHAs' financial interests for the beneficiary to improve quickly, so services whose primary purpose was to improve function, such as occupational therapy, were not encouraged in the plan of care.

In 2000, cost reimbursement was replaced with the *prospective payment system* (PPS), which is explained in **Appendix A, "Medicare as Payer."** HHAs now receive a lump-sum payment regardless of how many visits are made. Utilization statistics illustrate the effect of this change in payment methodologies on practice patterns. For example, the average number of visits per beneficiary was 74 in 1996, when the incentive for Medicare reimbursement was making visits; average visits per beneficiary dropped to 30 in 2001, when HHAs began receiving lump-sum payments (National Association for Home Care & Hospice, 2010).

Although the Medicare payment methodology has changed, the requirements for a beneficiary to qualify for the Medicare home health benefit have not changed and must be considered to understand current practice. One of the primary coverage criteria for ongoing home health services is that the Medicare beneficiary must continue to require skilled services that are reasonable and necessary to the treatment of the beneficiary's illness or injury (Centers for Medicare & Medicaid Services [CMS], 2014, § 40.2; see **Appendix A,** pp. 183–187). To justify maximizing visits during the previously cost-reimbursed Medicare home health services, the beneficiary had to demonstrate a need for continued skilled services. In **Appendix A,** the section "Medicare Coverage Under the Part A Home Health Benefit" (pp. 175–188) outlines all of the coverage criteria a Medicare beneficiary must meet to qualify for the home health benefit; familiarity with these criteria is necessary to understand the full effect of Medicare rules on occupational therapy practice in home health.

As explained in **Appendix A,** the need for occupational therapy alone does not initially qualify the beneficiary for the home health benefit. Although skilled nursing, physical therapy, or speech–language pathology initially qualifies the patient for the benefit, when occupational therapy begins at any time before the final visit by one of those disciplines, the need for occupational therapy continues to qualify the beneficiary for the home health benefit. The fact that occupational therapy alone cannot qualify a beneficiary for home health services has contributed to the perception of occupational therapy as a lesser or ancillary service. Changes in Medicare regulations are not as necessary to change this perception as is occupational therapy practitioners' ability to clearly demonstrate the value of occupational therapy to HHA outcomes.

Understanding *coverage criteria,* the criteria that must be met for Medicare to pay for services, is critical to understanding past, current, and emerging practice patterns. The home health Medicare coverage criteria detailed in **Appendix A** supplement the content found in the chapters of this text and Self-Paced Clinical Course (SPCC), and this and the other appendixes can serve as a future reference for readers. HHA interpretations of coverage criteria can vary, and when working with HHAs to develop or revise policies and procedures, occupational therapy practitioners are well served to have the source documents discussed in **Appendix A** as a reference.

Audience for and Contents of This Text and Self-Paced Clinical Course

Occupational therapy practitioners initially entering home health practice can benefit from all of the information provided in this text and SPCC. Practitioners who have experience in home health settings may find much of the information familiar, but they may also find that some of the information contradicts what they have held or been told to be true and thereby gain an important corrective learning experience.

This text and SPCC was written by occupational therapy practitioners for occupational therapy practitioners, but it also provides a resource for other stakeholders, such as HHAs, who want to know what to expect from occupational therapy practitioners in the home health setting. The following learning objectives for this text and SPCC are designed to guide practitioners toward the most accurate, effective, and enduring occupational therapy practice in the home.

Overall Learning Objectives

After completing this SPCC and reading this publication, learners and readers will be able to

- Identify the inherent advantages in practicing occupational therapy in the context of the physical and social environment of the client's own home;
- Differentiate the conditions of client populations receiving occupational therapy services in the home from the conditions of those treated in other practice settings;
- Identify all of the stakeholders in the efficient and effective practice of occupational therapy in the home;
- Differentiate the roles of Medicare as the major payer and regulator of home health services;
- Recognize how payer and regulatory requirements need to be integrated into daily occupational therapy home health practice;
- Identify the differences between regulatory requirements and HHA policies;
- Delineate how the occupational therapy home health evaluation based on the *Framework* differs from but can contribute to the accuracy of data reported using the Outcome and Assessment Information Set (OASIS); and
- Identify the similarities between the quality indicators measured by an HHA and the domain items of the *Framework*.

This text and SPCC frames occupational therapy in the context of the home health practice setting and provides the knowledge occupational therapy practitioners in home health need to explicitly practice and communicate the value of occupational therapy. Much of the material is based on information from current CMS publications, as cited in the "References" section of each chapter. Because these publications are periodically updated, it is recommended that readers make sure they are using the most recent version.

This text and SPCC is organized in three sections, as described in the paragraphs that follow.

Section I—"Stakeholder Context: Satisfying Stakeholders in Occupational Therapy Home Health Services"

Practicing occupational therapy in the rich context of home health can be very satisfying for occupational therapy practitioners. However, practitioners in this area of practice have obligations to many stakeholders in occupational therapy: clients and caregivers; agencies, the public, payers, and regulators; and the profession itself. The two chapters in Section I review the outcomes important to all those who have a stake in occupational therapy.

Chapter 1—"Stakeholders in Home Health: Agencies, the Public, Regulators, and Payers"—describes

- Entities other than clients and caregivers who have a stake in occupational therapy services
- Work arrangements between HHAs and occupational therapy practitioners
- The ways in which payers and regulators protect the public's stake in home health
- Strategies for moving from meeting to exceeding the expectations of patients, regulators, and payers
- The risk to home health occupational therapy practice when practitioners fail to understand and meet stakeholder expectations.

Chapter 2—"Stakeholders in Home Health: Clients and Caregivers"—explains

- The stake of clients and family caregivers in home health occupational therapy delivery and outcomes
- The elements of client- and caregiver-centered care
- Challenges in integrating family caregivers into the health care team and strategies to enhance collaboration and build partnerships
- Elements necessary for effective caregiver teaching
- Opportunities for reporting data on client and caregiver satisfaction with services.

Section II—"Occupational Therapy Practice in the Context of Home Health"

Persevering in understanding and complying with the layers of reimbursement requirements and regulations rewards home health occupational therapy practitioners with the honor and privilege of working with clients in the context of their own home. Section II describes the reimbursement and regulatory parameters of home health occupational therapy practice within the context of the *Framework*. The five chapters in this section describe the uniqueness of the home context and occupational therapy best practices in this setting.

Chapter 3—"Conditions in Home Health Care"—outlines

- The many types of conditions common in the population receiving home health care
- Why diagnosis alone provides inadequate information to describe the home health population
- The social and physical contexts of home health practice as critical components of the client's condition.

Chapter 4—"The Occupational Therapy Evaluation Process in Home Health"—covers

- The *Framework* as a guide to practice in the natural context of home health
- The components of the occupational therapy evaluation process in home health
- The components of the home health comprehensive assessment
- The best approach to the Medicare "therapy assessment" content requirements

- The importance of home health data accuracy to the occupational therapy evaluation process in home health and to the Home Health Quality Initiative (HHQI)
- Key occupational performance items in OASIS.

Chapter 5—"Home Health Plans of Care, Intervention, and Team Collaboration"—elaborates

- A process for identifying the need for occupational therapy and the outcomes of occupational therapy provided as part of home health services
- Pragmatic factors that must be considered in formulating an occupational therapy plan of care when providing home health services
- Elements of a home health plan of care that fulfill the requirements of CMS
- Strategies to enhance interdisciplinary communication and coordination that contribute to coherent care planning.

Chapter 6—"Sustainable Outcomes in Home Health"—examines

- Ways to identify sustainable outcomes in home health occupational therapy practice
- The client's perspective on outcomes and the significance of self-management in achieving desired home health outcomes
- Advantages and limitations of outcomes measured as end results in home health practice
- The relationship between trajectory and sustainable outcomes in home health practice
- Occupational therapy as OuTcomes.

Chapter 7—"Community Resources and Living Life to Its Fullest"—describes

- Challenges faced by clients and family caregivers in the transition from home health to "just plain home"
- The critical role of family caregivers in assisting a person in the community
- The significance of self-management in the ongoing well-being of clients and family caregivers
- The importance of connecting with community resources to help clients and family caregivers reengage and participate in their communities after the home health episode.

Section III—"Home Health and the Occupational Therapy Profession"

Practicing occupational therapy in the home health setting can be a very isolating, if rewarding, experience. Both occupational therapy practitioners and those who employ them are often unsure how to ensure best practices in this setting.

Section III has one chapter; Chapter 8—"Home Health Occupational Therapy Practitioners and the Occupational Therapy Profession"—delineates

- Qualifications and competencies necessary for a home health occupational therapy practitioner as outlined in federal and state regulations

- Roles in HHAs and in the home health industry available for occupational therapists and occupational therapy assistants on the basis of qualifications
- Ways that occupational therapy education, research, and practitioner preparation and professional development can sustain occupational therapy's stake in home health
- The benefits of a mentoring program to support the professional development of practitioners in home health
- Misperceptions about the extent of occupational therapy's role in the home health industry.

Appendixes

Home health occupational therapy services take place in the context of a daunting array of rules and regulations. Many of these are referred to in the chapters of this text and SPCC, but to allow the discussion to flow unencumbered by extensive attention to detail, appendixes are provided that focus at length on the rules and regulations related to four topics. **Appendixes A, B,** and **C** focus on the roles of Medicare in home health services as payer, regulator, and quality monitor, respectively, and **Appendix D** acquaints readers with OASIS, the repository of data whose collection not only is required of home health clinicians but also contributes to effective and efficient services at all levels of practice.

The sources of the rules and regulations in the appendixes are provided in each to enable home health occupational therapy practitioners to locate the exact language they need from the manuals to ensure proper application of these parameters within their own practice and within the context of their own employment setting. When practitioners find that HHA policies restrict occupational therapy practice because of improper application of regulations, having the source documents is helpful in advocating for positive changes to those policies. Because the appendixes to this book contain information that is essential to understanding the content of the chapters and to integrating that content into the context of occupational therapy practice, at specific points readers are directed to material in the appendixes that they should read before continuing with the chapter. This knowledge may be assessed in the exam questions.

Appendix content that is significantly important to chapter content will be brought to the reader's attention as shown in the following example. However, this content should not be considered the only appendix content to be reviewed. Appendix references throughout this text and SPCC will also be in **bold** and provide additional information or remind the reader of appendix content that has been addressed in more detail earlier.

 Stop here! Go to Appendix C and read the section "Empowerment of Consumers Through Public Disclosure" (pp. 207–208).

Any shaded rules and regulations in the appendixes are reproduced from current federal publications. However, because rules and regulations change, it is always a good idea for readers to confirm they are the most recent.

Appendix A, "Medicare as Payer," discusses

- An overview of Medicare as payer, including Parts A–D
- Medicare coverage under the Part A home health benefit, including conditions for coverage, assessment considerations for *homebound* status, plan of care, and covered services
- Medicare contractors
- The home health PPS, including payment rate, consolidated billing, home health resource groups, billing procedures, and Medicare as a secondary payer
- Part B outpatient therapy services provided by an HHA.

Appendix B, "Medicare as Regulator," provides

- An overview of Medicare as regulator
- Requirements for Medicare-certified HHAs
- Ways to locate and identify the Medicare Conditions of Participation (CoPs)
- Excerpts describing occupational therapist and occupational therapy assistant qualifications and supervision; coordination of patient services; acceptance of patients, plan of care, and medical supervision; therapy services; and comprehensive assessment of patients.

Appendix C, "Medicare as Quality Monitor," discusses

- An overview of Medicare as quality monitor
- The HHQI, including empowerment of consumers through public disclosure on the Home Health Compare website and support for providers' quality improvement efforts
- Outcome-Based Quality Improvement (OBQI), including outcome definition, measurement time points, and the two-stage framework of outcome analysis and outcome enhancement.

Appendix D, "Outcome and Assessment Information Set (OASIS)," describes

- An overview of OASIS
- Where to find and how to use the *OASIS Guidance Manual*
- Regulations governing OASIS data collection, including incorporating OASIS data into the comprehensive assessment, who may complete OASIS data collection, data collection time points, release of patient-identifiable OASIS information, and data transmission requirements
- Occupational therapy's role in accurate data collection for the agency, including collection of data during assessments, contributing to an accurate clinical picture, and offering agency training
- Conventions in OASIS data collection
- OASIS outcome measure item guidance
- OASIS process measure item guidance.

Finally, **Appendix E, "AOTA Fact Sheet: Occupational Therapy's Role in Home Health,"** is a resource for external audiences that occupational therapy practitioners are encouraged to use.

Terminology

Depending on where one practices, terminology that means one thing in a particular location may mean something else in another—the home health setting is no exception. Terms that occupational therapy practitioners use in their practice, education, and professional documents (e.g., the *Framework*) may not mean the same thing outside the profession. Practitioners in home health must understand the terminology used by other stakeholders to be able to fully participate and contribute according to the rules and regulations that guide practice in the home health setting. The sections that follow define Essential Terms, which are used across chapters and whose correct use is of critical importance in home health practice, and Key Terms, which are important to each chapter.

Essential Terms

Patient and Client

The *Framework* is referenced many times in this text and SPCC as an official document of AOTA (2014b) and as a guide for framing occupational therapy practice. The *Framework* states in its "Introduction" that

> The clients of occupational therapy are typically classified as *persons* (including those involved in care of a client), *groups* (collectives of individuals, e.g., families, workers, students, communities), and *populations* (collectives of groups of individuals living in a similar locale—e.g., city, state, or country—or sharing the same or like characteristics or concerns). (p. S3)

Although the *Framework* uses the term *client* to identify a person receiving occupational therapy services, that same person may also be referred to as a *patient,* depending on the type and location of the service and the language used to describe the services provided (e.g., that used in federal and state regulations and payer regulations). Therefore, both terms—*patient* and *client*—are used in this text and SPCC.

In Section I, "Stakeholder Context: Satisfying Stakeholders in Occupational Therapy Home Health Services," both terms are used because this section addresses both the delivery of occupational therapy services (to clients) and payer- and policymaker-related issues (affecting patients). In Section II, "Occupational Therapy Practice in the Context of Home Health," the term *client* is used throughout, consistent with the *Framework*. Section III, "Home Health and the Occupational Therapy Profession," also uses the term *client* because this section focuses on the profession itself in preparing and sustaining skill sets for service delivery in this practice setting. The appendixes use the term *patient* because they discuss Medicare-related issues, and Medicare documents refer to patients.

Evaluation and Assessment

The *Standards of Practice for Occupational Therapy* (AOTA, 2015c) defines the terms *evaluation* and *assessment* as follows:

- *Evaluation* is the "process of obtaining and interpreting data necessary for intervention. This includes planning for and documenting the evaluation process and results" (p. 2).

- *Assessment* refers to "specific tools or instruments that are used during the evaluation process" (p. 2).

The *Framework* makes a similar distinction between the terms *evaluation* and *assessment: Evaluation* begins the occupational therapy process and is "focused on finding out what a client wants and needs to do; determining what a client can do and has done; and identifying supports and barriers to health, well-being, and participation" (AOTA, 2014b, p. S13), whereas *assessment* refers to "tools designed to observe, measure, and inquire about factors that support or hinder occupational performance" (p. S14).

In many documents promulgated by payers and policymakers, the terms *evaluation* and *assessment* have meanings that are the reverse of those in the *Standards of Practice* and the *Framework*. In Medicare documents that set forth the reimbursement and regulatory context of home health occupational therapy, for example, *assessment* has the same meaning as *evaluation* does in the AOTA official documents and refers to the overarching process of obtaining data with specific timelines regarding what data are to be collected and by whom. It may appear that these terms are used interchangeably in this text and SPCC; however, that is not the case. Occupational therapy practitioners must understand and correctly use these terms to better frame the value of occupational therapy practice in home health for each type of stakeholder, including regulators and payers of home health services.

Practitioner and Clinician

This text and SPCC is directed toward both the occupational therapist and the occupational therapy assistant; the term *practitioner* is used to refer to both. *Clinician,* in contrast, refers to all health care professionals inclusively and is not discipline specific.

Although this text and SPCC is directed to both occupational therapists and occupational therapy assistants, their differing roles and responsibilities are the same as in other practice settings. As noted in the *Guidelines for Supervision, Roles, and Responsibilities During the Delivery of Occupational Therapy Services* (AOTA, 2014a), "occupational therapy assistants deliver occupational therapy services under the supervision of and in partnership with the occupational therapist. . . . [Together, they] are responsible for collaboratively developing a plan for supervision" (p. S17). In addition, occupational therapy practitioners deliver occupational therapy services in accordance with state and federal regulations, payer requirements, the AOTA *Standards of Practice for Occupational Therapy* (AOTA, 2015c), the *Occupational Therapy Code of Ethics (2015)* (AOTA, 2015a), the *Standards for Continuing Competence* (AOTA, 2015b), and the *Scope of Practice* (AOTA, 2014c). The current versions of these AOTA official documents, which are reviewed and updated as needed on a regular review cycle, are found at http://otjournal.net.

The home health CoPs specify definitions of *qualified occupational therapist* and *qualified occupational therapy assistant,* terms that are used often in the regulations. These qualifications are required agency-wide regardless of payer source (CMS, 2011) and are reprinted in **Appendix B.**

Caregiver and Family (or Informal) Caregiver

The terms *caregiver* and *family (or informal) caregiver* are used interchangeably in this text and SPCC and refer to unpaid spouses or partners, children and other relatives, friends, or members of the community who provide essential assistance to someone who has an acute or chronic illness or disability or is frail or has a cognitive impairment.

Key Terms

Each chapter has Key Terms important to that chapter that are bulleted at the beginning and defined in the chapter. Each Key Term appears in bold type on first use in a chapter. In some cases, a Key Term is also an Essential Term; this is noted as it occurs.

Conclusion

This text serves not only as an SPCC and an educational text but also as a resource for knowledge critical to occupational therapy practice in home health. One critical stakeholder affected by the lack of knowledge of a single occupational therapy practitioner is the profession itself. A profession needs access to appropriate settings in which to practice. A profession also depends on clinicians communicating to stakeholders, through effective practice and salient results, that its services have meaning and value. Practicing occupational therapy in a client's home is a perfect fit with practitioners' expertise in addressing the client's context, including the social and physical environment. Ensuring the satisfaction of all stakeholders with occupational therapy services provided in the home increases the profession's access to this practice setting.

References

American Occupational Therapy Association. (2014a). Guidelines for supervision, roles, and responsibilities during the delivery of occupational therapy services. *American Journal of Occupational Therapy, 68*(Suppl. 3), S16–S22. http://dx.doi.org/10.5014/ajot.2014.686S03

American Occupational Therapy Association. (2014b). Occupational therapy practice framework: Domain and process (3rd ed.). *American Journal of Occupational Therapy, 68*(Suppl. 1), S1–S48. http://dx.doi.org/10.5014/ajot.2014.682006

American Occupational Therapy Association. (2014c). Scope of practice. *American Journal of Occupational Therapy, 68*(Suppl. 3), S34–S40. http://dx.doi.org/10.5014/ajot.2014.686S04

American Occupational Therapy Association. (2015a). Occupational therapy code of ethics (2015). *American Journal of Occupational Therapy, 69*(Suppl. 3), 6913410030. http://dx.doi.org/10.5014/ajot.2015.696S03

American Occupational Therapy Association. (2015b). Standards for continuing competence. *American Journal of Occupational Therapy, 69*(Suppl. 3), 6913410055. http://dx.doi.org/10.5014/ajot.2015.696S16

American Occupational Therapy Association. (2015c). Standards of practice for occupational therapy. *American Journal of Occupational Therapy, 69*(Suppl. 3), 6913410057. http://dx.doi.org/10.5014/ajot.2015.696S06

Centers for Medicare & Medicaid Services. (2011). *Part 484: Home health services.* Washington, DC: Author. Retrieved from http://www.gpo.gov/fdsys/pkg/CFR-2011-title42-vol5/pdf/CFR-2011-title42-vol5-part484.pdf

Centers for Medicare & Medicaid Services. (2014). *Medicare benefit policy manual: Chapter 7—Home health services.* Retrieved from https://www.cms.gov/Regulations-and-Guidance/Guidance/Manuals/downloads//bp102c07.pdf

Merriam-Webster. (2015). *Context.* Retrieved from http://www.merriam-webster.com/dictionary/context

National Association for Home Care & Hospice. (2010). *Basic statistics about home care.* Washington, DC: Author. Retrieved from http://www.nahc.org/assets/1/7/10HC_Stats.pdf

Schell, B. A. B. (2008). Pragmatic reasoning. In B. A. B. Schell & J. W. Schell (Eds.), *Clinical and professional reasoning in occupational therapy* (pp. 169–187). Baltimore: Lippincott Williams & Wilkins.

Section I: Stakeholder Context: Satisfying Stakeholders in Occupational Therapy Home Health Services

INTRODUCTION TO

"Stakeholder Context: Satisfying Stakeholders in Occupational Therapy Home Health Services"

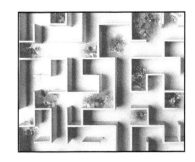

Carol Siebert, MS, OTR/L, FAOTA, and
Karen Vance, BSOT

A *stakeholder* is "one who is involved in or affected by a course of action" or one who has "an interest or share in an undertaking or enterprise" (Merriam-Webster, 2013). The most obvious stakeholder and the one most directly affected by a home health occupational therapy course of action—that is, intervention—is the client receiving occupational therapy services. The client would arguably be the only stakeholder in occupational therapy services if such services did not require operational support, protection of the interests of all parties involved, and financial resources. The reality, however, is that there are many stakeholders in home health occupational therapy services.

This section describes who the stakeholders are and why it is imperative that occupational therapy practitioners know the expectations of these stakeholders. Moreover, in this section practitioners are encouraged not only to meet but to exceed those expectations to secure the stake occupational therapy has as a profession in home health practice. Chapter 1 focuses on agencies, the public, regulators, and payers, setting the stage for Chapter 2, which turns to clients and caregivers. Before walking through a client's door, a home health occupational therapy practitioner must be prepared to follow the requirements of the agency, payers, and regulators and to capture it all adequately in documenting the visit.

Naming the Stakeholders

Stakeholders in home health occupational therapy services, beyond the client, include caregivers, home health agencies (HHAs), the public, regulators, and payers of home health services.

- *Caregivers:* The caregiver is included with the client receiving occupational therapy services. The caregiver (also called *family caregiver* or *informal caregiver*) may be an unpaid spouse or partner, relative, friend, or member of the community who provides assistance to the client. Caregivers' stake in the success of occupational therapy services is often as critical as that of the client.

- *Agencies:* HHAs share a stake with occupational therapy practitioners in cost-efficient and effective plans of care that achieve good outcomes for their clients. Agencies depend on practitioners to follow policies and procedures and to demonstrate compliance with regulations and payer requirements.

- *The public and regulators:* Regulators have a stake in the health care enterprise to protect the public interest. Regulations are the minimum health and safety standards with which HHAs must comply to be Medicare certified. Regulators of occupational therapy services require agencies to meet minimum health and safety standards.

- *Payers:* Payers have a stake in ensuring the best value of occupational therapy services for the dollars paid. Payers expect providers to show evidence that they have met coverage criteria and have achieved good clinical outcomes in a cost-efficient manner.

The relationships among stakeholders are formal: The client receives specified types and amounts of services, the agency provides those services, the payers fund the services, and the regulators govern the relationships among the stakeholders and preserve the public interest in the health and safety of its members. Occupational therapy practitioners' role in these relationships is to act on behalf of the HHA to provide services that satisfy the expectations of all of the stakeholders.

Elevating Practice to Satisfy Stakeholders

The two chapters in Section I encourage occupational therapy practitioners to elevate their practice beyond the level of practice that currently exists. *Elevating practice* means being aware of all stakeholders and not just meeting their expectations, but exceeding them. Elevating practice requires not just doing something differently, but thinking differently. The stakeholder that stands to benefit the most from elevated practice is the occupational therapy profession itself.

The shift from complying with expectations to exceeding expectations begins with a change in mind-set that then leads to a change in behavior (Prochaska & Velicer, 1997). When expectations or requirements are presented, the response "Do I have to do this?" indicates a minimal compliance mind-set. Even worse, the response "How can I avoid doing this?" indicates a noncompliance mind-set. A minimal or noncompliance mind-set will certainly not lead to a change in behavior needed for practice that exceeds expectations rather than just meeting them. With broader knowledge, the mind-set shift leads to a response that takes a more analytical approach: "What behaviors do I need to change to meet and exceed these expectations and requirements?" "What do these expectations or requirements mean for my practice?"

The occupational therapy practitioner's shift in mind-set begins with an openness to understanding the stakeholders' expectations and requirements. An open mind-set reflects a willingness to appreciate the circumstances associated with the expectations and requirements and to move beyond a rote or minimal response to a response that is based on comprehension (Bloom, Engelhart, Furst, Hill, & Krathwohl, 1956). The chapters of Section I emphasize the importance of investigating and understanding the whys of stakeholder expectations in the home health practice setting generally and in home health occupational therapy practice specifically.

The practitioner's shift in mind-set continues as his or her knowledge expands. With a more comprehensive understanding of the needs and expectations of clients, caregivers, the public, regulators, and payers, practitioners will find that agency policies and procedures make more sense. Such understanding results in strong connections between the individual practitioner's day-to-day practice and its broader effect on the agency and the home health industry and in the lives of those receiving services. With heightened awareness, connections between policy and practice become apparent.

The final shift in mind-set occurs when this broader and deeper perspective leads to an evaluative and anticipatory mind-set: What is the best way to address the stakeholders' needs? How can I contribute? How does my contribution fit within the broader effort? Section I facilitates occupational therapy practitioners' journey through these mind-set shifts to reflect on and evaluate the potential for elevating their practice and exceeding stakeholder expectations.

References

Bloom, B. S. (Ed.), Engelhart, M. D., Furst, E. J., Hill, W. H., & Krathwohl, D. R. (1956). *Taxonomy of educational objectives: The classification of educational goals. Book 1: Cognitive domain.* New York: David McKay.

Merriam-Webster. (2013). *Stake, stakeholder.* Retrieved from http://www.merriam-webster.com/dictionary/stakeholder

Prochaska, J. O., & Velicer, W. F. (1997). The Transtheoretical Model of health behavior change. *American Journal of Health Promotion, 12,* 38–48. http://dx.doi.org/10.4278/0890-1171-12.1.38

CHAPTER 1

Stakeholders in Home Health: Agencies, the Public, Regulators, and Payers

Carol Siebert, MS, OTR/L, FAOTA, and
Karen Vance, BSOT

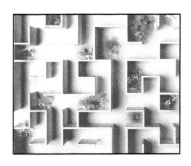

Learning Objectives

After completing this chapter, readers will be able to

- Identify the various work arrangements between agencies and occupational therapy practitioners seeking to provide occupational therapy services in home health;
- Recognize the formal relationships among patient, agency, and payer and among patient, agency, and practitioner;
- Identify how regulations and payer requirements protect the public interest;
- Identify the risk to home health occupational therapy practice when practitioners fail to understand and meet stakeholder expectations; and
- Identify the connections among the expectations of patients, regulators, and payers and the opportunities for occupational therapy practitioners to satisfy those expectations beyond minimum requirements.

Introduction

For many occupational therapy practitioners, working with **patients** and caregivers is what practice is all about. Working one-to-one with a patient and caregiver and effecting changes that make a difference for the patient can be satisfying and rewarding. However, occupational therapy services have **stakeholders** other than the patient and caregiver. A *stakeholder* is a person, group, or organization that has a **stake,** or interest, in the success of an endeavor—in the case of occupational therapy in home health, in providing services in the home to promote clients' health and engagement in meaningful occupations.

To be compensated for working with patients in the home, occupational therapy practitioners must satisfy agency **policies and procedures,** making the home health agency (HHA) a major stakeholder. *Agency policies and procedures* (i.e., the

Key Terms

- **beneficiary**
- **compliance**
- **Conditions for Coverage**
- **Conditions of Participation**
- **home health benefit**
- **Home Health Compare**
- **Medicaid**
- **Medicare**
- **Outcome and Assessment Information Set (OASIS)**
- **Outcome-Based Quality Improvement (OBQI)**
- **patient** (Essential Term—see definition in the "Introduction" to this text and SPCC)
- **payer**
- **policies and procedures**
- **provider**
- **the public**
- **quality measures**
- **regulations**
- **regulator**
- **stake**
- **stakeholder**
- **standard**
- **value**

written rules and guidelines that govern the actions and decisions that take place within the agency) originate from the requirements of **regulators** and **payers** who have a stake in the services and outcomes of occupational therapy and HHAs.

Practitioners in home health must understand and meet the expectations of agencies, **the public,** payers, and regulators if occupational therapy is to continue to have a role in home health. In our experience, occupational therapy's role has been limited in home health because of misunderstandings and misapplications of **regulations** to agency policies by both practitioners and agencies. If occupational therapy practitioners choose to do the minimum required by regulations or seek opportunities to do less than the minimum, occupational therapy is perceived as delivering minimal **value,** and occupational therapy's role and position within the home health industry will fade. Occupational therapy practitioners have a duty to understand and act on the expectations of all home health stakeholders; if they fail to do so, occupational therapy practice in home health settings "is ours to lose" (Zahoransky, Vance, Siebert, & Kohl, 2010).

Success in home health depends on doing more than meeting patients' and caregivers' expectations. In this chapter, we address the important stake that agencies, the public, regulators, and payers have in home health because satisfying these stakeholders opens the door to providing services to patients. This chapter also addresses how agencies, regulators, and payers affect, and are affected by, the day-to-day actions of home health occupational therapy practitioners. Occupational therapy practitioners must understand the relationships among and exceed the expectations of all stakeholders if occupational therapy is going to thrive in home health.

> Occupational therapy practitioners must understand the relationships among and exceed the expectations of all stakeholders if occupational therapy is going to thrive in home health.

Agencies as Stakeholders

Occupational therapy practitioners' duty to their own practice and to the profession, as stated in the *Occupational Therapy Code of Ethics (2015)* (American Occupational Therapy Association [AOTA], 2015) is to "collaborate with employers to formulate policies and procedures in **compliance** with legal, regulatory, and ethical standards and work to resolve any conflicts or inconsistencies" (p. 5). Occupational therapy practitioners must

- Know the regulations and payer requirements that inform agency policies and procedures and
- Advocate with agencies to ensure that policies and procedures do not limit occupational therapy practice more than do current regulations or payer requirements.

Occupational therapy practitioners' duty to the agency that employs them includes *compliance with* (i.e., fulfillment of) the regulations and payer requirements, which constitute the minimum **standard** an HHA must meet. Similarly, adherence to agency policies and procedures is a minimum standard an occupational therapy practitioner—or any clinician—must meet. Failure to adhere to policies and procedures may jeopardize an agency's participation in the **Medicare** program, the U.S. government–administered health insurance program for older adults and people with disabilities (Centers for Medicare & Medicaid Services [CMS], 2015).

Home health offers more ways for occupational therapy practitioners to be employed than most other practice settings. The combination of practice in patients' homes and limited contact with the agency can limit a practitioner's awareness not only of the agency's stake in the care being provided but also of the stake of regulators and payers. Although the different models for arranging occupational therapy staffing have different implications for practitioner training, support, and accountability, all practitioners must be mindful of their obligation to the agency as stakeholder.

One way for occupational therapy practitioners to provide services in home health is as a regular employee of an HHA. Under this model, practitioners may be paid either a salary or an hourly rate. Another common model involves the agency hiring practitioners to work per diem or per visit, meaning that the practitioner is paid on the basis of services provided and is engaged only when those services are needed. In either case, the practitioner is an employee of the agency and receives an Internal Revenue Service Form W-2 reporting salary and benefits the agency provides to the practitioner.

A third model of service is contracting. The HHA may contract with a staffing company that supplies clinicians to the agency. Under this model, the occupational therapy practitioner is an employee not of the HHA but rather of the staffing company, which provides them with Form W-2. The staffing company has a contract with the HHA that defines the services to be provided. The practitioner has no direct relationship with the HHA but provides services on its behalf.

In some cases, practitioners are independent contractors who subcontract with HHAs either through a staffing company or directly with the agency. In either case, the practitioner is employed by neither the staffing company nor the HHA. The contractor receives an Internal Revenue Service Form 1099 from the contracting entity that reports compensation paid. The relationship between the practitioner and the contracting entity is not an employer–employee relationship; the terms of the relationship are defined by the contract. As in the other employment arrangements, however, the practitioner provides services on behalf of the agency.

The system under which HHAs are paid is described in **Appendix A,** "Medicare as Payer."

Stop here! Go to Appendix A and read the section "Home Health Prospective Payment System" on pages 189–193.

Under that system, agencies must deploy resources while avoiding expenditures that do not add value (Institute of Medicine, 2001). The **Conditions of Participation** (CoPs) do not require HHAs to offer occupational therapy services (CMS, 2011, § 484.14[a]); the existence of occupational therapy positions depends on agencies perceiving occupational therapy not as an optional service, but as a valuable and essential agency resource. Occupational therapy practitioners must understand the stake and exceed the expectations of the HHA that employs them because agencies decide whether occupational therapy positions in home health will exist.

> Occupational therapy practitioners must understand the stake and exceed the expectations of the HHA that employs them because agencies decide whether occupational therapy positions in home health will exist.

The Public as Stakeholder

Medicare and **Medicaid** (the U.S. government–administered health insurance for people with low income and resources) are funded with public dollars. Thus, *the public*—the people of the United States as a whole—is a stakeholder in the home health enterprise. Medicare is both a payer and a regulator, as described in **Appendix A,** "Medicare as Payer," and **Appendix B,** "Medicare as Regulator." Regulations are developed to ensure that **providers** who receive public funds meet minimum criteria as service providers and that public funds are used prudently. Thus, the relationship between HHAs and payers is defined primarily by regulations to protect the interest of the public and the interests of those receiving services (i.e., patients or **beneficiaries**).

Regulators as Stakeholders: Conditions of Participation

The creation of Medicare and Medicaid in the 1960s introduced public dollars into the health care enterprise. To protect the interests of the public, the U.S. Department of Health and Human Services created regulators, principally the CMS (originally the Health Care Financing Administration), to develop and enforce *regulations,* or specific rules for implementing laws related to the health care system. These regulators established conditions for the use of public dollars allocated to health care—specifically, CoPs (CMS, 2015).

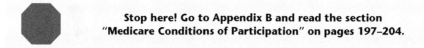

Stop here! Go to Appendix B and read the section "Medicare Conditions of Participation" on pages 197–204.

Compliance with these conditions is a minimum requirement for a health care agency to participate in the Medicare (or Medicaid) program. HHAs are scrutinized in a process called a *survey* to determine their compliance with the CoPs; **Appendix A** describes the role of Medicare Program Integrity Contractors in ensuring compliance (p. 188). Agencies found to be in compliance are identified as Medicare-certified HHAs. The CoPs apply to all operations of the agency and affect all patients who receive services from the agency, regardless of the source of payment for those services. Thus, the CoPs pertaining to patient rights protect not only Medicare beneficiaries but all patients served by the agency.

Payers as Stakeholders: Conditions for Coverage

Until the second half of the 20th century, health care could be described as a dyadic relationship between the provider of services and the patient or recipient of services. In that relationship, the provider rendered services to the patient. In return, the patient paid the provider directly for the services rendered. Figure 1.1 represents that relationship graphically.

Beginning in the 1960s, health insurance, including Medicare, became an important part of health care, altering the relationship from a dyad to a triad, as shown in Figure 1.2. In this triadic relationship, the provider renders services to a patient. The patient may pay all, part, or none of the fees associated with the services received. An insurer or third-party payer pays the provider on the basis of the terms of the benefit or policy (contract between patient and payer) and of the provider agreement (contract between payer and provider).

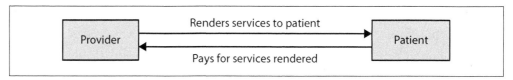

Figure 1.1. **Before the 1960s: Provider–patient dyad.**

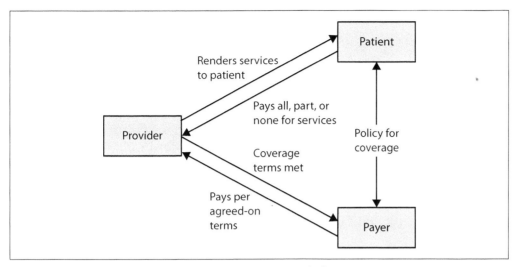

Figure 1.2. From the 1960s on: Provider–patient–payer triad.

Medicare and Medicaid are the dominant sources of payment for home health care (National Association for Home Care & Hospice, 2010). The **home health benefit** defines the circumstances that make a *beneficiary* (i.e., one who receives the benefit stipulated for Medicare recipients) eligible for home health and the services that will be covered (paid for) on behalf of the beneficiary. For nearly all services covered by the home health benefit, Medicare pays 100% of the amount due the provider. **Appendix A** includes the conditions for eligibility to receive benefits from the *Medicare Benefit Policy Manual* (CMS, 2014a). All home health clinicians must know and understand these conditions to ensure adequate payment for the services they provide.

 Stop here! Go to Appendix A and read the section "Medicare Coverage Under the Part A Home Health Benefit" on pages 175–188.

Federal regulations govern the relationship between the payer and the provider. Under the home health benefit, the provider is the HHA. The home health CoPs, described in **Appendix B,** define the conditions HHAs must meet to participate in the Medicare program: "The existing CoPs are the minimum health and safety standards that home health agencies (HHAs) must comply with in order to qualify for reimbursement under the Medicare program" (CMS, 2015, "Brief Description of Documents" section, para. 1).

Other federal regulations define additional requirements HHAs must meet to receive payment for services rendered to eligible beneficiaries. Federal regulations defining skilled occupational therapy services are reviewed in Chapter 4, "The Occupational Therapy Evaluation Process in Home Health," and Chapter 5, "Home Health Plans of Care, Intervention, and Team Collaboration."

Health insurers, including Medicare, identify the circumstances under which they will make payments on behalf of a beneficiary. These circumstances include when a beneficiary is eligible for a specific benefit or coverage, what services will be covered under the benefit, and how payment for the services will be determined. These circumstances are known as the **Conditions for Coverage** (CfCs). Medicare benefits are determined by Congress as amendments to Title XVIII of the Social

Security Act (Pub. L. 89–97), and CMS is responsible for operationalizing these benefits. CMS codifies some aspects of the benefits in federal regulations. This operationalization is addressed in detail in the *Medicare Benefit Policy Manual* (CMS, 2014a; see **Appendix A,** "Medicare Coverage Under the Part A Home Health Benefit," pp. 175–188). The manual defines the conditions the beneficiary must meet to be eligible for a given Medicare benefit and the conditions a provider must meet to be paid for service under that benefit. These are the Medicare CfCs.

Other payers also establish CfCs. Some payers adopt the Medicare CfCs in part or in entirety, and other payers establish conditions that differ significantly from those of Medicare. If a provider expects to be paid by any payer—Medicare, Medicaid, or other insurance—the burden is on the provider to determine what the home health CfCs are for each payer the provider will be billing.

> If a provider expects to be paid by any payer—Medicare, Medicaid, or other insurance—the burden is on the provider to determine what the home health CfCs are for each payer the provider will be billing.

Interactions Among the Key Stakeholders in Home Health

Figure 1.3 illustrates the relationships among three key stakeholders in the home health enterprise: (1) HHAs (providers), (2) Medicare (payer), and (3) beneficiaries (home health patients). *Providers* (i.e., agencies) are responsible for rendering services. *Patients* (also called *clients* or *beneficiaries*) receive services or benefits from providers. *Payers*—in the case of home health, primarily Medicare—pay for the services rendered.

In home health, no formalized relationship exists between individual clinicians and patients or between individual clinicians and the payer: The provider entity is the HHA. The agency must meet the CoPs and comply with the CfCs. An individual clinician (of any discipline) cannot be a home health provider under the CoPs, nor can a clinician bill Medicare, Medicaid, or most private insurers for home health services. Individual clinicians, whether employees or contractors, act as agents of the HHA. Thus, although the agency is recognized as the provider entity, the actions of employees or contractors determine whether the agency meets or adheres to the CoPs and CfCs. **Appendix B** contains CoPs that home health clinicians must follow and provide evidence of in their documentation.

Regardless of the relationship between an occupational therapy practitioner and the employing agency, the practitioner's financial stake is directly dependent on the agency's financial stake. If an agency fails to adhere to payer requirements for delivery of services, the payer may withhold payment (i.e., deny a claim), which affects the agency financially. If an agency is deficient in meeting a condition or standard in the

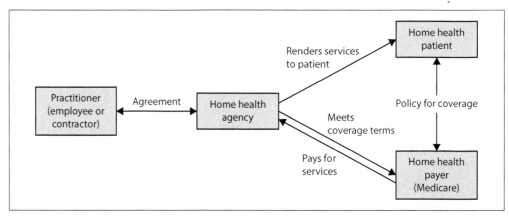

Figure 1.3. **Relationships among practitioner, home health agency, patient, and payer.**

CoPs, the agency's participation in the Medicare program is jeopardized. The effect on the agency of no longer participating in the Medicare program may be financial losses or even inability to exist as a going concern. In either circumstance, the effect on the agency will also have an effect on the practitioner and the practitioner's livelihood.

Agencies expect that clinicians will meet regulations and payer requirements in their daily performance in delivering services on behalf of the agency. Agencies must comply with regulations and payer conditions to exist, and compliance with regulations and payer conditions is dependent on the behavior of practitioners. Complying with agency policies and procedures is a minimum standard. Exceeding expectations means understanding and demonstrating value to HHAs, regulators, and payers.

> Agencies must comply with regulations and payer conditions to exist, and compliance with regulations and payer conditions is dependent on the behavior of practitioners.

From Meeting to Exceeding Stakeholder Expectations

Agency policies and procedures set minimum standards of practice based on regulations and other quality principles. All clinicians providing services on behalf of the agency must comply with the standards set in these policies and procedures. Demonstrating *value* means going beyond minimal standards to provide optimal value to stakeholders—the patient, the public, the regulator, and the payer—by delivering results that matter and that last and by using resources prudently to achieve those results.

What are the meaningful, lasting results that stakeholders expect? Patients and families want patients to be able to stay in their homes, and to do this patients must manage daily tasks, get around safely, and avoid falls and other injuries. Some meaningful results include the ability to

- Get around the house,
- Get in and out of bed,
- Take a bath,
- Not be in pain during activities, and
- Breathe easily.

The public and regulators expect practitioners to use their skills and best practices to deliver safe and effective care. These practices include

- Monitoring patients' pain and treating it when it is present,
- Monitoring and treating symptoms of high-risk conditions such as heart failure,
- Monitoring and reducing the risk of pressure ulcers,
- Initiating care promptly,
- Teaching patients and caregivers about their medications and supporting them in taking medications properly,
- Monitoring fall risk and reducing that risk when it is present,
- Monitoring patients for signs of depression,
- Monitoring patients' risk of developing flu or pneumonia, and
- Teaching patients with diabetes to take care of their feet.

Payers want to avoid costly complications and hospitalizations. Results that matter to payers include

- Improvement or healing of wounds after an operation,
- Reduction in pressure ulcers,

- Patients taking their medications to manage their conditions,
- Reduced need for unplanned or emergency care, and
- Reduced hospital admissions.

These meaningful results are among the measures included in **Home Health Compare** (HHC), a CMS website that helps consumers make informed choices about home health providers (http://www.medicare.gov/homehealthcompare). **Appendix C** (Box C.1) lists outcome measures publicly reported in HHC.

**Stop here! Go to Appendix C and read Box C.1,
"List of Home Health Compare Measures Publicly Reported"
on page 208.**

HHC is available to the public and allows the public to compare an agency's performance with that of its competitors, so agencies have a stake in how their outcomes look on HHC. The more important point, though, is that HHC exists to report on **quality measures** that are important to the other stakeholders: the patient, the public, and the payer. According to CMS,

> Quality measures are tools that help us measure or quantify healthcare processes, outcomes, patient perceptions, and organizational structure and/or systems that are associated with the ability to provide high-quality health care and/or that relate to one or more quality goals for health care. These goals include: effective, safe, efficient, patient-centered, equitable, and timely care. (CMS, 2014b, para. 2)

The quality measures listed in HHC are but a few measured by the **Outcome and Assessment Information Set (OASIS)** and monitored in the **Outcome-Based Quality Improvement (OBQI)** process. The OASIS consists of data elements (e.g., sociodemographic, environmental, and functional characteristics of patients) that home health practitioners collect at specified times during service provision (e.g., start of care, follow-up, discharge) and submit electronically to a central database operated by CMS. HHAs are required to submit OASIS data to retain their Medicare certification. **Appendix D** describes OASIS in detail.

**Stop here! Go to Appendix D and read the section
"Overview of OASIS" (pp. 222–224).**

The OBQI is a process in which OASIS data are used to generate reports that analyze the agency's outcomes, which the agency can use to focus its quality improvement activities. **Appendix C** explains the OBQI.

**Stop here! Go to Appendix C and read the section
"Outcome-Based Quality Improvement" (pp. 209–219).**

Many of the measures that agencies target for improvement are related to aspects of the domain of occupational therapy (AOTA, 2014), particularly areas of occupation. Occupational therapy practitioners demonstrate value to an HHA by explicitly considering the targeted measures when developing and implementing intervention plans. Occupational therapy intervention plans addressing various areas of occupation thus have an influence on agency outcome measures related to areas of occupation. All stakeholders expect that when home health services are provided, they will make a meaningful difference in the life and health of the patient.

How does a practitioner explicitly demonstrate that expectations have been met? What does delivering value look like in day-to-day practice? Table 1.1 lists actions home health occupational therapy practitioners can implement to exceed their agency's expectations and deliver value to home health stakeholders. The table also provides links to chapters and appendixes in this text and Self-Paced Clinical Course (SPCC) that provide more information on how to implement these actions.

Delivering value also means ensuring that agency expectations are never less than the expectations of the other stakeholders. The CoPs require that agencies follow their own policies and procedures. Therefore, revisions to policies and procedures may be necessary before occupational therapy practitioners' responsibilities can be expanded consistent with regulations and payer conditions. Practitioners can work with their agency to ensure that the agency's expectations reflect those of regulators and payers and that agency policies and procedures are consistent with regulations and payer conditions. AOTA has developed a fact sheet titled *Occupational Therapy's Role in Home Health* that addresses key federal regulations and Medicare CfCs that have been prone to misinterpretation either by agencies or by practitioners; this fact sheet is reproduced in **Appendix E** of this text and SPCC. The fact sheet can

> **Practitioners can work with their agency to ensure that the agency's expectations reflect those of regulators and payers and that agency policies and procedures are consistent with regulations and payer conditions.**

- Help practitioners work with their agencies to resolve any confusion about what services occupational therapy can provide under current federal regulations and Medicare CfCs,
- Help HHAs review agency policies and procedures to ensure that the expectations of occupational therapy practitioners are consistent with the expectations of other stakeholders, and
- Help both practitioners and agencies ensure that occupational therapy services deliver enhanced value to all stakeholders.

Participation in this process helps practitioners ensure that occupational therapy will thrive in home health and be seen as delivering value to all home health stakeholders.

 Stop here! Go to Appendix E and review its contents (pp. 255–257).

Conclusion

Patients and caregivers are the most obvious but not the only stakeholders in home health. Agencies, the public, regulators, and payers are equally important stakeholders. Thus, the success of occupational therapy in home health depends on more than a sole focus on the needs and expectations of patients and caregivers; success

Table 1.1. Practitioner Actions That Meet or Exceed Stakeholder Expectations

Topic	Actions That Meet Expectations	Actions That Exceed Expectations	More Information
Agency policies	• Improve and support regulatory compliance • Improve occupational therapy utilization in home health	Advocate for agency policies to be consistent with (and not more restrictive than) current federal and state regulations	Appendix A Appendix B
Agency and the public	• Improve patient outcomes • Improve patient satisfaction • Improve efficiency • Improve agency best practices • Improve occupational therapy utilization in home health	Review information on the employing agency and its competitors on Home Health Compare to understand the agency's strengths, challenges, and standing in relation to competitors	Appendix C
Aide services and care processes	• Improve patient outcomes • Improve efficiency • Improve occupational therapy utilization in home health	Advocate for agency policy to permit occupational therapy practitioners to supervise aides on non-nursing cases	Chapter 5
	• Improve patient outcomes • Improve efficiency • Improve and support regulatory compliance • Improve agency best practices • Improve occupational therapy utilization in home health	Collaborate with the discipline supervising aides to ensure that the aide care plan corresponds to the needs and progress addressed by occupational therapy	Chapter 5
Start-of-care procedures	• Improve efficiency • Improve and support regulatory compliance • Improve data accuracy (for outcomes) • Improve occupational therapy utilization in home health	Advocate for agency policy to permit occupational therapy to conduct start-of-care procedures when the payer deems that the patient's need for occupational therapy constitutes eligibility for home health	Chapter 4 Appendix B
	• Improve patient outcomes • Improve agency best practices • Improve data accuracy (for outcomes) • Improve occupational therapy utilization in home health	Contact the clinician who conducted the initial comprehensive assessment to inform him or her of occupational therapy findings	Chapter 6 Appendix B
Comprehensive assessment with integrated OASIS	• Improve efficiency • Improve and support regulatory compliance • Improve occupational therapy utilization in home health	Advocate for agency policy to permit occupational therapy practitioners to conduct a comprehensive assessment, including OASIS, at all time points subsequent to start of care	Appendix D
	• Improve patient outcomes • Improve efficiency • Improve and support regulatory compliance • Improve agency best practices • Improve data accuracy (for outcomes) • Improve occupational therapy utilization in home health	Advocate (or volunteer) to attend or participate in trainings focused on OASIS competencies	Chapter 4 Appendix D
	• Improve patient outcomes • Improve efficiency • Improve and support regulatory compliance • Improve agency best practices • Improve data accuracy (for outcomes) • Improve occupational therapy utilization in home health	Volunteer for or participate in efforts to optimize OASIS data accuracy by sharing strategies for effective assessment with other members of the clinical team	Chapter 4 Appendix D
Comprehensive assessment and medication regimen review	• Improve efficiency • Improve and support regulatory compliance • Improve agency best practices • Improve data accuracy (for outcomes) • Improve occupational therapy utilization in home health	Volunteer for or participate in any trainings related to accurate completion of the medication regimen review	Chapter 3 Chapter 4 Appendix D

(Continued)

Table 1.1. Practitioner Actions That Meet or Exceed Stakeholder Expectations *(cont.)*

Topic	Actions That Meet Expectations	Actions That Exceed Expectations	More Information
Evaluation and care planning	• Improve patient outcomes • Improve patient satisfaction • Improve and support regulatory compliance • Improve occupational therapy utilization in home health	Elicit patient and caregiver needs, concerns, and goals, and address them in the care plan	Chapter 2 Chapter 4 Chapter 7
	• Improve efficiency • Improve and support regulatory compliance • Improve agency best practices • Improve occupational therapy utilization in home health	Advocate for forms and templates to be used in evaluation or care planning that accurately reflect the domain and process of occupational therapy	Chapter 4
	• Improve patient outcomes • Improve patient satisfaction • Improve occupational therapy utilization in home health	Find opportunities to improve patient outcomes regardless of diagnosis or condition	Chapter 3 Chapter 4 Chapter 6
Care planning	• Improve patient outcomes • Improve patient satisfaction • Improve occupational therapy utilization in home health	Be familiar with OASIS items, OBQI-reported outcomes, and publicly reported outcomes Make the linkage between the occupational therapy care plan and outcomes explicit	Chapter 5 Appendix C Appendix D
Care planning and care processes	• Improve patient outcomes • Improve patient satisfaction • Improve occupational therapy utilization in home health	Include medication routines in ADL assessment to assist nursing in teaching medication management and improving the medication regimen	Chapter 5
Care processes: scheduling	• Improve efficiency • Improve and support regulatory compliance • Improve occupational therapy utilization in home health	Be familiar with the required content and schedule for therapy reassessments, and ensure that reassessment home visits are completed on time	Chapter 5 Appendix A
Care processes: communication	• Improve patient outcomes • Improve patient satisfaction • Improve occupational therapy utilization in home health	Participate consistently in case conferences or other collaboration efforts to offer the occupational therapy perspective and contribute to care delivery	Chapter 6
Regulatory compliance	• Improve and support regulatory compliance • Improve occupational therapy utilization in home health	Participate in policy and procedure review processes to ensure the least restrictive application to occupational therapy services	Chapter 1 Chapter 8
	• Improve and support regulatory compliance • Improve occupational therapy utilization in home health	Participate in peer review chart audits for improved documentation and opportunities to suggest occupational therapy interventions in plans of care	Chapter 1 Chapter 8
Professional development	• Improve occupational therapy utilization in home health	Be a mentor, formally or informally	Chapter 8
	• Improve agency best practices • Improve occupational therapy utilization in home health	Expect setbacks but channel frustration toward specific, achievable accomplishments that benefit both occupational therapy and one or more stakeholders	All chapters and appendixes
	• Improve patient outcomes • Improve efficiency • Improve agency best practices • Improve occupational therapy utilization in home health	Expand the repertoire of intervention approaches and techniques appropriate to the setting and population served	Chapter 3 Chapter 5 Chapter 7 Chapter 8

Note. ADL = activity of daily living; OASIS = Outcome and Assessment Information Set; OBQI = Outcome-Based Quality Improvement.

depends on individual occupational therapy practitioners recognizing the stake they and all other stakeholders have in the home health enterprise:

- Occupational therapy practitioners have a stake because HHAs decide whether occupational therapy positions exist in home health. Agencies also decide the number of and roles available for occupational therapy practitioners.
- The public's stake in the effectiveness of home health services is protected by public policy. Regulators protect the public interest by establishing conditions that agencies must meet. Compliance with these regulations is essential for the agency to operate as a Medicare-certified agency.
- Payers create coverage conditions that determine the circumstances under which payment is made to the agency for services rendered. The financial viability of the agency is dependent on adherence to these conditions.
- Agency compliance with both regulations and payer conditions is dependent on the behavior of individual clinicians. Occupational therapy practitioners have a stake in the agency's compliance because failure to comply can result in financial losses or even the closing of the agency. Home health occupational therapy positions and practitioner livelihoods depend on agencies that are regulatory compliant and financially healthy.

All stakeholders expect that when practitioners provide home health services, they will make a meaningful difference in the life and health of patients. For occupational therapy to thrive in home health, occupational therapy practice must deliver value to all home health stakeholders.

References

American Occupational Therapy Association. (2014). Occupational therapy practice framework: Domain and process (3rd ed.). *American Journal of Occupational Therapy, 68*(Suppl. 1), S1–S48. http://dx.doi.org/10.5014/ajot.2014.682006

American Occupational Therapy Association. (2015). Occupational therapy code of ethics (2015). *American Journal of Occupational Therapy, 69*(Suppl. 3), 6913410030. http://dx.doi.org/10.5014/ajot.2015.696S03

Centers for Medicare & Medicaid Services. (2011). *Part 484: Home health services.* Washington, DC: Author. Retrieved from http://www.gpo.gov/fdsys/pkg/CFR-2011-title42-vol5/pdf/CFR-2011-title42-vol5-part484.pdf

Centers for Medicare & Medicaid Services. (2014a). *Medicare benefit policy manual: Chapter 7—Home health services.* Retrieved from https://www.cms.gov/Regulations-and-Guidance/Guidance/Manuals/downloads//bp102c07.pdf

Centers for Medicare & Medicaid Services. (2014b). *Quality measures.* Retrieved from http://www.cms.gov/Medicare/Quality-Initiatives-Patient-Assessment-Instruments/QualityMeasures/index.html?redirect=/QUALITYMEASURES/

Centers for Medicare & Medicaid Services. (2015). *Conditions of participation, Brief description of documents.* Retrieved from https://www.cms.gov/Regulations-and-Guidance/Legislation/CFCsAndCoPs/homehealth.html

Institute of Medicine. (2001). *Crossing the quality chasm: A new health system for the 21st century.* Washington, DC: National Academy Press.

National Association for Home Care & Hospice. (2010). *Basic statistics about home care.* Washington, DC: Author. Retrieved from http://www.nahc.org/assets/1/7/10HC_Stats.pdf

Social Security Amendments of 1965, Pub. L. 89–97, 42 U.S.C. §§ 1395-1395kkk1 (Medicare) and 42 U.S.C. §§ 1396-1396w5 (Medicaid).

Zahoransky, M., Vance, K., Siebert, C., & Kohl, R. (2010, April 30). *OT in home care: It's ours to lose.* Short course presented at the AOTA Annual Conference & Expo, Orlando, FL.

CHAPTER 2

Stakeholders in Home Health: Clients and Caregivers

Ann O'Sullivan, OTR/L, LSW, FAOTA

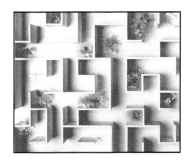

Learning Objectives

After completing this chapter, readers will be able to

- Identify the stake of clients and family caregivers in home health occupational therapy delivery and outcomes;
- Recognize the challenges in integrating family caregivers into the intervention team and identify strategies to enable better integration;
- Recognize the unique advantages and challenges for occupational therapy practitioners in providing intervention in the home;
- Identify the elements of client-centered care;
- Identify strategies to enhance collaboration and build partnerships with clients and family caregivers;
- Identify elements necessary for effective caregiver teaching; and
- Recognize the opportunities for reporting data on client and caregiver satisfaction with services.

Key Terms

- **client-centered care**
- **collaboration**
- **culturally appropriate care**
- **family (informal) caregiver** *or* **caregiver** (Essential Term— see definition in the "Introduction" to this text and SPCC)

Introduction

Occupational therapy practitioners' perspective emphasizes the recognition of, respect for, and appreciation of clients' opinions, preferences, experiences, and knowledge about their life situations. Increasingly, **family (informal) caregivers** of people who are sick or disabled assume responsibility for their care after an episode of professional care (United Hospital Fund [UHF], 2008). The client's continued health and well-being depend on the family caregiver, especially when the client is elderly or chronically ill. The family caregiver must be willing and able to handle potentially complex health, financial, legal, and social needs, possibly over a period of months or years. Therefore, both clients and family caregivers have a stake in the success of occupational therapy services in improving or maintaining long-term health. Not every client has or needs

Helping clients and caregivers make the connection between past successful strategies and current challenges improves their sense of control and reinforces their ability to problem solve and manage their current and future situations.

a caregiver, and not every family member is a caregiver. Although this chapter's focus is on the client–caregiver unit, all of the concepts presented may also be applied to clients who do not have a family caregiver and thus coordinate their own care.

By emphasizing clients' and caregivers' personal assets and coping skills, practitioners support self-efficacy and resilience and help them regain a sense of control over their lives (Stevens-Ratchford, 2005). Helping clients and caregivers make the connection between past successful strategies and current challenges improves their sense of control and reinforces their ability to problem solve and manage their current and future situations.

Integrating Caregivers Into Health Care Delivery

Development of partnerships between clinicians and clients and their family caregivers is increasingly being recognized as an essential component of health care quality improvement. Beyond addressing such partnerships at the clinician level, research is pointing to the need to support this thinking at the administrative and policy levels through professional and consumer education, accreditation standards, and payer recognition of the role of partnership in positive outcomes (Johnson et al., 2008).

Public policy has traditionally viewed family caregivers' service as a personal, moral obligation and not as an extension of the workforce. One consequence of this view is that research has not provided a systematic accounting of the numbers, qualifications, and competence of family caregivers (Institute of Medicine [IOM], 2008). Families and friends of older adults with disabilities are the predominant providers of long-term care and in general are thought to provide task assistance that is low in cost, high in quality, and consistent with older adults' preferences. A more explicit recognition of family caregivers as providers and partners in health care processes could benefit both clients and caregivers in managing the health needs of older adults in the community (IOM, 2008).

Why are caregivers not more integrated into the current health care delivery system? Levine (2007) suggested several factors behind this "(dis)-integration":

- The sole focus in insurance and medical practice has traditionally been on the client or beneficiary, not on the family member providing care.
- Providers say that they do not have time to talk to or train family caregivers, possibly because they are not paid to do so.
- Poor communication skills on the part of both providers and family caregivers break down trust.
- Privacy rules under the Health Insurance Portability and Accountability Act of 1996 (HIPAA; Pub. L. 104–191) have been misinterpreted and misapplied, leaving families without sufficient information to be full members of the care team.
- The culture of medicine and health care may perceive families as intrusive and time consuming.

As the predominant health insurance program of older Americans, Medicare is relevant to and, in many ways, reliant on family caregivers. Yet aside from covering respite care through the hospice benefit, the Medicare program does not currently consider informal caregivers in formal policy (IOM, 2008). Medicare, however, has begun to educate physicians about caregiver teaching during clients' face-to-face visits being part of the counseling and coordination of care to be provided (Centers for Medicare & Medicaid Services [CMS], n.d.). In addition, new, more effective models of chronic care management involve clients and their families to a much greater degree.

Health care involves frequent moves by patients from one setting to another, each carrying the possibility of miscommunication between the sending and receiving care providers. With each change of setting, clients and families must meet new staff, learn new rules, and adapt to a new culture. The family caregiver may be the only person who knows the client, can interpret his or her cues, and has followed the course of the illness from the beginning (Levine, 2007). Research on care transitions has made it clear that these junctures are critical to ongoing client health and well-being (Coleman & Williams, 2007). Evidence-based programs have been developed to support transitions from the hospital to the community. National standards and guidelines are needed for transitions from the formal to the informal care system, particularly for evaluating client and caregiver readiness and providing training and ongoing support (Raphael & Cornwell, 2008).

Caregivers' occupational needs and role demands must be incorporated into occupational therapy practitioners' therapeutic interventions with clients (Moghimi, 2007). Practitioners should provide information on community services, take time to follow through with both the client and the family, and encourage both the client and caregivers to ask questions and participate in problem solving.

> Caregivers' occupational needs and role demands must be incorporated into occupational therapy practitioners' therapeutic interventions with clients.

Effective communication is key to care coordination, prevention of errors and adverse events, and better outcomes (Center for Home Care Policy and Research, 2009). Occupational therapy practitioners can support client and caregiver behaviors that will facilitate their becoming better recognized as team members. For example, clients and caregivers can be encouraged to make lists of questions to ask health care providers, to understand the client's health insurance coverage, to work with the provider to learn the best treatments for the client's illness, to maintain a personal medical summary record, and to be specific about what treatments the client does or does not want (Warshaw, 2007).

Context of the Home Environment

Providing services in the home is different from providing them in a medical or community-based setting. Both benefits and challenges should be considered. Many occupational therapy practitioners who work in home health have observed that the home is the ideal environment in which to address activities in the context in which they are performed. The home context allows adaptation of tasks and routines that are home based (e.g., activities of daily living [ADLs], many instrumental activities of daily living [IADLs]) without trying to re-create in the clinic the conditions that will be present during ongoing daily performance. Providing care in a client's home gives the practitioner a window into the social, physical, and emotional environment in which the client dwells. Client interests and skills that may be helpful in adapting to a disability or illness may more easily become obvious in the surroundings of the home. Understanding the client's unique environment enables practitioners to customize recommendations to the specific concerns and contexts of that client's activity performance and care provision (Toth-Cohen et al., 2001).

In a hospital environment, clients and families must adapt to an unfamiliar culture, and they may feel obligated to give priority to the demands of the facility rather than to their own personal preferences and schedules. In the home, the practitioner is an invited guest, and interactions are thus typically guided by the client and caregiver, who can more easily direct the type of services and information they want to receive (Toth-Cohen et al., 2001). In addition, home health clients may be more comfortable refusing to participate in specific interventions or with specific clinicians.

Most important, home health clients are better able to incorporate interventions into their existing and adapted routines, which presents opportunities and challenges for clinicians. Occupational therapy practitioners can use clients' already established routines to help them succeed with new or changed tasks, and health care services provided in the home can be a great convenience to clients and caregivers, who avoid the burden of obtaining health care outside the home.

Home health clients are better able to incorporate interventions into their existing and adapted routines, which presents opportunities and challenges for clinicians.

Providing services in the home may, however, require the practitioner to offer more flexibility in scheduling and to show greater respect for client priorities, which may not seem as important to the practitioner as therapy. For example, clients may strongly prefer to schedule therapy visits around cherished TV shows or the expected arrival of the Meals on Wheels volunteer. In addition, clients and families may struggle with scheduling a variety of care providers while adjusting to the increased demands of managing new routines. Practitioners must work collaboratively with clients and families to ensure that the home health experience is the least exhausting and stressful possible.

Toth-Cohen and colleagues (2001) suggested that providers take four factors into account when providing services in the home:

1. The personal meaning of home for the family can be used to support intervention strategies that are consistent with the values of the client and caregiver.
2. The caregiver's beliefs and values about disability and care are important in building intervention strategies that are acceptable and meaningful.
3. The demands of the intervention influence caregiver well-being; services provided in the home require time and energy from the caregiver and may call for behavior change, resulting in further stress or fatigue.
4. A view of caregivers as lay practitioners entails a shift in the practitioner's role from expert to partner in collaborative problem solving and recognizes the caregiver's expertise and knowledge of the client's routines and history and the likelihood of success of any given strategy.

A major challenge home health clients and caregivers face is the level of performance expectation that may be placed on them at home and the resulting pressure they feel. A discrepancy may exist between the formal organizational structure of long-term care and the tasks expected of family caregivers (Hunt, 2007). Many health economists, providers, and policymakers have agreed that a mismatch exists between how the current health care system defines and pays for services and how care is actually being delivered. Third-party payers and providers view health care as time limited, discrete, and necessitated by acute or catastrophic illness rather than as long term, continuous, and provided to prevent the need for more costly care. This view places additional pressure on friends and family to provide care after formal care stops, especially when managing chronic conditions. Most payers and providers do not acknowledge that family caregivers are an extension of the care delivery team and may need care themselves (Raphael & Cornwell, 2008). Yet substantial evidence has indicated that patient safety can be compromised by miscommunication and failure to adequately prepare health care providers when the client transitions from inpatient care to home health (UHF, 2008).

Client-Centered Care

Because this chapter considers the client and caregiver as a unit, the term *client-centered care* includes the caregiver. The core principles of client-centered care are dignity and respect, information sharing, participation, and **collaboration** (Warshaw, 2007). Key attributes of client-centered care include education and shared knowledge, involvement of family and friends, collaboration and team management, sensitivity to the nonmedical and spiritual dimensions of care, respect for client needs and preferences, and free flow and accessibility of information (Shaller, 2007). Both clients and caregivers are important members of the health care team, yet often little is done to teach them the knowledge or skills they need to be full team members. Any plan to enable clients and family caregivers to become more capable members of the health care team is likely to require increased training and greater support from and integration with the formal health care system (IOM, 2008).

One of the challenges in working with family caregivers, particularly when it comes to their obtaining outside help, is that they may not self-identify as caregivers, instead seeing themselves as meeting their responsibilities as spouse or adult child. Helping people recognize the additional roles and occupations the caregiver role entails can be a first step toward connecting them with needed resources and supports.

Family caregivers take on elements of the roles of both client and provider (IOM, 2008). In the role of client, they may take responsibility for logistics, care management, and medical decision making. For example, they may schedule medical appointments, provide transportation, and handle billing questions. They may assume responsibility for presenting the client's history and listening to clinicians' assessments or instructions. They may make or influence decisions regarding the appropriate course of intervention. They also take on a health status monitoring function, as envisioned under the self-management concept described in Chapter 7 of this text and Self-Paced Clinical Course (SPCC), "Community Resources and Living Life to Its Fullest." In the health care provider role, caregivers perform many of the functions that direct care workers perform on a paid basis, including support for ADLs and IADLs.

Client-centered practitioners understand that older adults and their caregivers come with a lifetime of values, learning, and experiences. Adults bring to the health care encounter a life story of occupational engagement, participation, and all the problem-solving and other life skills that have contributed to the achievement of their developmental tasks and life goals (Stevens-Ratchford, 2005). These experiences can support successful self-management and caregiving or, negatively, erode the person's confidence in the possibility of success.

Some key concepts of client-centered practice for occupational therapy practitioners include facilitation of client participation in all aspects of occupational therapy services and provision of information, physical comfort, and emotional support. Clients and families have the ultimate responsibility for decisions about daily

Key attributes of client-centered care include education and shared knowledge, involvement of family and friends, collaboration and team management, sensitivity to the nonmedical and spiritual dimensions of care, respect for client needs and preferences, and free flow and accessibility of information.

occupations and occupational therapy services. Client-centered practice ensures that practitioners give caregivers the respect and attention they need to promote successful outcomes for both the client and the caregiver (Moghimi, 2007).

Care should be based on the best available evidence and then individualized for each client and caregiver. Individualizing care allows each client's unique characteristics and goals to drive planning and implementation. The diversity of health risks and care preferences, combined with clinical complexity, require that care decisions be founded on evidence "combined with clinical judgment that is balanced by patient-specific information based on that individual's life circumstances and personal values" (Durso, 2006, as cited in Center for Home Care Policy and Research, 2009, p. 5). In addition, interventions tailored to specific risk factors and other patient characteristics have proved beneficial in situations such as managing dementia, encouraging adherence to medications, and preventing falls (Alkema & Frey, 2006; Day, 2011; Gitlin, Winter, Dennis, Hodgson, & Hauck, 2010).

Culturally appropriate care, an element of client-centered care, responds to clients' and family caregivers' traditions, history, values, and family systems. Cultural experiences influence how clients and caregivers receive information and make choices, how symptoms are expressed, what type of treatment is preferred, and who provides care. Sometimes, the degree of difference between the client's and the caregiver's perception of appropriate care is based on how much of their life was spent in the United States and how strongly they value their cultural background (Given, Sherwood, & Given, 2008). Cultural differences can exacerbate communication issues among clients, caregivers, and providers and contribute to the failure of an ongoing plan of care (POC).

Collaboration is an ongoing process characterized by active listening; honest, clear, and jargon-free communication; mutual respect; accessibility and responsiveness; and reciprocal sharing of information. It requires the practitioner's understanding, empathy, and recognition and support of individual and family values, customs, and beliefs. Collaboration between practitioners and clients and their families entails shared evaluation, planning, and decision making, without judgment or labeling (Walens & Rockwell-Dylla, 1996). Recognition of and respect for the client's and caregiver's knowledge, skills, and experience are key to collaboration. Simply put, collaboration involves practitioners and clients working jointly to identify problem areas and develop a corresponding intervention plan (Gitlin & Corcoran, 2005). Collaboration in the home environment is based on an approach in which the caregiver's perspective is considered equal to that of the occupational therapy practitioner and helps direct the treatment process (Law, 1998, as cited in Gitlin & Corcoran, 2005).

Promoting Mastery, Preparedness, and Competence

Most studies do not organize or classify interventions according to caregivers' tasks or the knowledge and skills they require, but this information is vital in planning and implementing effective interventions. The concepts of mastery, preparedness, and competence are necessary components of effective decision making and problem solving by family caregivers, but the formal care system has paid little attention to these concepts (Given et al., 2008). To support caregivers' sense of mastery and self-efficacy, practitioners can emphasize caregiver strengths and show appreciation of their opinions, preferences, experiences, and knowledge about their life situation (Stevens-Ratchford, 2005).

A respect for the range and level of skill demanded by caregiving is also important. Requisite caregiver skills described by Schumacher, Stewart, Archbold, Dodd, and Dibble (2000) include monitoring, interpreting, making decisions, taking action, adjusting to changing needs, comforting with hands-on care, accessing resources, working with the ill person, and negotiating the health care system. Skills such as monitoring and interpreting require complex reasoning (Given et al., 2008), and caregivers are likely to need education, guidance, and reinforcement to develop these skills and incorporate them into existing and new routines.

Occupational therapy practitioners can help clients and caregivers develop their problem-solving skills to enhance their ability to provide continued and effective care. Problem-solving skills offer an enduring technique for aiding clients and caregivers in managing newly emerging problems after a formal intervention is completed (Gitlin & Corcoran, 2005). Practitioners can help clients and caregivers learn to build on their existing knowledge and help them explore their own thinking to address specific situations. Helping a caregiver identify the underlying triggers for problematic behaviors related to dementia, for example, can help him or her structure the environment to minimize their occurrence.

Clearly, enhanced teaching for family members is needed. The Caregiving in the U.S. study found that only 1 in 5 caregivers said they had obtained formal caregiver training and that three-quarters said they felt they needed more help or information (National Alliance for Caregiving, 2009). In another national survey, 20% of family caregivers who assisted with medication management and 30% of those who assisted with changing dressings had received no instruction from a health care professional regarding how to perform the task (IOM, 2008). In the Caregiving in the U.S. study, caregivers identified their greatest information needs as strategies for keeping the care recipient safe at home, managing their own stress, doing easy activities with the care recipient, finding time for themselves, and balancing work and family responsibilities. An increasing number identified managing challenging behaviors and moving and lifting the care recipient as priorities (National Alliance for Caregiving, 2009).

Occupational therapy practitioners can provide targeted caregiver education, training, and skill building. Effective caregiver interventions share some common features (Gitlin, 2007):

- Customized strategies to fit specific person–environment constellations or caregiver needs
- Focus on the specific contextual needs of caregivers
- Client-driven rather than prescriptive framework
- Emphasis on change in behavioral, psychosocial, and environmental factors and reduction of modifiable factors that place family caregivers at risk.

The overall goals of caregiver education are the reduction of excess disability in care recipients; the reduction of caregiver burden; and the promotion of safety,

> To support caregivers' sense of mastery and self-efficacy, practitioners can emphasize caregiver strengths and show appreciation of their opinions, preferences, experiences, and knowledge about their life situation.

It is important for occupational therapy practitioners to provide caregivers with the skills they will need to handle future care challenges.

health, and well-being for both caregivers and care recipients (Behr, Gray, Horowitz, & O'Sullivan, 2005). Caregivers must continue to manage day-to-day care on their own after discharge, making adjustments as the situation changes. Thus, it is important for occupational therapy practitioners to provide caregivers with the skills they will need to handle future care challenges (Gitlin & Corcoran, 2005).

Recognizing the Challenges of Caregiving

Caregiving challenges include both the care tasks themselves and the stresses and demands they place on the caregiver. Caregivers need to perform complex medical tasks, coordinate care, supervise care recipients, administer medications, handle medical equipment, and provide direct care such as wound care and lifting and turning, as well as manage the household; plan and provide meals; make decisions; solve problems; and provide emotional support and comfort, custodial care, transportation, and advocacy. Some tasks are merely time consuming; others are difficult to perform. In addition, to improve function and safety for the client, caregivers may need to modify the environment and acquire equipment and assistive devices (Given et al., 2008). Health care professionals go to school to learn many care tasks that caregivers must provide without such training.

An additional consideration is that care tasks may be performed by people who are themselves elderly, ill, or disabled. They require training and other support to safely perform more physically strenuous care tasks such as moving, lifting, and turning very ill adults (Moghimi, 2007).

Care demands depend on factors such as the client's personality; the type or stage of illness; and the caregiver's physical, cognitive, social, organizational, and psychological knowledge and skills. Occupational therapy practitioners must assess care demands and their match with the caregiver's availability, capacity, knowledge, skills, competing family roles, and resources. The predictability and routine nature of the care, as well as its duration (weeks or months) and quantity (daily hours of care), must be considered when developing and implementing therapeutic POCs with the family (Given et al., 2008).

Learning Caregivers' Priorities

When asked to identify their learning priorities, 40 caregivers in a focus group interview study (Yedidia & Tiedermann, 2008) identified the following areas of need:

- Information about available services and activities
- Stress management and coping strategies
- Information on the care recipient's condition
- Training in care tasks
- Education on communication and behavior strategies for care recipients with dementia
- Training in medication management
- Assistance in realistic goal setting
- Help with prioritizing goals
- Ways to engage clients in care.

In addressing learning needs, it is important to take health literacy into account. Nearly half of American adults have problems accessing, reading, understanding, and using health care information (Moghimi, 2007). Information must be tailored to be meaningful and useful to each client and caregiver. Extensive information is available about effective teaching strategies to address all levels of health literacy (National Network of Libraries of Medicine, 2015).

Caregivers also face the need to be critical thinkers when assessing problems, developing solutions, and mobilizing resources. Education and practice in critical thinking and problem solving prepare caregivers to handle the unexpected and to gain confidence in their ability to do so (Moghimi, 2007).

Client and Caregiver Satisfaction With Services

Most practitioners want to offer interventions that meet clients' needs and leave them feeling well served. Health care in general, and home care in particular, has evolved to look more closely at clients' perceptions of care as a measure of quality. Clients and caregivers can report on and evaluate their experiences with health care through the Home Health Consumer Assessment of Healthcare Providers and Systems (HHCAHPS; Agency for Healthcare Research and Quality, 2015). This information is reported to help inform clients' and families' decisions about what provider to use. Data are incorporated into the Home Health Compare website (http://www.medicare.gov/homehealthcompare/) to complement the clinical measures reported there. CMS requires that all home health agencies use the HHCAHPS to measure Medicare and Medicaid patients' perceptions of care (U.S. Department of Health and Human Services, 2010). Results are reported publicly on five composite outcome measures:

1. Overall rating of care
2. Likelihood of recommending
3. Care of patients
4. Communications
5. Specific care issues.

> Health care in general, and home care in particular, has evolved to look more closely at clients' perceptions of care as a measure of quality.

Stop here! Go to Appendix C and read the section "Empowerment of Consumers Through Public Disclosure" (pp. 207–208).

As described in **Appendixes C** and **D,** data are also collected from the Outcome and Assessment Information Set (OASIS) to report aggregate outcomes (change or lack of change in patient condition) achieved by home health providers, which allows consumers to compare and choose providers. The availability of these comparative data responds to the growing expectation of accountability from individual providers and agencies.

Caregiver and care recipient satisfaction are interrelated; one influences the other. The challenge for the practitioner is to hear and respect both voices. Research has shown that caregivers report more satisfaction if the everyday care they provide matches the values and preferences of the care recipient (Family Caregiver Alliance, 2000); thus, practitioners should use a holistic approach to identify and help achieve this care goal and increase caregiver satisfaction. A holistic approach to both caregiver and care recipient is especially important when the client has dementia because the challenges facing both people are so intimately related. For example, the agitated behavior of a person with dementia may distress the caregiver, and caregiver distress may increase agitation in the person with dementia (Toth-Cohen et al., 2001).

Another contributor to caregiver satisfaction (and to effective treatment) is practitioners valuing the caregiver's experience and expertise as a lay practitioner. Practitioners must adjust their communication approach to the caregiver's level of expertise in the caregiver role, knowledge of the client's medical conditions, and emotional response to ensure that the intervention addresses the caregiver's unique needs and abilities.

Donovan and Corcoran (2010) found that long-term caregivers of people with dementia reported higher levels of well-being after learning to incorporate into their caregiving simplified daily routines and organization, task choice and adaptation for the care recipient, self-care, and social engagement and support (including recognizing and adjusting social demands). Learning to adapt communication strategies, take a more positive approach, and understand the limitations imposed by dementia were shown to be beneficial to both the caregiver and the care recipient. Occupational therapy practitioners in home health can help caregivers maintain their quality of life, balance caregiving responsibilities with other demands and needs, and create opportunities to address personal needs, all identified as common caregiver goals (Heart and Stroke Foundation of Ontario, 2011).

> Occupational therapy practitioners in home health can help caregivers maintain their quality of life, balance caregiving responsibilities with other demands and needs, and create opportunities to address personal needs, all identified as common caregiver goals.

Conclusion

Family caregivers provide assistance with ADLs and IADLs, but their role has expanded to include care coordination and performing complex medical tasks once provided only in the hospital (Reinhard, Levine, & Samis, 2012). The evidence that caregivers have a profound effect on long-term care processes and outcomes is strong (IOM, 2008). Engaging families in client care has been shown to improve outcomes in dementia and schizophrenia care and to postpone institutionalization (IOM, 2008). In assuming specific tasks and responsibilities, family caregivers become part of the health care delivery team and contribute directly to health outcomes, although this contribution is not always recognized in the health care community.

Caregiver support allows older people to remain in their communities as long as possible, and the importance of family caregivers in reducing the risk of nursing home entry has been well documented (Feinberg, Reinhard, Houser, & Choula, 2011; Reinhard et al., 2012). The availability of a family caregiver has been linked to shorter hospital stays, and the absence of adequate caregiving has been associated with problematic hospital discharges and readmissions (IOM, 2008). Family caregivers are thus vital partners in occupational therapy intervention and follow-through for clients who live at home.

References

Agency for Healthcare Research and Quality. (2015). *Home Health Care CAHPS Survey*. Retrieved from https://homehealthcahps.org/Home.aspx

Alkema, C. G., & Frey, D. (2006). Implications of translating research into practice: A medication management intervention. *Home Health Care Services Quarterly, 25*(1–2), 33–54.

Behr, S., Gray, K., Horowitz, B., & O'Sullivan, A. (2005). *Families and caregivers across the lifespan* (Report to the Executive Board). Bethesda, MD: American Occupational Therapy Association.

Center for Home Care Policy and Research. (2009). *Framework for geriatric home health care*. New York: Visiting Nurse Service of New York. Retrieved from http://www.champ-program.org/static/CHAMP-Overall%20Brief.pdf

Centers for Medicare & Medicaid Services. (n.d.). *Tip sheet for providers: Caregiving education* (Publication No. 11390-P). Baltimore: Author. Retrieved from http://www.caregiving.org/data/CMS_Tip_Sheet_for_Providers_Caregiving_Education.pdf

Coleman, E., & Williams, M. (2007). Executing high-quality care transitions: A call to do it right. *Journal of Hospital Medicine, 2,* 287–290. http://dx.doi.org/10.1002/jhm.276

Day, L. (2011). Systematic review with meta-analysis: The Otago strength and balance exercise programme lowers the risk of death and falls in the older people at 12 months. *Evidence-Based Nursing, 14,* 76–78. http://dx.doi.org/10.1136/ebn1157

Donovan, M. L., & Corcoran, M. A. (2010). Description of dementia caregiver uplifts and implications for occupational therapy. *American Journal of Occupational Therapy, 64,* 590–595. http://dx.doi.org/10.5014/ajot.2010.09064

Durso, S. C. (2006). Using clinical guidelines designed for older adults with diabetes mellitus and complex health status. *JAMA, 295,* 1935–1940.

Family Caregiver Alliance. (2000). *Helping families make everyday care choices* (Fact Sheet). San Francisco: National Center on Caregiving. Retrieved from http://www.caregiver.org/helping-families-make-everyday-care-choices

Feinberg, L., Reinhard, S. C., Houser, A., & Choula, R. (2011). *Valuing the invaluable: 2011 update—The growing contributions and costs of family caregiving.* Washington, DC: AARP Public Policy Institute. Retrieved from http://assets.aarp.org/rgcenter/ppi/ltc/i51-caregiving.pdf

Gitlin, L. (2007). New models for caring for the caregiver: What, how, when, and where should we intervene? In Family Caregiver Alliance (Ed.), *Family caregiving: State of the art, future trends* (pp. 63–68). San Francisco: Family Caregiver Alliance. Retrieved from http://www.caregiver.org/sites/caregiver.org/files/pdfs/2007_asa_preconference_proceedings.pdf

Gitlin, L. N., & Corcoran, M. A. (2005). *Occupational therapy and dementia care: The Home Environmental Skill-Building Program for individuals and families.* Bethesda, MD: AOTA Press.

Gitlin, L. N., Winter, L., Dennis, M. P., Hodgson, N., & Hauck, W. W. (2010). A biobehavioral home-based intervention and the well-being of patients with dementia and their caregivers. *JAMA, 304,* 983–991. http://dx.doi.org/10.1001/jama.2010.1253

Given, B., Sherwood, P., & Given, C. (2008). What knowledge and skills do caregivers need? *American Journal of Nursing, 108*(9), 28–33. http://dx.doi.org/10.1097/01.NAJ.0000336408.52872.d2

Health Insurance Portability and Accountability Act of 1996 (HIPAA), Pub. L. 104–191, 42 U.S.C. § 300gg, 29 U.S.C § 1181-1183, and 42 U.S.C. § 1320d-1320d9.

Heart and Stroke Foundation of Ontario. (2011). *Community re-integration and long-term care.* Retrieved from http://www.heartandstroke.on.ca/site/c.pvI3IeNWJwE/b.5346783/k.DBAD/HCP__Community_Reintegration.htm

Hunt, G. (2007). Interface between family caregivers and direct care workers. In Family Caregiver Alliance (Ed.), *Family caregiving: State of the art, future trends* (pp. 42–44). San Francisco: Family Caregiver Alliance. Retrieved from http://www.caregiver.org/sites/caregiver.org/files/pdfs/2007_asa_preconference_proceedings.pdf

Institute of Medicine. (2008). *Retooling for an aging America: Building the health care workforce.* Washington, DC: National Academies Press.

Johnson, B., Abraham, M., Conway, J., Simmons, L., Edgman-Levitan, S., Sodomka, P., . . . Ford, D. (2008). *Partnering with patients and families to design a patient- and family-centered health care system.* Bethesda, MD: Institute for Patient- and Family-Centered Care. Retrieved from http://www.ipfcc.org/pdf/PartneringwithPatientsandFamilies.pdf

Law, M. (1998). *Client-centered occupational therapy.* Thorofare, NJ: Slack.

Levine, C. (2007). (Dis)-integration of caregivers in the health care system. In Family Caregiver Alliance (Ed.), *Family caregiving: State of the art, future trends* (pp. 77–80). San Francisco: Family Caregiver Alliance. Retrieved from http://www.caregiver.org/sites/caregiver.org/files/pdfs/2007_asa_preconference_proceedings.pdf

Moghimi, C. (2007). Issues in caregiving: The role of occupational therapy in caregiver training. *Topics in Geriatric Rehabilitation, 23,* 269–279. http://dx.doi.org/10.1097/01.TGR.0000284770.39958.79

National Alliance for Caregiving. (2009). *Caregiving in the U.S. 2009.* Bethesda, MD: Author. Retrieved from http://www.caregiving.org/data/Caregiving_in_the_US_2009_full_report.pdf

National Network of Libraries of Medicine. (2015). *Health literacy.* Bethesda, MD: National Library of Medicine. Retrieved from http://nnlm.gov/outreach/consumer/hlthlit.html

Raphael, C., & Cornwell, J. (2008). Influencing support for caregivers. *American Journal of Nursing, 108*(9), 78–82. http://dx.doi.org/10.1097/01.NAJ.0000336428.73064.f4

Reinhard, S. C., Levine, C., & Samis, S. (2012). *Home alone: Family caregivers providing complex chronic care.* Washington, DC: AARP Public Policy Institute. Retrieved from http://www.aarp.org/home-family/caregiving/info-10-2012/home-alone-family-caregivers-providing-complex-chronic-care.html

Schumacher, K. L., Stewart, B. J., Archbold, P. G., Dodd, M. J., & Dibble, S. L. (2000). Family caregiving skill: Development of the concept. *Research in Nursing and Health, 23,* 191–203.

Shaller, D. (2007). *Patient-centered care: What does it take?* New York: Commonwealth Fund. Retrieved from http://www.commonwealthfund.org/usr_doc/Shaller_patient-centeredcare-whatdoesittake_1067.pdf?section=4039

Stevens-Ratchford, R. (2005). Occupational engagement: Motivation for older adult participation. *Topics in Geriatric Rehabilitation, 21,* 171–181.

Toth-Cohen, S., Gitlin, L., Corcoran, M., Eckhardt, S., Johns, P., & Lipsitt, R. (2001). Providing services to family caregivers at home: Challenges and recommendations for health and human service professions. *Alzheimer's Care Quarterly, 2,* 23–32.

United Hospital Fund. (2008). *Assessing family caregivers: A guide for health care providers.* New York: Author. Retrieved from http://www.nextstepincare.org/uploads/File/Guides/Provider/Assessing_Family_Caregivers.pdf

U.S. Department of Health and Human Services, Centers for Medicare & Medicaid Services. (2010). Medicare program; Home Health Prospective Payment System rate update for calendar year 2011; changes in certification requirements for home health agencies and hospices; final rule. 75 *Fed. Reg.* 70372–70486.

Walens, D., & Rockwell-Dylla, L. (1996). Client– and family–practitioner relationships: Collaboration as an effective approach to treatment. In K. O. Larson, R. G. Stevens-Ratchford, L. W. Pedretti, & J. L. Crabtree (Eds.), *ROTE: The role of occupational therapy with the elderly* (pp. 826–855). Bethesda, MD: American Occupational Therapy Association.

Warshaw, G. (2007). Health care system trends: Families as care partners. In Family Caregiver Alliance (Ed.), *Family caregiving: State of the art, future trends* (pp. 16–20). San Francisco: Family Caregiver Alliance. Retrieved from http://www.caregiver.org/sites/caregiver.org/files/pdfs/2007_asa_preconference_proceedings.pdf

Yedidia, M., & Tiedermann, A. (2008). How do family caregivers describe their needs for professional help? *American Journal of Nursing, 108*(9, Suppl.), 35–37. http://dx.doi.org/10.1097/01.NAJ.0000336411.37624.2b

Section II: Occupational Therapy Practice in the Context of Home Health

INTRODUCTION TO

"Occupational Therapy Practice in the Context of Home Health"

Karen Vance, BSOT

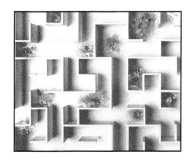

Photographs in old frames dot the walls, advancing in time as they continue around the corner to the adjacent wall. Smiling, posed faces within the frames increase in number every few feet as the family grows. The couple in the first picture stands tall with uncertain but happy expressions, he in a uniform, she in a fitted dark suit snug around a trim waist and a small brimmed fedora tilted over her right brow. Her eyes are bright and determined as she clutches the modest wedding bouquet.

Those same eyes sparkle now through the wrinkles of years as she points to the pictures with a gnarled finger. Her life story unfolds with little prompting, painting a clear picture of where she has been, her priorities, and her desires. She also provides a clear image of how she sees herself now and in the foreseeable future: agile, strong, mobile, and capable of caring for herself and her small ranch house without help. To any observer, the tiny, fragile frame of this woman belies her self-image, but her intentions are clear: This is where she belongs.

Occupational therapy practitioners may not always so easily elicit an occupational profile, a key piece in the occupational therapy evaluation process (American Occupational Therapy Association [AOTA], 2014). Home health practice, however, provides a rich context for natural cues that often can open the floodgate of disclosure essential to compiling clients' occupational profile. The challenge for practitioners is to translate this rich context and shared expectations to an intervention that supports clients' ability to achieve the desired outcomes they want. Section II describes the unique elements of the home health setting, the performance of occupational therapy practice in the context of home health, and the many important opportunities for occupational therapy practitioners to assist home health clients in living life to its fullest.

Chapter 3, "Conditions in Home Health Care," provides a frame for considering the client's whole condition—that is, the many aspects of the client's context.

The types of clients in home health care differ from those in many other settings, even though they may be in a similar age group. Aspects of the whole condition of home health clients certainly include advanced age, but diagnosis and impairment of body function, chronicity and multiple diagnoses, and the presence of family or other caregivers are other conditions that may help or hinder the occupational therapy process. In addition, the homebound status of Medicare beneficiaries who receive home health services has implications for the condition of the home health client and for occupational therapy practice. Chapter 3 provides occupational therapy practitioners with information to better manage this rich context for a better-informed plan of care and a more effective client–practitioner relationship.

Chapter 4, "The Occupational Therapy Evaluation Process in Home Health," focuses on what occupational therapy evaluation can and should look like in home health care. The *Occupational Therapy Practice Framework: Domain and Process* (3rd ed.; AOTA, 2014) structures the home health evaluation process, including the occupational profile and analysis of occupational performance, to inform goals and shared expectations. Recording the evaluation is critical not only to aid the practitioner in directing the intervention but also to satisfy the other stakeholders in home health care that rely on documentation to ensure compliance with their own expectations, such as regulatory or coverage requirements. Chapter 4 makes clear the connection between the occupational therapy evaluation and both Medicare's Home Health Quality Initiative (HHQI; described in **Appendix C, "Medicare as Quality Monitor"**) and clients' priorities of remaining at home and out of the hospital.

Chapter 5, "Home Health Plans of Care, Intervention, and Team Collaboration," guides occupational therapy practitioners in envisioning the outcomes of occupational therapy practice in home health care and developing an occupational therapy intervention plan that fits with the agencywide home health plan of care in a way that meets the requirements of the Centers for Medicare & Medicaid Services (CMS). Chapter 5 also discusses essential elements in documenting the interventions outlined in the occupational therapy plan. Among the unique elements of home health care is the challenge of team collaboration when all members are in different places at all times. Chapter 5 reinforces the need for communication and collaboration among team members to practice effectively and to provide opportunities to demonstrate the value of effective occupational therapy interventions as a part of a coherent agency home health plan of care.

Chapter 6, "Sustainable Outcomes in Home Health," describes outcomes from the client's perspective and from Medicare's perspective. Outcomes in home health care are a prevailing metric used in comparing performance among agencies and between time points for an individual agency. Although a client's desired outcomes may be essentially the same as Medicare's, the outcomes clients desire are much farther-reaching in time than those measured by Medicare. Outcomes selected in the context of home health must be relevant to the client. In addition, the value of these outcomes to clients and caregivers is greatest when they can be sustained after home health care has ended. Achieving desired outcomes may mark the end of a home health occupational therapy plan of care, but it is usually far from the end of the journey for the client.

Chapter 7, "Community Resources and Living Life to Its Fullest," addresses what happens after home health services finish. Successful return from the role of client to that of person often relies on the effectiveness of the support network, with the role of the caregiver being key, and adequate caregiver assessment and attention to caregiver needs are necessary to promote reengagement of the client and family in the community. Successful return from the role of client to that of person also relies on connecting with community resources to improve long-term outcomes and support living life to its fullest. Active engagement in occupation promotes, facilitates, and maintains the person's health and participation into the future (AOTA, 2014), and the occupational therapy process supports reengagement in continued meaningful occupations.

Section II describes how occupational therapy practice can look in home health care. Regardless of how general practice currently exists in a home health agency, occupational therapy practitioners can elevate their own practice by using clinical reasoning, communicating effective outcomes, and facilitating clients' ability to live life to its fullest.

Reference

American Occupational Therapy Association. (2014). Occupational therapy practice framework: Domain and process (3rd ed.). *American Journal of Occupational Therapy, 68*(Suppl. 1), S1–S48. http://dx.doi.org/10.5014/ajot.2014.682006

CHAPTER 3

Conditions in Home Health Care

Carol Siebert, MS, OTR/L, FAOTA

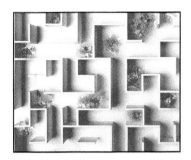

Learning Objectives

After completing this chapter, readers will be able to
- Identify the many types of conditions common in the population receiving home health care;
- Delineate why diagnosis alone provides inadequate information to describe the home health population; and
- Recognize the social and physical context of home health practice as it relates to the whole condition of the client.

Introduction: Conditional Reasoning in Home Health

Who receives home health services? People who receive home health care typically experience multiple **conditions**—that is, factors and circumstances—that may or may not fit neatly into diagnostic categories. These conditions drive the need for home health care, inform the practice of clinicians providing home health services, and influence the ultimate outcomes of home health care.

The term *condition* is more appropriate than *diagnosis* when discussing the home health population. Most home health clients have more than one health problem, so diagnosis alone does not adequately capture the health condition of a given client. The home, including its physical, social, and cultural contexts, influences the client and the needs and services provided. Each client's unique home situation is an environmental condition that is integral to the provision of home health care. Given the multiple conditions present for any one home health client, it is helpful to first consider the concept of **conditional reasoning** as a framework for thinking about the home health population.

Conditional reasoning is one of several modes of clinical reasoning identified by Mattingly and Fleming (1994) in their landmark study of clinical reasoning. Fleming (1994) posited that "this reasoning style moves beyond specific concerns about the

Key Terms

- conditional reasoning
- conditions
- homebound
- primary home health diagnosis
- self-management
- self-management support

person and the physical problems and places them in broader social and temporal contexts" (p. 133). Home health practice involves a similar, multidimensional perspective.

Fleming (1994) explained that the term *condition* has three meanings:

> One is that therapists think about the whole condition; this includes the person, the illness, the meanings the illness has for the person, the family, and the social and physical contexts in which the person lives. A second is that therapists need to imagine how the condition could change and become a revised condition. The imagined new state is a condition, that is, a proposed state, which may or may not be achieved. The third sense is that the success or failure of reaching a point in life that approximates that future image is very much contingent upon (or conditional upon) the client's participation. The client must participate, not only in the therapeutic activities themselves, but also in the construction of the image of the possible outcome, the revised condition. (p. 133)

This chapter addresses primarily the first aspect of conditional reasoning: What is the whole condition of the client?

Fleming's definition of *conditional reasoning* and the three meanings of *condition* provide a framework for thinking about clients who receive home health care and about the role of home health services in a given client's life. This chapter addresses primarily the first aspect of conditional reasoning: What is the whole condition of the client?

Older Adult Population

Medicare is by far the biggest payer for home health services (Centers for Medicare & Medicaid Services [CMS], 2012). Thus, most home health recipients are Medicare beneficiaries: Either they are older adults who have attained the age to qualify for Social Security (and, thus, Medicare), or they are adults who have qualified for Social Security after a determination that they are permanently disabled and thus unable to earn a living by working. Figure 3.1 depicts the proportion of the home health population in each age group.

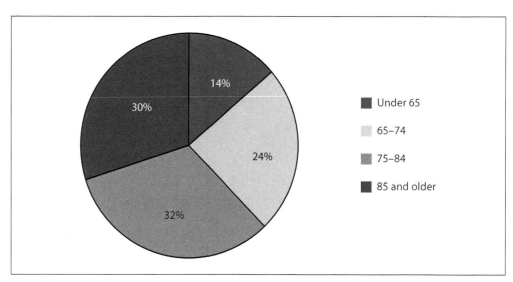

Figure 3.1. Age of Medicare home health patients, 2012.

Source. Data from *Medicare and Medicaid Statistical Supplement, 2013 Edition* (Table 7.2), by Centers for Medicare & Medicaid Services, 2013, Baltimore: Author. In the public domain.

In the home health practice setting, the term *young* is often used for clients younger than age 65. Clients ages 85 or older, often referred to as "the oldest old," comprise nearly a third of the home health population (CMS, 2013; see Figure 3.1). The demographics of the home health population suggest two conditions important to occupational therapy practitioners. The first is that many home health clients are no longer involved in paid employment. For this population, work as an area of occupation is focused primarily on adjustment to retirement, volunteer exploration, and volunteer participation. The absence of paid work influences this population's roles and routines.

The second condition associated with age is the experience of age-related changes in body structures and functions. This condition requires occupational therapy practitioners to be aware of age-related changes and to be able to discriminate between the normal effects of aging versus impairment not associated with aging. The condition also demands that practitioners appreciate that when assessing various body systems, norms for older or very old adults are different from those for young or middle-aged adults.

Diagnosis and Impairment of Body Function

Although diagnosis alone offers limited information about any given home health client, data related to diagnoses in the home health client population offer some perspective on differences between the home health population and populations encountered in other settings. The most common diagnoses in home care can be determined from aggregate client data collected as part of the mandated Outcome and Assessment Information Set (OASIS; Shaughnessy, Schlenker, & Crisler, 2002); OASIS is described in **Appendix D** of this text and Self-Paced Clinical Course (SPCC; pp. 221–254).

The *OASIS–C1/ICD–10 Version Guidance Manual* specifies that the **primary home health diagnosis** is the diagnosis that best describes the reason home health care is needed—that is, the condition that is the primary focus of home care (CMS, 2015). Specifically, the primary diagnosis is the diagnosis most related to the patient's current plan of care, the chief reason home care is needed, and the most acute.

The six most commonly reported home health diagnoses are diabetes, heart failure, essential hypertension, chronic ulcer of the skin, osteoarthrosis and related conditions, and cardiac dysrhythmias (CMS, 2013). Table 3.1 lists the percentage of home health beneficiaries with each of these primary diagnoses. The most common diagnostic categories triggering a need for home health (musculoskeletal

Table 3.1. Most Common Principal Diagnoses of Medicare Home Health Beneficiaries, 2012

Primary Diagnosis	% of Total Beneficiaries Served
Diabetes	9.5
Heart failure	7.5
Essential hypertension	6.6
Chronic ulcer of the skin	4.5
Osteoarthrosis and allied disorders	4.1
Cardiac dysrhythmias	2.7
Total	**34.9**

Source. From *Medicare and Medicaid Statistical Supplement, 2013 Edition* (Table 7.6), by Centers for Medicare & Medicaid Services, 2013, Baltimore: Author. In the public domain.

Table 3.2. Percentage of Total Medicare Home Health Beneficiary Care Episodes by Major Diagnostic Category, 2010

Major Diagnostic Category	% of All Beneficiary Care Episodes
Infectious and parasitic diseases	0.8
Neoplasms	3.2
Endocrine, nutritional, and metabolic diseases and immunity disorders	10.5
Diseases of the blood and blood-forming organs	1.7
Mental disorders	2.8
Diseases of the nervous system and sense organs	4.7
Diseases of the circulatory system	27.6
Diseases of the respiratory system	9.3
Diseases of the digestive system	2.7
Diseases of the genitourinary system	3.2
Diseases of the skin and subcutaneous tissue	6.7
Diseases of the musculoskeletal system	13.0
Congenital abnormalities	0.1
Symptoms, signs, and ill-defined conditions	6.5
Injury and poisoning	6.3
Supplementary classification of factors influencing health status and contact with health services	36.3

Source. From *Medicare and Medicaid Statistical Supplement, 2013 Edition* (Table 7.6), by Centers for Medicare & Medicaid Services, 2013, Baltimore: Author. In the public domain.

and neurological conditions) are not those usually associated with rehabilitation. Table 3.2 lists the percentage of care episodes related to the major diagnostic categories, offering a snapshot of the Medicare home health population through the lens of body system impairments. Circulatory, metabolic, respiratory, and integumentary conditions account for more than half of primary home health diagnoses for Medicare beneficiaries (54%), and musculoskeletal and nervous system disorders account for almost 18% of such services.

> The conditions inherent in home health clients' diagnoses have implications for the knowledge and competencies needed by home health occupational therapy practitioners.

The conditions inherent in home health clients' diagnoses have implications for the knowledge and competencies needed by home health occupational therapy practitioners. Impairments in cardiovascular (circulatory), respiratory, or metabolic functions are assessed through lab values or by direct assessments such as blood pressure, blood glucose testing, pulse oximetry, and daily weights. These assessments differ significantly from assessments such as joint range of motion, strength, postural alignment, tone, or coordination typically used to quantify musculoskeletal or neurological impairments. Practitioners working in home health must be familiar with the assessment procedures for cardiovascular, respiratory, and metabolic function and, more important, must recognize the effect of occupational therapy interventions on these measures.

Chronicity

The most common home health diagnoses are characterized by chronicity. Conditions associated with cardiovascular, respiratory, and metabolic functions may present with periods of acute exacerbation, but they are chronic conditions. These conditions are also associated with complications or sequelae that can be disabling or even life threatening. As a result, these conditions require day-to-day management to keep them controlled. Chronicity and the need for day-to-day management are also associated with many musculoskeletal and neurological conditions, but these conditions are less likely to be associated with emergent or life-threatening exacerbations.

The need to manage chronic conditions is an important aspect of home health care. When home health services are initiated, the agency may take on all or most of the responsibility for managing the client's condition, a responsibility typically shared by the client's physicians. However, home health is a transitional service: One of the important goals of home health is to transfer management of the condition to (or back to) the client or caregiver. Day-to-day management of a chronic condition by the person experiencing the condition is one aspect of **self-management.**

Home health is a transitional service: One of the important goals of home health is to transfer management of the condition to (or back to) the client or caregiver.

Multiple Chronic Conditions and Acute Hospitalizations

A factor not captured by the data on primary diagnosis is that many home health recipients have multiple chronic conditions and disabilities associated with those chronic conditions. For these clients, a home health referral may be precipitated by an acute event (e.g., stroke, amputation), but regaining or maintaining control of the underlying condition or conditions is as much a priority as addressing the newly acquired condition.

More than half of all home health clients are admitted to home care from an inpatient setting (U.S. Department of Health and Human Services, 2001), either directly from a hospital or from a postacute care facility after hospitalization. Data from much of the past decade have indicated that more than 1 in 4 home health clients have experienced an acute hospitalization while receiving an episode of home health services (CMS, 2012; Jencks, Williams, & Coleman, 2009). Beginning in 2007, CMS initiated various efforts to encourage home health agencies to focus on reducing the rate of hospitalization during home health services and specifically to reduce "avoidable" hospitalizations. A variety of practice tools were developed to prevent avoidable hospitalizations, but even after several years of these efforts, the rate of hospitalization remained at more than 25%. Hospitalization rates are shown on Home Health Compare (http://www.medicare.gov/HomeHealthCompare), which is explained in **Appendix C** (see "Home Health Quality Initiative" section, pp. 206–209). Reducing avoidable hospitalizations continues to be a challenge and a priority in home health care.

How do data on acute hospitalization contribute to an understanding of the home health population? For more than half of home health clients, receiving home health is part of going home. Returning to the hospital is not a desired event but instead a circumstance to be avoided. For some home health clients, acute hospitalizations are a familiar occurrence because inadequate management of chronic conditions results in exacerbations or events that require hospitalization. Although not all hospitalizations are avoidable, clients and their families, agencies, and payers all have a stake in avoiding hospitalizations that can be prevented.

Some home health clients and their families exhibit anxiety about the possibility of hospitalization. Clients who have had many hospitalizations, however, may come to assume that hospitalization is inevitable and that there is nothing they can do to avoid another trip to the hospital. Caregivers and family members may or may not share the client's attitude toward their ability to manage the client's conditions successfully or the inevitability of hospitalization. Attitude toward hospitalization influences the client's and caregiver's expectations of home health care and interactions with home health clinicians.

Self-Management

Self-management is defined as "the tasks that individuals must undertake to live well with one or more chronic conditions. These tasks include having the confidence to deal with medical management, role management, and emotional management of their conditions" (Institute of Medicine [IOM], 2004, p. 57). **Self-management support** is defined as "the systematic provision of education and supportive interventions by health care staff to increase patients' skills and confidence in managing their health problems, including regular assessment of progress and problems, goal setting, and problem-solving support" (IOM, 2003, p. 52).

The role of home health, and of each home health clinician, is to support self-management. This role has important implications for occupational therapy. Management of a chronic condition or conditions may include tasks to monitor the condition, new activities to prevent worsening of the condition, or modification of existing activities to prevent worsening of the condition. One of the challenges of self-management is that it is not enough for the client to demonstrate the new or modified tasks in isolation: The client must be able to incorporate or integrate these tasks and activities into daily life, and in this critical aspect of managing chronic conditions, occupational therapy practitioners' focus on performance patterns is essential to clients' achieving self-management.

Presence and Influence of Caregivers

The presence and influence of family and other unpaid caregivers is another important factor in understanding the condition of the home health client. For clients returning home from an inpatient setting, the assurance that caregivers would be available—even 24 hours a day—may have been a condition for discharge. Some home health clients may have paid aides or companions in the home, but most of the assistance or caregiving provided to home health clients is delivered by family members, friends, or other unpaid caregivers. Having care provided by unpaid caregivers contributes to several important aspects of the home health client's overall condition: the existing relationship between client and caregiver, caregiver limitations in the caregiving experience, lack of a formal caregiving contract or agreement, and, at times, discontinuity in caregiving.

The relationship dynamic between many clients and caregivers was established before the client needed caregiving. When a spouse, child, friend, or neighbor becomes a caregiver, the caregiving relationship is added to but does not replace the existing relationship. The dynamics of the existing relationship, however, may be exaggerated by the addition of the caregiver–care recipient dynamic. Unpaid caregivers may have goals for the client that are different from those expressed by the client. Caregivers also have their own wants and needs that may affect their caregiving and their relationship with home health clinicians.

> The role of home health, and of each home health clinician, is to support self-management.

Unlike settings in which caregiving is provided by trained aides, companions, or care managers, in home health the unpaid caregivers who take on these responsibilities may have little or no caregiving training or experience. Any education or training by clinicians before the client is discharged to home typically occurs during a stressful time, while a loved one is hospitalized, and once the client is at home even attentive caregivers may find they recall little of such training. Unpaid caregivers may be anxious about knowing what to expect and what to do. For clients with a long-standing condition, the caregiver is experienced and thus may not be anxious about caregiving, but the caregiver may be resistant to trying new approaches to better manage the condition or may infer that new approaches are an indictment of the caregiver's methods. Even if a client wants to implement new approaches to care, buy-in by unpaid caregivers will be necessary.

Unpaid caregivers usually have no defined agreement regarding their caregiving responsibilities. This lack of a formalized agreement can, at times, make circumstances difficult when caregiver and client disagree about care or any other aspect of either's life. In most cases, unpaid caregivers have work, family, and other responsibilities in addition to being a caregiver. Any of these other responsibilities may have a bearing on the caregiver's availability, attentiveness, and investment in caregiving.

Problems with continuity of caregiving also arise in home health practice. Often the stipulation that a client must have 24-hour care to be discharged home is fulfilled by recruiting any willing friend, neighbor, or relative to participate in caregiving. The practitioner may arrive in the home and find that a caregiver who is a neighbor, a distant relative, or an acquaintance is assisting or "sitting" with the client. The practitioner cannot assume that occasional caregivers will be present on future visits or that the client wants personal health information to be shared with such caregivers.

Unpaid caregivers' knowledge and abilities are part of the condition of the home health client. Occupational therapy practitioners must account for unpaid caregivers' needs and wants when considering a possible revised condition for the client. The participation of unpaid caregivers, not just the client, is critical to achieving any desired revised condition.

Client Status as *Homebound*

Being ***homebound***, or confined to the home, is one criterion a beneficiary must meet to receive services under the Medicare Part A home health benefit. Box 3.1 provides the definition of *homebound* from the *Medicare Benefit Policy Manual* (CMS, 2014). Other payers, including many private insurers, also include *homebound* as a criterion for coverage of services provided in the home and use the Medicare definition or a similar one. Although some payers may make exceptions, in general, clients receiving home health services are confined to the home, with the exception of the circumstances outlined in the final paragraph of the *Medicare Benefit Policy Manual* definition in Box 3.1.

What does this coverage provision indicate about the population receiving home health? Those receiving home health are medically stable enough to be at home but have functional or medical limitations that make leaving the home difficult and infrequent and typically require the assistance of others to accomplish.

Those receiving home health are medically stable enough to be at home but have functional or medical limitations that make leaving the home difficult and infrequent and typically require the assistance of others to accomplish.

Box 3.1. Definition of *Homebound* in the *Medicare Benefit Policy Manual*

Patient Confined to the Home

For a patient to be eligible to receive covered home health services under both Part A and Part B, the law requires that a physician certify in all cases that the patient is confined to his/her home. For purposes of the statute, an individual shall be considered "confined to the home" (homebound) if the following two criteria are met:

1. Criteria-One:

The patient must either:

- Because of illness or injury, need the aid of supportive devices such as crutches, canes, wheelchairs, and walkers; the use of special transportation; or the assistance of another person in order to leave their place of residence

OR

- Have a condition such that leaving his or her home is medically contraindicated.

If the patient meets one of the Criteria-One conditions, then the patient must ALSO meet two additional requirements defined in Criteria-Two below.

2. Criteria-Two:

- There must exist a normal inability to leave home;

AND

- Leaving home must require a considerable and taxing effort.

If the patient does in fact leave the home, the patient may nevertheless be considered homebound if the absences from the home are infrequent or for periods of relatively short duration, or are attributable to the need to receive health care treatment. Absences attributable to the need to receive health care treatment include, but are not limited to:

- Attendance at adult day centers to receive medical care;
- Ongoing receipt of outpatient kidney dialysis; or
- The receipt of outpatient chemotherapy or radiation therapy.

Any absence of an individual from the home attributable to the need to receive health care treatment, including regular absences for the purpose of participating in therapeutic, psychosocial, or medical treatment in an adult day-care program that is licensed or certified by a State, or accredited to furnish adult day-care services in a State, shall not disqualify an individual from being considered to be confined to his home. Any other absence of an individual from the home shall not so disqualify an individual if the absence is of an infrequent or of relatively short duration. For purposes of the preceding sentence, any absence for the purpose of attending a religious service shall be deemed to be an absence of infrequent or short duration. It is expected that in most instances, absences from the home that occur will be for the purpose of receiving health care treatment. However, occasional absences from the home for nonmedical purposes, e.g., an occasional trip to the barber, a walk around the block or a drive, attendance at a family reunion, funeral, graduation, or other infrequent or unique event would not necessitate a finding that the patient is not homebound if the absences are undertaken on an infrequent basis or are of relatively short duration and do not indicate that the patient has the capacity to obtain the health care provided outside rather than in the home.

Source. From "Patient Confined to the Home," § 30.1.1, in Chapter 7, *Medicare Benefit Policy Manual,* by Centers for Medicare & Medicaid Services, 2014, Baltimore: Author. In the public domain.

For some clients, being homebound is a new condition. Other clients may have been functionally homebound for weeks, months, or even years. In either case, the homebound client is typically unable to do things that most people take for granted, such as make a quick trip to the grocery store, see a new movie, or take a walk around the block. The inability or the extensive effort required to leave the home may be a source of frustration or a condition the client has grown accustomed to. Whether long-standing or newly imposed, being homebound means that the home and the immediate vicinity are the client's world for much of the day or week or month. When the practitioner offers a casual "have a good weekend" or "how was your holiday?" to a home health client, he or she must be aware that the client may have remained in the home, or even in the same room, for the duration of the interval or occasion.

Homebound status also implies functional limitations. If a person is normally unable to leave the home or if leaving the home requires assistance or is a considerable and taxing effort, then it reasonably can be inferred that the person's impairment or disability contributes to that inability or effort or need for assistance. It is important to recognize that the inability may not result solely from a mobility or motor limitation; other recognized causes include pain, cognitive limitations, anxiety or fear, cardiopulmonary limitations, visual impairments, or any other client factor that makes the client normally unable to leave his or her own home. If a client qualifies for home health services, being homebound is part of that person's experience.

From the perspective of Medicare and other payers, professional health care provided in the home occurs when the client is medically stable enough not to need inpatient care. As noted in the Medicare definition of *homebound* (see Box 3.1), the client's lack of or limited ability to leave the home is a key factor that qualifies the client for home health care. Some practitioners assume that if it is at all feasible for a client to access outpatient services, such as an outpatient therapy clinic, the client should no longer receive home health services. However, the Medicare definition of *homebound* acknowledges that a client may leave the home on infrequent occasions for short durations and still be considered homebound. It is important to consider the overall effect on the client of going out and his or her overall service needs when determining whether a client is homebound and in the ongoing reassessment of homebound status.

The Home: More Than a Location

Home health service delivery is distinct in that it is provided not in a facility but in the client's home. This uniqueness, though, pertains not just to where practitioners provide their services. That the home health client is home is more than simply a statement about location: It is a statement about being. Awareness of this fact is an essential aspect of thinking about the whole condition of the client.

The home is not solely a physical environment. The home is also a reflection of the lives of those who dwell within its walls (Cooper Marcus, 1997). Meeting a client in his or her home is an opportunity to become acquainted with that person, his or her family, and his or her culture in ways that are not possible in other settings. The client's possessions, the arrangement and tidiness of the environment, and even the way the practitioner is greeted on arrival all convey information about the client and his or her life (Goffman, 1959). The home is a place filled with meanings and history (Tuan, 1977). It is to this place that the client returns on discharge from an inpatient setting, and it is in this place that the client seeks to remain.

The home offers the practitioner an abundance of information about the client's current condition. Although the home may provide little information about the client's health condition, it offers much understanding about his or her roles and valued occupations (Hasselkus, 2011). The conditions in the home also offer indications of the client's social or economic circumstances. Eliciting stories about photos or other artifacts offers a window into the client's experience.

Although the home may provide little information about the client's health condition, it offers much understanding about his or her roles and valued occupations.

Living Arrangements Outside the Client's Own Home

In some instances, home health is provided to clients who are not in their own home or residence. This circumstance often arises when a client is able to be discharged from an inpatient setting, but the client's own home is either inaccessible to the client or inconvenient for those providing intensive unpaid caregiving. The client may live with a relative or other caregiver for the duration of the episode. Such clients may or may not understand why they are unable to go home and may express the desire to be in their own home instead of an alternative arrangement. In these situations, it is important for practitioners to recognize that the client is not at home and is either adjusting to or resisting adjusting to the new living situation. For clients who are staying in a new location, disruption of habits and routines may be attributable as much to relocation as to any change in the client's skills.

Importance of Place and Control

Although the home offers much information to help the practitioner make sense of the client's condition, it is also important to understand what the home is not. It is not a clinic. It is not the practitioner's turf. It is a practice environment that is not under the control of the practitioner but is instead under the control of the client or his or her family. Understanding that the control in this environment lies with the client and his or her support network is a critical aspect of understanding the client's whole condition. Respect for how the client chooses to relate to practitioners coming into the home and handles potential disruptions to the home and routines of the home is critical to establishing an effective client–practitioner partnership in home health.

Conclusion

People are referred to home health care for a variety of reasons. The most frequently reported diagnoses supporting the need for home health care are conditions associated with impairment of cardiovascular, metabolic, integumentary, musculoskeletal, and respiratory functions. Many home health clients have multiple conditions, and often these conditions are chronic. The referral to home health care may follow an exacerbation of one or more of these conditions. An important goal of home health care is to assist the client and caregivers in managing or better managing these chronic conditions.

Diagnostic information, however, does not adequately capture or describe client conditions in home health. One way to better understand the home health population is to consider the commonalities in what Fleming (1994) described as the whole condition of the client. These common circumstances or factors help paint a more useful picture of the population served by home health care.

First, Medicare is the dominant payer in home health. Thus, most Medicare clients are either older adults or adults with significant disabilities. Second, home health is unique in that unpaid caregivers play a critical role. It is rare to encounter a home health client who does not have unpaid caregivers involved. Practitioners must negotiate the relationship between clients and their caregivers and work with caregivers who have other roles and priorities that may compete with caregiving. Caregivers influence the client's expectations and the course of home health care.

Finally, home health is provided in the client's home or a home setting. Home is where most clients want to be and to stay. The home can provide an abundance of clues about the client's social, economic, and cultural context and about roles and valued occupations. One of the challenges of home health is to appreciate being in a client's home and delivering services in an environment in which the practitioner is a guest.

References

Centers for Medicare & Medicaid Services. (2012). *National health expenditure data, historical, 2010.* Baltimore: Author.

Centers for Medicare & Medicaid Services. (2013). *Medicare and Medicaid statistical supplement: 2013 edition.* Baltimore: Author.

Centers for Medicare & Medicaid Services. (2014). *Medicare benefit policy manual: Chapter 7— Home health services.* Retrieved from https://www.cms.gov/Regulations-and-Guidance/ Guidance/Manuals/downloads//bp102c07.pdf

Centers for Medicare & Medicaid Services. (2015). *OASIS–C1/ICD–10 version guidance manual.* Retrieved from http://www.cms.gov/Medicare/Quality-Initiatives-Patient-Assessment-Instruments/HomeHealthQualityInits/HHQIOASISUserManual.html

Cooper Marcus, C. (1997). *House as a mirror of self: Exploring the deeper meaning of home.* Berkeley, CA: Conari Press.

Fleming, M. H. (1994). The therapist with the three-track mind. In C. Mattingly & M. H. Fleming (Eds.), *Clinical reasoning: Forms of inquiry in a therapeutic practice* (pp. 119–136). Philadelphia: F. A. Davis.

Goffman, E. (1959). *The presentation of self in everyday life.* New York: Doubleday.

Hasselkus, B. (2011). *The meaning of everyday occupation* (2nd ed.). Thorofare, NJ: Slack.

Institute of Medicine. (2003). *Priority areas for national action: Transforming health care quality.* Washington, DC: National Academies Press.

Institute of Medicine. (2004). *First annual Crossing the Quality Chasm Summit: A focus on communities.* Washington, DC: National Academies Press.

Jencks, S. F., Williams, M. V., & Coleman, E. A. (2009). Rehospitalizations among clients in the Medicare fee-for-service program. *New England Journal of Medicine, 360,* 1418–1428. http://dx.doi.org/10.1056/NEJMsa0803563

Mattingly, C., & Fleming, M. H. (1994). *Clinical reasoning: Forms of inquiry in a therapeutic practice.* Philadelphia: F. A. Davis.

National Center for Health Statistics & Centers for Medicare & Medicaid Services. (2015). *International classification of diseases, 10th revision, clinical modification.* Hyattsville, MD: National Center for Health Statistics.

Shaughnessy, P., Schlenker, D., & Crisler, K. (2002). *Outcome and Assessment Information Set (OASIS).* Colorado Springs: Center for Health Services Research.

Tuan, Y.-F. (1977). *Space and place: The perspective of experience.* Minneapolis: University of Minnesota Press.

U.S. Department of Health and Human Services, Office of Inspector General. (2001). *Medicare home health care community beneficiaries 2001* (Publication No. OEI-02-01-00070). Washington, DC: Author. Retrieved from http://www.oig.hhs.gov/oei/reports/oei-02-01-00070.pdf

CHAPTER 4

The Occupational Therapy Evaluation Process in Home Health

Carol Siebert, MS, OTR/L, FAOTA

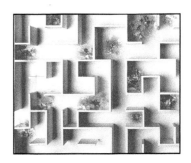

Learning Objectives

After completing this chapter, readers will be able to

- Delineate how the *Occupational Therapy Practice Framework: Domain and Process* can be used to guide the occupational therapy evaluation process in home health;
- Identify the components of the occupational therapy evaluation process in home health;
- Identify the components of the home health comprehensive assessment;
- Identify the relationship between occupational therapy evaluation in home health and home health data accuracy and the Home Health Quality Initiative; and
- Identify key Outcome and Assessment Information Set items of interest in the occupational therapy evaluation process.

Introduction

In occupational therapy, **evaluation** is defined as the "process of obtaining and interpreting data necessary for intervention . . . [including] documenting the evaluation process and results" (American Occupational Therapy Association [AOTA], 2014, p. S42). In home health, occupational therapy evaluation may inform not only occupational therapy intervention but also the interventions of other professionals on the home health care team. Data obtained and interpreted by occupational therapy professionals may inform the home health **comprehensive assessment,** which includes the **Outcome and Assessment Information Set (OASIS)** data (Centers for Medicare & Medicaid Services [CMS], 2015), even when an occupational therapist is not directly responsible for conducting the comprehensive assessment. Additionally, the occupational therapy evaluation process may help improve data accuracy, specifically the accuracy of outcome measures. Public reporting of outcome measures (and, by inference, the accuracy of such measures) is a key aspect of national efforts to improve home health quality.

Key Terms

- **analysis of occupational performance**
- **assessment** (Essential Term—see definition in the "Introduction" to this text and SPCC)
- **comprehensive assessment**
- **evaluation** (Essential Term—see definition in the "Introduction" to this text and SPCC)
- **Home Health Quality Initiative**
- **level of assistance**
- **occupational profile**
- **occupational therapy domain**
- *Occupational Therapy Practice Framework: Domain and Process*
- **occupational therapy process**
- **Outcome and Assessment Information Set (OASIS)**

Home health practice is a specific subset of occupational therapy practice. Home health care is strongly shaped by Medicare regulations and Medicare benefit coverage criteria. Home health care is also shaped by its primary service population, older adults who are homebound. Two additional factors shaping home health care are less obvious—(1) the location of service, the home, and (2) the history of home health care even before the existence of the Medicare benefit; these influences were described in Section I.

Home health as a practice setting is often categorized on the basis of one or sometimes both of these factors. Those who focus on the population consider home health to be gerontological practice. Those who focus on the setting may characterize home health as community practice. Others consider home health to be one aspect of postacute care. Still others view home health as nursing care. Although each of these characterizations has some basis in truth, in reality none is adequate to fully describe home health care or home health practice.

However, these partial descriptions and practitioners' prior experiences often shape how occupational therapy practitioners come to understand home health care. For example, a practitioner interested in working with older adults may consider home health practice because of its population. A practitioner who has worked in inpatient rehabilitation may view home health as a continuation of the rehabilitation process. A practitioner who has worked in inpatient acute care may perceive home health as community practice. And practitioners new to home health are often puzzled by those who order or receive home health services who perceive all home health care as nursing.

The result of these multiple characterizations of home health and home health practice is that what occupational therapy addresses in home health and what occupational therapy practitioners do in home health may not always be clear. This lack of clarity often frustrates occupational therapy practitioners working in home health, but it also confuses those requesting occupational therapy services, agencies providing occupational therapy services, and the practitioners providing occupational therapy services in home health. This confusion leads to occupational therapy being misunderstood and underused in home health. It is therefore essential that occupational therapy practitioners in home health be able to communicate clearly what they address and what they do. How to communicate occupational therapy clearly—to clients, in documentation, and to coworkers—is a recurrent theme throughout this chapter.

Occupational Therapy Practice Framework

Occupational therapy practice—what is addressed (domain) and what is done (process)—is articulated in the **Occupational Therapy Practice Framework: Domain and Process** (3rd ed.; referred to as the *Framework*; AOTA, 2014). The *Framework* communicates occupational therapy practice in a generic way that applies across all populations and settings.

The *Framework* is more than terminology. In home health, which is shaped by regulation, population, and service location, the *Framework* offers a means to frame practice that is grounded in the core tenets of occupational therapy and tailored to address the unique population and service delivery, regulatory, and reimbursement contexts of home health care. By framing their discussion using the constructs of

In home health, which is shaped by regulation, population, and service location, the *Framework* offers a means to frame practice that is grounded in the core tenets of occupational therapy and tailored to address the unique population and service delivery, regulatory, and reimbursement contexts of home health care.

Table 4.1. The Domain of Occupational Therapy: What Does Occupational Therapy Address?

Occupations	Client Factors	Performance Skills	Performance Patterns	Contexts and Environments
Activities of daily living (ADLs)[a]	Values, beliefs, and spirituality	Motor skills	Habits	Cultural
Instrumental activities of daily living (IADLs)	Body functions	Process skills	Routines	Personal
Rest and sleep	Body structures	Social interaction skills	Rituals	Physical
Education			Roles	Social
Work				Temporal
Play				Virtual
Leisure				
Social participation				

Source. From "Occupational Therapy Practice Framework: Domain and Process," 3rd ed., by the American Occupational Therapy Association, 2014, *American Journal of Occupational Therapy, 68*(Suppl. 1), p. S4, Bethesda, MD: Author. Copyright © 2014 by the American Occupational Therapy Association. Used with permission.
[a]Also referred to as *basic activities of daily living* (BADLs) or *personal activities of daily living* (PADLs).

the *Framework,* practitioners can effectively communicate to all home health stakeholders the expertise of occupational therapy and the contributions of occupational therapy to home health outcomes.

The **occupational therapy domain** is the "profession's purview and the areas in which its members have an established body of knowledge and expertise" (AOTA, 2014, p. S3). This domain includes occupations, client factors, performance skills, performance patterns, and contexts and environments, as outlined in Table 4.1. The aspects of the domain do not form a hierarchy; all aspects of the domain are of equal value. The aspects "interact to affect the client's occupational identity, health, well-being, and participation in life" (AOTA, 2014, p. S4).

As noted in the *Framework,*

> The *occupational therapy process* is the client-centered delivery of occupational therapy services. The process includes evaluation and intervention to achieve targeted outcomes, occurs within the purview of the occupational therapy domain, and is facilitated by the distinct perspective of occupational therapy practitioners when engaging in clinical reasoning, analyzing activities and occupations, and collaborating with clients. (AOTA, 2014, pp. S9–S10)

The **occupational therapy process** involves evaluation, intervention, and targeting of outcomes. Many professions use a process of evaluation–intervention–outcomes, but "only occupational therapy practitioners focus on the use of occupations to promote health, well-being, and participation in life" (AOTA, 2014, p. S11). The occupational therapy process is not linear; rather, it is dynamic. Figure 4.1 depicts the occupational therapy process and illustrates its dynamic aspects.

The *Framework* has much richness and detail that cannot be addressed in this chapter; readers seeking more information on or study of the *Framework* are directed to the *Framework* itself (AOTA, 2014) and to continuing education resources that address the *Framework* (e.g., Amini, 2014). The brief review of the *Framework* in this chapter can help practitioners communicate what occupational therapy addresses and what practitioners do with each population and in each practice arena. In addition, this review provides a context to guide practitioners as they work with other disciplines in conducting evaluations with home health clients.

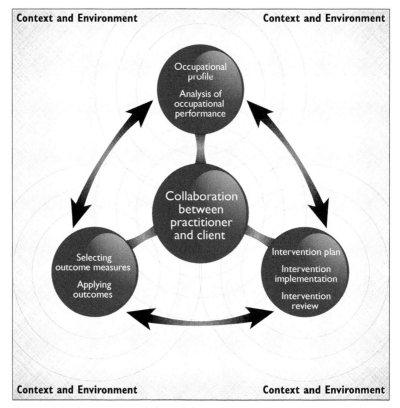

Figure 4.1. **Occupational therapy's process.**

Source. From "Occupational Therapy Practice Framework: Domain and Process," 3rd ed., by the American Occupational Therapy Association, 2014, *American Journal of Occupational Therapy, 68*(Suppl. 1), p. S10. Copyright © 2014 by the American Occupational Therapy Association. Used with permission.

Occupational Therapy Evaluation Process

Although the occupational therapy process is not linear, it always begins with evaluation. Evaluation has two stages: (1) development of an **occupational profile** and (2) an **analysis of occupational performance.** The *occupational profile* is "a summary of a client's occupational history and experiences, patterns of daily living, interests, values, and needs" (AOTA, 2014, p. S13). Development of an occupational profile includes eliciting the client's history, strengths, needs, desires, and preferences from the perspective of the client. In a nutshell, this aspect of the evaluation involves finding out who the client is and what the issues are from his or her perspective. The analysis of occupational performance may include observing the client's performance of activities, noting the effectiveness of performance skills and patterns, selecting and administering **assessments** to identify factors (context, activity demands, client factors) that may be influencing performance patterns and skills, conducting activity analysis, interpreting assessment data to identify facilitators of and barriers to performance, developing and refining hypotheses about the client's occupational performance strengths and weaknesses, collaborating with the client to establish goals, and delineating areas for intervention on the basis of best practice and evidence (AOTA, 2014).

In general, it makes the most sense to develop the occupational profile, or at least to begin this aspect of evaluation, before initiating the analysis of performance.

Although the occupational therapist may develop the occupational profile while conducting some aspects of the analysis of performance, it is prudent to first elicit information about the client to appreciate circumstances and problems from the client's perspective and to avoid focusing the analysis of occupational performance on factors that may not be relevant to the client's needs or priorities.

The findings of the evaluation inform the intervention plan. An intervention plan includes objective and measurable goals with realistic time frames, identifies occupational therapy intervention approaches, and specifies mechanisms for service delivery. The intervention plan addresses the client's potential and expected discharge needs and plan and identifies recommendations or referrals to other health professionals as needed. The intervention plan also specifies the targeted outcomes selected (AOTA, 2014).

Occupational Therapy Evaluation Process in Home Health

So far, this description of the initial aspects of the occupational therapy process has been generic. How does the occupational therapy evaluation process contribute to home health practice?

Occupational Profile

For home health clients, the occupational therapy evaluation typically occurs during the occupational therapist's first visit to the client's home. Clients usually have already been admitted to home health care and may also be receiving services from other home health disciplines. The client may or may not have received occupational therapy services previously. In this first encounter, the therapist has the opportunity and the duty to describe to the client what home health occupational therapy is and what the client can expect. Even, and perhaps especially, if the client has previously received occupational therapy in another service setting, it is important to address what occupational therapy is about in home health. Framing home health occupational therapy as being about "finding ways for you to do your daily activities and to be able to stay at home" resonates with both clients and their caregivers and loved ones. This simple explanation connects occupational therapy to the client's goals, frames expectations, and clearly distinguishes occupational therapy from other home health services.

An advantage of explaining occupational therapy in this way is that it segues easily into a discussion of the client's history, strengths, and needs. Eliciting baseline performance (and how long ago this baseline was derived), identifying daily activities and routines, and establishing client priorities follow easily from this brief explanation of occupational therapy; thus, the occupational profile is begun. As the profile emerges, the therapist can begin to form hypotheses and select relevant assessments even while continuing to elicit information from the client. Eliciting the occupational profile and understanding the client's priorities and circumstances are an important investment of effort that will support both time management and episode management as the care episode progresses.

Analysis of Occupational Performance

The analysis of occupational performance is the step in the evaluation process during which "the client's assets and problems or potential problems are more specifically

Although the occupational therapist may develop the occupational profile while conducting some aspects of the analysis of performance, it is prudent to first elicit information about the client to appreciate circumstances and problems from the client's perspective and to avoid focusing the analysis of occupational performance on factors that may not be relevant to the client's needs or priorities.

identified through assessment tools designed to observe, measure, and inquire about factors that support or hinder occupational performance. Targeted outcomes also are identified" (AOTA, 2014, p. S14). In the home, many skills, client factors, and environmental factors can be assessed. As occupational therapists conduct the analysis of occupational performance, they must bear in mind that it is not an effective use of resources to collect and record data that are not relevant to the client's priorities or to an effective and appropriate care plan to address the client's functional needs.

Conducting Skilled Observations

The home provides a natural context for skilled observation. In the home, skilled observation takes two forms: (1) observation of performance elicited by prompting from the occupational therapist and (2) observation of performance that is spontaneous. In the home, spontaneous performance is typically *habitual performance*—that is, action shaped by weeks, months, or even years of repetition involving an unconscious transaction among person, environment, and activity. Spontaneous performance is not available for observation in most other settings; even spontaneous performance in a clinical setting occurs in an unfamiliar or contrived environment.

Unlike spontaneous performance, prompted performance always has an aspect of assessment or testing. Whenever an occupational therapist initiates skilled observation by saying "show me," the result will have at least some aspect of performance in the theatrical sense—a conscious, deliberate action that may or may not be congruent with the same action performed spontaneously. At times, a "show-me" prompt may result in performance that is far from the habitual action and that may even seem reckless, especially in situations in which a client believes that his or her ability to manage in the home is being questioned. By eliciting the client's concerns in the occupational profile before analyzing performance, the therapist can frame a show-me prompt as a request to understand performance of concern to the client rather than as an unintentional challenge of the client's capacities.

> By eliciting the client's concerns in the occupational profile before analyzing performance, the therapist can frame a show-me prompt as a request to understand performance of concern to the client rather than as an unintentional challenge of the client's capacities.

After eliciting the client's priorities and concerns during the occupational profile, the occupational therapist can ask the client, or the caregiver if the client is unable, to show the therapist the areas of the home in which performance occurs and that are most relevant to the client's concerns and thus to the client's goals. As this tour of the home proceeds, the therapist can conduct skilled observation of both prompted and spontaneous performance and, when appropriate, can conduct specific assessments relevant to the observed or reported performance. If the occupational therapy evaluation visit coincides with a home health comprehensive assessment time point (discussed later in this chapter), the tour of the home also provides opportunities to specifically assess functional or clinical status indicators that are mandated aspects of the comprehensive assessment. Box 4.1 lists examples of items to assess in context while touring the home with the client and suggested prompts and opportunities to observe spontaneous performance.

Selecting and Administering Assessments

During and after the tour of the home, the occupational therapist has the opportunity to select specific aspects of performance and factors influencing performance for further assessment. This selection is driven by the practice context, the priorities and concerns of the client, and the hypotheses formed by the therapist.

Box 4.1. Observations to Make While Touring the Home

On arrival to the home:

1. Does the client meet you at the door? Does the client hear and respond to the bell or knock?

2. Did the client remember the appointment?

3. To what room does the client (or caregiver) lead you for the initial assessment? What cues are present in this room (use all of your senses)?

While eliciting the occupational profile:

1. How does the client describe his or her condition and the reason for the home care referral?

2. Can the client describe what has happened in the past few days?

3. Who is in the home, and what assistance is provided while you are present? Does the assistance provided correspond to the needs and care being reported? Does the caregiver corroborate the client's reports?

4. Does the client initiate activity or wait for assistance?

After eliciting at least a basic occupational profile, ask to see the areas of the home relevant to the client's activities. Ask the client to show them to you or join you.

In the bedroom (or where the client sleeps):

1. If the room where the client sleeps is not a bedroom, ask why the client is not sleeping in a bedroom and how long he or she has been sleeping in the current room.

2. Does the client sleep well at night? If not, what interrupts sleep (e.g., pain, urinary urgency)?

3. Is the client able to describe usual routines? Ask whether he or she has changed part of the routines and, if so, why and how long ago.

4. Ask the client to sit or lie down on the bed. Is assistance needed? Conduct a head-to-toe integumentary assessment (if required).

5. Ask how often the client gets up at night. How far away is the bathroom (or bedside commode, if used)? Ask whether the client makes it in time. Is there evidence (especially olfactory or visual) that the client experiences incontinence?

In the bathroom:

1. Note the state of the tub or shower. Is there evidence that it is used? If so, how regularly? Ask about bathing and follow up on any earlier reports or concerns about bathing. Verify whether and how the client enters the tub or shower. Verify current and preferred bathing (sponge bath, bath, shower [seated or standing]). If assisted, by whom and how much? Ask whether the client has concerns about safety while bathing or accessing the tub or shower and toilet.

2. Note the spontaneous use of handholds such as doorknobs, towel racks, or fixtures. Request that the client demonstrate toilet transfer (if he or she uses a toilet). Note evidence of incontinence (visual or olfactory). Tactfully ask about the client's ability to make it in time or experiences with accidents.

3. Ask whether the client avoids any activities or has had any close calls with falls that have led him or her to avoid or lessen activities. Avoid asking directly whether the client has had a fall. If the client acknowledges near-falls or close calls, ask him or her to elaborate on where, when, and other circumstances.

4. Note the presence of over-the-counter products, especially topical products, for pain or other problems. Does the client use them? If so, how often? If medications have not yet been addressed, ask where medications are kept and where the client is when taking medications; ask to go to these areas.

Before leaving the bedroom and bathroom area:

1. Ask where the client spends most of his or her time. How would the client call for assistance (routine or emergency) from that location? How would the client exit the home in an emergency?

While moving between rooms:

1. If the client has a cane or walker, does he or she use it spontaneously, or are prompts required? Is the device used properly and safely?

2. How does the client move? Is there evidence of problems with balance, pain, endurance, or dyspnea?

3. How steady is the client with and without an ambulation device? Does the client use furniture or walls for support?

(Continued)

Box 4.1. Observations to Make While Touring the Home *(cont.)*

4. Do obstructions or narrow pathways impede passage? Does the client remark on or refer to such problems, or does he or she seem unconcerned or unaware?

5. Does the client get distracted while moving about? Does he or she have to stop to talk because of dyspnea or the need to concentrate on mobility?

Where medications are stored:

1. Note whether medications are in prescription vials or a medication organizer or are stored in some other system.

2. Ask the client to show you which medications he or she takes in the morning. If medications are stored in prescription vials, ask the client to tell you the name of each medication and the phone number of the pharmacy. Does the client recall this information or read it? If the client reads it, does he or she need glasses?

3. Verify how many times a day the client takes medications. If medications are not stored in the area in which the client spends time, ask whether the client ever gets busy and forgets to take his or her medications. Does the client choose not to take any medications? Why? Does the client report any concerns about medications or the effects of medications?

In the kitchen:

1. How does the client get meals? Who prepares them? How many meals does the client consume on most days? Are accommodations available to simplify meal preparation (e.g., microwave meals, cold foods only, delivered meals)?

2. Can the client transport food items from the refrigerator to the table or counter? Can transport be accomplished while using cane or walker, or does the client abandon the device while managing kitchen tasks? Where does the client usually eat meals? How does he or she transport items to the eating area and transport dirty dishes and waste to the appropriate areas?

3. Are nonrefrigerated foods accessible to the client (in cupboards or the pantry or left accessible on counters or tables)?

4. Is the client aware of any dietary restrictions and requirements? Does the client indicate that he or she follows this diet? If not, why not?

In all areas of the home:

1. Observe for evidence of the priorities, problems, and concerns identified by the client while eliciting the occupational profile.

2. Observe for evidence of roles and occupations valued by the client (e.g., family photos, work memorabilia, crafts, certificates, trophies). Note how the client responds when you comment on these items.

3. Observe for evidence of fatigue. Does the client exhibit dyspnea while moving about? How much movement or what activity triggers the dyspnea?

On return to the area where the visit began:

1. Corroborate observations with the client and caregivers and discuss any reported concerns and priorities.

2. Identify and seek feedback on any safety concerns identified during the tour.

For Medicare home health clients, the following minimum requirement applies to assessment and the related documentation:

> The patient's clinical record must demonstrate that the method used to assess a client's function included *objective measurements of function in accordance with accepted professional standards of clinical practice enabling comparison of successive measurements to determine the effectiveness of therapy goals* [italics added]. Such objective measurements would be made by the qualified therapist using measurements which assess activities of daily living (ADLs) that may include but are not limited to eating, swallowing, bathing, dressing, toileting, walking, climbing stairs, or using assistive devices, and mental and cognitive factors. (CMS, 2011a, p. 336)

Box 4.2. Selecting Assessment Tools and Methods

The Centers for Medicare & Medicaid Services do not require occupational therapy practitioners and other clinicians to use standardized assessments. If the occupational therapist wants to use a standardized assessment, he or she should consider the following factors when selecting an instrument:

- Has the assessment been validated for use in the home setting?
- Has the assessment been validated for use with the population to which a given client belongs?
- Is administration of the assessment compatible with home health service delivery? For example, will sufficient time to administer the assessment and the proper equipment and supplies be available? Will the occupational therapist have enough control of the environment? Is the assessment compatible with software or documentation systems in the therapist's agency?
- Does the instrument assess aspects of the domain of occupational therapy?
- Does the instrument assess aspects of occupational performance that are relevant to the client's needs and goals?

If the occupational therapist does not follow the standardized protocol, it cannot be assumed that the results are valid. If the protocol is modified, the therapist is obligated to document the modification and note that the applicability of the findings is limited because of the nonstandardized protocol (American Occupational Therapy Association, 2015).

There is no federal requirement to use a specific assessment tool or methodology when services are being provided under the Medicare Part A home health benefit. However, federal requirements do provide criteria for choosing from the available occupational therapy assessment tools or methodologies. The key requirements are as follows:

- Assessment tools or methodologies must be consistent with accepted occupational therapy professional standards of clinical practice.
- Measurements must be objective (i.e., discernible to others and not influenced by personal feelings, interpretations, or prejudice) and repeatable.

Standardized assessments are not required. Selection of assessment tools and methodologies must be consistent with the setting and the population served by home health. Box 4.2 lists factors to consider in selecting formal or standardized assessment tools.

Some assessments measure performance skills and performance patterns. Others identify or measure contexts and environments, activity demands, and client factors that influence performance skills and performance patterns. The information gathered should not only be objective and measurable but should also relate to the client's performance (function), identify what supports and what hinders performance, and establish the basis for goals and outcomes of intervention.

Creating Goals and Measuring Outcomes on the Basis of Evaluation Data

The occupational profile and analysis of occupational performance enable the occupational therapist to work with the client to formulate goals and identify means to measure the outcomes of intervention. This step is critical to establishing a collaborative relationship with clients and caregivers. An experienced therapist may complete the evaluation and have a clear picture of what can be accomplished through home health occupational therapy, but goal creation is incomplete without the client's contribution. Creating a shared expectation of outcomes is essential to integrating the client's investment in treatment with the practitioner's clinical expertise.

Creating a shared expectation of outcomes is essential to integrating the client's investment in treatment with the practitioner's clinical expertise.

Creating a shared vision begins with the way the occupational therapist frames home health occupational therapy at the beginning of the first visit. Taking the time to elicit an occupational profile places the focus on what is meaningful and relevant to the client. Judiciously selecting assessment tools reflects attention to what the client has reported and demonstrated. Summarizing findings and seeking clarification emphasize the importance of a shared understanding.

These steps segue easily into a conversation about expectations and outcomes and clearly convey that outcomes depend on investment by both the practitioner and the client in a collaborative relationship. Discussing the means to measure outcomes ensures that the measures selected are relevant to the client. Finally, a shared understanding of outcomes facilitates the development of an intervention plan.

Recording the Evaluation: Documentation

The content of the occupational therapy evaluation and the documentation (record) of the evaluation are the means by which the domain of occupational therapy and the clinical reasoning of the occupational therapist are communicated to all other home health stakeholders. Other home health disciplines, clinical supervisors and managers, and payers look to this documentation to substantiate the need for occupational therapy. These parties also look to the evaluation documentation to relate the factors analyzed and assessed to the client's performance, safety, and health status.

IADLs are also within the scope of home health occupational therapy, and to support clients' ability to manage daily activities and stay in the home, the home health occupational therapy evaluation should reflect aspects of performance relevant to IADLs.

In the author's experience, home health agencies' (HHAs') occupational therapy evaluation forms and software templates are dominated by measures of upper-extremity function and performance of basic ADLs (e.g., dressing, bathing, toileting, feeding, functional mobility). Specific analysis of and collection of data on upper-extremity function are relevant only when upper-extremity impairment contributes to the identified occupational performance problems. ADLs may be a priority of a significant number of home care clients, but they are only a small portion of the activities that any given client must manage to live at home. Instrumental activities of daily living (IADLs) are also within the scope of home health occupational therapy, and to support clients' ability to manage daily activities and stay in the home, the home health occupational therapy evaluation should reflect aspects of performance relevant to IADLs.

Home health providers' growing reliance on comprehensive home health software means that forms or software for the occupational therapy evaluation are often mandated by corporate policy or by default when software is adopted. Most of these forms or software templates were not created by occupational therapists, and many have had little or no input from or review by occupational therapy practitioners.

If a mandated form or software template restricts an occupational therapist's ability to adequately and accurately document the evaluation process, it is imperative that the therapist advocate for changes to the form or software so that evaluations can be documented appropriately. The content of the evaluation form or template reflects the role and philosophy of occupational therapy in the setting and agency. Occupational therapy forms that are nearly indistinguishable from physical therapy forms, for example, suggest to other stakeholders that occupational therapy duplicates services provided by another discipline. Templates that are limited to basic ADLs imply that the scope of occupational therapy is limited to personal care.

Home health occupational therapy documentation forms and software should reflect the domain of occupational therapy within the context of home health practice. If they do not, it is the responsibility of the occupational therapy practitioners working within the agency to actively advocate for change. The *Framework* and this chapter can be helpful resources for such advocacy efforts.

Describing Performance

Chapter 3 discussed the client conditions typically seen in the home health setting. Describing the performance of clients with these conditions in the home should be very different from describing the performance of clients in other settings. One of the most common methods for measuring and recording performance in other settings is to specify the **level of assistance** needed, and this practice is often applied to home health. Measures of levels of assistance are addressed later in this section. In home health care, however, intensity of assistance is not the most appropriate parameter by which to measure performance. Framing a client's problem in terms of the assistance he or she requires implies that intervention will be directed to reducing the intensity of assistance. However, not all occupational performance problems can be addressed or resolved in this way. The sections that follow describe other important ways to describe a client's performance.

Trajectory

An aspect of performance that is important to document is trajectory. As the occupational therapist elicits information about past and current performance for the occupational profile, a performance trajectory emerges, providing information about changes in performance. For example, three clients currently need moderate assistance to dress and bathe. One client has needed this same intensity of assistance for many months. The second client was independent in dressing and bathing until 2 weeks ago. The third client has needed assistance for at least 6 months, but the assistance needed has increased from setting up the task to hands-on assistance to the current level over this 6-month period. Including the temporal dimension of performance in information about level of assistance provides a more complete picture of performance. The additional information provided by these three very different performance trajectories is necessary to develop individualized approaches to addressing performance problems.

Circumstances That Affect Performance

Given the conditions common among the home health population (see Chapter 3), there are three common circumstances in which level of assistance (or the expectation of improving level of assistance) is not sufficient to capture the nature of the occupational performance problem: (1) when performance is affected by pain, (2) when performance is isolated from routines, and (3) when performance is incompatible with disease management.

First, when the client's performance is affected by pain, measuring the frequency and duration of the activity is a more appropriate means to measure performance than is assistance needed. If pain limits an activity, the client may be unable to tolerate the activity or may refuse to attempt it. The number of refusals to participate or the number of attempts to participate over a specified interval offers a more accurate

> When the client's performance is affected by pain, measuring the frequency and duration of the activity is a more appropriate means to measure performance than is assistance needed.

means to establish the baseline for such performance. Once such a baseline is established, fewer refusals, more attempts to initiate or participate, or longer duration of performance may offer an objective measure of progress.

Second, measuring level of assistance is typically based on scoring the client's performance of isolated activities (e.g., dressing, bathing, toileting) or even subsets of such activities (e.g., upper-body dressing, chair transfers). However, these activities do not occur in isolation but are typically performed as part of a continuous routine. Even isolated activities may involve preparation or setup and may require cleanup afterward. Assessing the level of assistance required for specific subsets of an activity or required for an activity without regard to setup or cleanup fails to accurately determine whether assistance is needed to manage the routine safely and effectively. Because managing routine tasks in the home is an important expectation of home health clients and their families, it is important to assess each routine as a whole, not just its components.

It is also important to identify when a discrepancy exists between performance of the components of a routine and performance of the routine as a whole. For example, a client is able to prepare and eat simple meals independently if the ingredients are set up but is not able to wash the dishes, put the ingredients away, or clean up the work area. Although the client may be independent in the tasks of preparation, feeding, and drinking, he or she cannot perform the entire routine without the involvement of another person for setup and cleanup. Accurate assessment of this circumstance establishes a baseline and supports intervention designed to add or integrate a new task into the full meal routine.

The third circumstance in which level of assistance fails to capture the occupational performance problem involves clients, especially those with multiple chronic conditions (see Chapter 3), for whom performance is incompatible with the requirements of health and disease management. Management of many conditions involves the regular performance of specific tasks or modification of usual activities to incorporate new tasks. Assessing such clients' level of performance must include gathering complete information regarding self-management of the chronic conditions.

One example is a client with diabetes who is able to bathe without assistance in usual bathing tasks but either is unable to perform adequate diabetic foot care, which includes washing the feet, or does not perform the foot care consistently. Scoring the client as independent in bathing masks the problem of inadequate or inconsistent foot care. In another example, a client with congestive heart failure (CHF) routinely prepares meals, but the meals are frozen prepackaged meals with high levels of sodium. For this client, simplifying meal preparation to conserve energy makes sense, but the high sodium intake is likely to exacerbate the CHF. Thus, scoring the level of assistance in meal preparation as low is an inadequate assessment of the situation. Designating the problem as the need to simplify the task while incorporating the appropriate diet accurately identifies the need and supports an intervention plan that addresses both energy conservation and dietary adherence.

Disease Management

An aspect of performance related to chronic disease management is learning new disease management activities and incorporating them into existing routines. Examples of such activities include obtaining daily weights and performing nebulizer treatments. Assessment may involve analyzing the client's ability to perform the new task and obtaining the baseline frequency of performance and compatibility with existing routines. This assessment supports an intervention plan that addresses proficient performance of the task and incorporation of the task into existing daily routines.

Definition of Terms

Another aspect of documenting performance is defining measurement terms. Even when intensity of assistance is an appropriate means to measure performance, it is essential that the gradations of assistance be well defined so that those reading the documentation can clearly understand the performance beyond shorthand terms. *Moderate assistance* (or shorthand such as *mod assist*) means nothing unless three conditions are met: (1) The term is applied consistently by every therapist conducting assessments, (2) the level is defined to account for both physical and cognitive assistance, and (3) the definition is accessible and understandable to those who did not witness the performance.

For example, the statement "dresses lower body with min assist and verbal cues" suggests limited caregiver involvement. A reviewer might conclude that only limited intervention is needed to help the client achieve independent performance. If, however, the client needs continual verbal cuing to maintain attention and sequence each task step, caregiver involvement is in reality extensive, and significant intervention may be needed to eliminate the involvement of a caregiver, an outcome that may not even be feasible.

Definitions of *levels of assistance,* which have historically been an integral part of determining many of the services Medicare has covered, have undergone some changes. Before the current system of determining which services would be covered—the Medicare local coverage determinations (LCDs)—was established, CMS (then called the Health Care Financing Administration, or HCFA) explicitly defined levels of assistance (HCFA, 2000). Although these definitions are no longer used for medical review, they continue to be relevant and may be useful for agencies seeking to adopt a level-of-assistance scale that accounts for physical and cognitive assistance and has a history of accepted use in Medicare reviewing. Table 4.2 summarizes these definitions of levels of assistance.

The definitions of levels of assistance listed in Table 4.2 accounted for the intensity of both physical and cognitive assistance. Because the HCFA (2000) guidelines were applied across all Medicare settings, these definitions were used almost universally across Medicare-dominated practice settings. The guidelines specifically recognized that experiencing a change in level of assistance (e.g., a reduction in assistance required) and adding a new activity to a sequence or routine were ways to document progress. Additionally, the guidelines recognized that in some circumstances, usually associated with the presence of pain or certain cognitive or behavioral health impairments, a decrease in refusals to perform an activity was also a legitimate means by which to document progress.

The definitions of level of activity were superseded by the LCDs in the early 2000s. An unintended consequence of this change was the loss of a uniform system for documenting levels of assistance that was recognized and understood across practice settings and geographic locations. Now, practitioners coming from other

> Even when intensity of assistance is an appropriate means to measure performance, it is essential that the gradations of assistance be well defined so that those reading the documentation can clearly understand the performance beyond shorthand terms.

Table 4.2. Definitions of Levels of Assistance From a Past Version of the *Medicare Program Integrity Manual*

Level of Assistance	Description
Total assistance	The patient requires 100% assistance. The patient is able to initiate only minimal voluntary motor actions, and external stimuli are required to elicit automatic actions such as swallowing or responding to auditory stimuli.
Maximum assistance	The patient requires 75% assistance by one person to physically perform any part of a functional activity or cognitive assistance to perform gross motor actions in response to direction. A patient requires maximum assistance if maximum physical support and proprioceptive stimulation are needed for performance of each step of an activity every time it is performed.
Moderate assistance	The patient requires 50% assistance by one person to perform physical activities or constant cognitive assistance to sustain or complete simple, repetitive activities safely. Moderate assistance is needed when the therapist or caregiver needs to be in the immediate environment to assist the patient through a sequence to complete a functional activity. Such assistance may halt continuing repetition of a task or prevent unsafe, erratic, or unpredictable actions that interfere with appropriate sequencing.
Minimum assistance	The patient requires 25% assistance by one person for physical activities or periodic cognitive assistance to perform functional activities safely. A physically impaired patient requires minimum assistance if he or she can perform activities only after physical setup by the therapist or caregiver and if he or she needs physical help to initiate or sustain an activity. A patient with cognitive impairment requires minimal assistance if he or she needs help in performing known activities to correct repeated mistakes, to follow established safety procedures, or to solve problems posed by unexpected hazards.
Standby assistance	The patient requires supervision by one person to perform new activity procedures the therapist has adapted to enable safe and effective performance. A patient requires standby assistance when he or she does not always anticipate the potential for errors and the need for safety precautions.
Independent status	The patient requires no physical or cognitive assistance to perform functional activities. He or she is able to implement the selected courses of action, consider potential errors, and anticipate safety hazards in familiar and in new situations.

Source. From "Intermediary Medical Review Guidelines for Specific Services: Change in Level of Assistance," in the *Medicare Program Integrity Manual,* Chapter 6, § 7.3.4.1, by the Health Care Financing Administration, 2000, Baltimore: Author. In the public domain.

practice settings to home health may use conventions or terminology developed in those other settings that are not appropriate for home health or have not been adopted by the HHA in its policies and procedures.

The Evaluation Process in Relation to the Comprehensive Assessment

In accordance with federal regulations and agency policies, occupational therapists may conduct the comprehensive assessment at specified time points. As shown in Box 4.3, the comprehensive assessment includes discipline-specific content, agency-specific content, and OASIS data items. *Discipline-specific content* is that content appropriate to the scope of the discipline conducting the comprehensive assessment. Thus, a comprehensive assessment conducted by the occupational therapist includes aspects of any occupational therapy evaluation or reevaluation. *Agency-specific content* refers to patient, household, or other factors the agency has chosen to incorporate into the comprehensive assessment of its patients. *OASIS data items* are those assessed regardless of which discipline conducted the comprehensive assessment. The specific items included in the comprehensive assessment vary depending on the time point of the comprehensive assessment, but all items for that time point must be addressed.

Completion of the comprehensive assessment is the responsibility of the clinician who conducts the assessment. That clinician may rely on other clinicians who have assessed the client to ensure or verify the accuracy of data before the comprehensive assessment is finalized. The clinician who conducts the in-home visit associated with the comprehensive assessment is individually responsible for signing the documentation and, thus, attesting to its accuracy.

Box 4.3. Comprehensive Assessment Requirements

Every Medicare-certified home health agency must conduct a comprehensive assessment, including incorporation of Outcome and Assessment Information Set (OASIS) data set items, at specific time points:

- At start of care
- On transfer to an inpatient facility
- On resumption of care after an inpatient stay
- When the patient is recertified for an additional episode of care
- Within 48 hours of a change in condition
- On discharge from home care
- In the event of death while receiving home care.

The contents of a comprehensive assessment are as follows:

OASIS items
+
Agency-specific content
+
Discipline-specific content
_____
Comprehensive assessment

Occupational therapy distinguishes between *evaluation,* "the process of obtaining and interpreting data necessary for intervention," and *assessment,* or use of "specific tools or instruments . . . during the evaluation process" (American Occupational Therapy Association, 2015, p. 2). In contrast, the Centers for Medicare & Medicaid Services (CMS) uses the terms *assess* and *assessment* to refer to the evaluation process a health professional conducts. *Assess* and *assessment* are the terms used in regulations, Medicare coverage policies, and all documents related to the Home Health Quality Initiative (discussed later in this chapter). To be consistent with these documents, the terms *assess* and *assessment* are used when discussing the comprehensive assessment.

The relevant requirements for the comprehensive assessment are codified at 42 *Code of Federal Regulations* [CFR] § 484.55: Condition of participation: Comprehensive assessment of patients, subsections b, d, and e (CMS, 2011b, p. 129):

(b) *Standard: Completion of the comprehensive assessment.*

(1) The comprehensive assessment must be completed in a timely manner, consistent with the patient's immediate needs, but no later than 5 calendar days after the start of care.

(2) Except as provided in paragraph (b)(3) of this section, a registered nurse must complete the comprehensive assessment and for Medicare patients, determine eligibility for the Medicare home health benefit, including homebound status.

(3) When physical therapy, speech–language pathology, or occupational therapy is the only service ordered by the physician, a physical therapist, speech–language pathologist or occupational therapist may complete the comprehensive assessment, and for Medicare patients, determine eligibility for the Medicare home health benefit, including homebound status. The occupational therapist may complete the comprehensive assessment if the need for occupational therapy establishes program eligibility. . . .

(d) *Standard: Update of the comprehensive assessment.* The comprehensive assessment must be updated and revised (including the administration of the OASIS) as frequently as the patient's condition warrants due to a major decline or improvement in the patient's health status, but not less frequently than—

(1) The last five days of every 60 days beginning with the start-of-care date, unless there is a—

(i) Beneficiary elected transfer;

(ii) Significant change in condition; or

(iii) Discharge and return to the same HHA [home health agency] during the 60-day episode.

(2) Within 48 hours of the patient's return to the home from a hospital admission of 24 hours or more for any reason other than diagnostic tests;

(3) At discharge.

(Continued)

Box 4.3. Comprehensive Assessment Requirements *(cont.)*

(e) *Standard: Incorporation of OASIS data items.* The OASIS data items determined by the Secretary must be incorporated into the HHA's own assessment and must include: clinical record items, demographics and patient history, living arrangements, supportive assistance, sensory status, integumentary status, respiratory status, elimination status, neuro/emotional/behavioral status, activities of daily living, medications, equipment management, emergent care, and data items collected at inpatient facility admission or discharge only.

What Does This Mean?

Because occupational therapy does not establish initial eligibility for the Medicare Part A home health benefit, occupational therapists are not permitted to conduct the start-of-care comprehensive assessment for patients for whom Medicare Part A is the payer. However, occupational therapy may establish eligibility for patients with other payers. An occupational therapist may conduct the comprehensive assessment on a therapy-only (i.e., no nursing orders) patient when the need for occupational therapy is deemed to establish eligibility by that patient's payer (§ 484.55[b][3]).

After the start-of-care time point, no requirement specifies who may or shall conduct the comprehensive assessment at subsequent time points (§ 484.55[d]), so an occupational therapist may do so. All clinicians must incorporate OASIS items into the comprehensive assessment at all time points (§ 484.55[e]).

If occupational therapy is the skilled discipline present at the final visit in the episode of care, the occupational therapist must conduct the discharge comprehensive assessment, including OASIS, at the final occupational therapy home visit. If occupational therapy is going to continue into another certification period (i.e., beyond the initial 60 days), the occupational therapist may conduct the recertification comprehensive assessment. If occupational therapy is the only skilled discipline continuing into a subsequent recertification period, then occupational therapy must conduct the recertification comprehensive assessment.

Conducting the comprehensive assessment and completing the OASIS data items included in the comprehensive assessment are both closely associated with the **Home Health Quality Initiative** (HHQI). The importance of understanding OASIS data items and issues relevant to collecting OASIS data in relation to the HHQI is addressed in the following section.

The Evaluation Process in Relation to the Home Health Quality Initiative

In the 1990s, CMS (then HCFA) initiated efforts to improve the quality of care provided to Medicare and Medicaid beneficiaries across a range of service settings; in home health, this effort is referred to as the *Home Health Quality Initiative.* HHQI was established with the purpose of "moving the [Medicare home health] program towards rewarding better value, outcomes, and patient-focused care instead of the volume of services provided" (U.S. Department of Health and Human Services, 2012, p. 4). HHQI focuses on promoting quality care across the entire home health client population. The OASIS data set is the measurement tool developed and piloted during that time to monitor and to support improvement in the quality of home health care (CMS, 2012). In the 21st century, HHQI has become a top priority for policymakers and payers and, thus, for HHAs. **Appendix C, "Medicare as Quality Monitor,"** reviews the history of Medicare's quality improvement efforts, including the HHQI.

Stop here! Go to Appendix C and read the section "Overview of Medicare as Quality Monitor" on pages 205–206.

Thus far, this chapter has addressed evaluation and assessment of the individual client. The HHQI effort involves measuring outcomes of care and identifying processes of care across the home health population. HHQI enables home health providers to identify and direct interventions to problems that are particularly relevant to the home health population using best practices. Every home health clinician, regardless of discipline, has a responsibility to advance home health quality and value through the care he or she provides to each and every client. Assessment is part of that responsibility, specifically understanding and accurately assessing client status indicators that have been prioritized by HHQI.

HHQI is the reason that occupational therapists must be familiar with the OASIS. Federal regulations and agency policy dictate which clinician is responsible for conducting the comprehensive assessment, which includes the OASIS, at each mandated time point (see Box 4.3). However, HHQI is not the responsibility of a specific clinician or discipline: HHQI is the responsibility of all disciplines and all clinicians. Regardless of whether an occupational therapist is responsible for conducting a given comprehensive assessment, occupational therapy contributes accurate assessment data necessary to complete the OASIS and advance HHQI. Accurate data also contribute to obtaining appropriate agency payment and identifying effective care processes. So it is essential that occupational therapists become competent in assessing all the client status indicators reflected in OASIS data items.

Some OASIS items, such as performance of personal care activities and routine mobility, are already part of a routine occupational therapy evaluation. Other items are less routinely assessed or may be unfamiliar to some occupational therapists, especially those new to home health. For client status indicators that are familiar, occupational therapists must understand the specific activity being scored in each OASIS item; any inclusions, exclusions, or conditions applied to the activity; and the conventions of OASIS data collection for accurate scoring. For indicators that are less familiar, therapists must educate themselves on how to accurately assess and score client status in these indicators using expertise that is within the scope of occupational therapy practice.

> Some OASIS items, such as performance of personal care activities and routine mobility, are already part of a routine occupational therapy evaluation.

OASIS Occupational Performance Items and Scoring Conventions

The *OASIS–C1/ICD–10 Version Guidance Manual* (CMS, 2015) provides item-by-item details and conventions for completion of all OASIS items. It is freely available as a download from the CMS website as a resource for occupational therapists when conducting the comprehensive assessment. **Appendix D** provides guidance on how to retrieve and navigate the *OASIS Guidance Manual*.

 Stop here! Go to Appendix D and read the sections "How to Retrieve the *OASIS Guidance Manual*" and "How to Navigate the *OASIS Guidance Manual*" on page 225.

The OASIS uses a level-of-assistance scoring system for a subset of items pertaining to functional status (e.g., dressing, bathing, transfers). However, the levels of assistance used in the OASIS items are not the same as those familiar to occupational therapists, nor are they consistent with those listed in Table 4.2. It is essential that occupational therapists become familiar with the unique conventions used in the OASIS functional status items so that they score each functional status item accurately. The sections that follow describe the conventions specific to ADL and IADL items that occupational therapists must understand so the information they collect aligns with the OASIS (see Box D.1 in **Appendix D** for a full list of conventions).

Ability

By convention, *ability* as used in OASIS items refers to the physical, cognitive, and emotional ability to perform the specified activity safely. If a client is physically, cognitively, or emotionally unable to perform the specified activity, the occupational therapist must report this inability in scoring the item. For example, emotional inability includes fear; if a client sponge bathes because she or he is afraid to get into the tub or shower as the result of a previous fall, this is inability, not preference, and should be scored as such.

Usual Performance

Unlike some other assessment protocols, which use a standardized environment, OASIS scoring is based on the client's usual environment or attire. If a client's bathroom or bathtub is in an area of the home that is inaccessible to the client, then the client cannot be scored as able to bathe in a tub or shower because the environment precludes this activity. Similarly, dressing is scored on the basis of the client's usual attire. If the client's usual attire is slacks and a button-down top, then the ability to don a sweatshirt and sweatpants does not merit scoring the client as independent on the OASIS dressing items.

Definition of the Activity

Each OASIS ADL and IADL item defines the activity to be assessed and scored. Some of these definitions involve explicit inclusions or exclusions. The OASIS dressing items, for example, include retrieval of garments from their usual location as well as donning and doffing and fastening. If a client is able to dress once the garments are available but needs assistance to retrieve clothing from closets or dresser drawers, then dressing cannot be scored as independent. Similarly, the OASIS grooming item includes shaving or applying makeup, washing the face and hands, nail care, and teeth and denture care, and the therapist must provide information on all of these activities. The OASIS bathing item, however, includes washing the body but does not include washing the face and hands, shampooing hair, drying oneself, or setting up the bathing activity. In addition, the item on use of the telephone must be scored on the basis of effectively placing as well as receiving calls.

Medical Precautions and Restrictions

Items must be scored with consideration of the medical precautions and restrictions in effect at the time of the assessment. For example, if a client cannot perform a toilet transfer while maintaining ordered joint range-of-motion restrictions, then the toilet transfer item must be scored as inability. If a client has a cast or wound dressing that cannot contact water but he or she is otherwise able to bathe or shower, the bathing item must be scored on the basis of what the client can do while adhering to the medical restrictions.

Caregiving Intensity and Device Use

The OASIS ADL and IADL items are scored on the basis of the intensity of caregiving required to perform the specified activity safely and adequately. However, the intensities of assistance differ from those typically found in most assessments. In general, the scoring follows these gradations:

- No other human need be present for the activity to be performed.
- Another human must set up the activity or be present while it is performed.
- Another human must participate in the activity.
- Another human must perform the activity.

These intensities correspond to the involvement that may be required from a caregiver. For some OASIS items, such as dressing and grooming, scoring as independent (i.e., no other human involved) is the same regardless of whether the client uses an assistive device or not. For other items, notably bathing, mobility, and transfers, the scoring must account for both the use of specific devices and the intensity of assistance. In **Appendix D,** the section "Implications of ADL and IADL Data for Allocating Resources" (pp. 241–247) provides additional insight into assessing the level of need for caregiver assistance with ADLs and IADLs on the OASIS as a means of identifying resource allocation.

  Stop here! Go to Appendix D and read the section "K. Activities of Daily Living and Instrumental Activities of Daily Living" on pages 241–247.

Addressing Discrepancies in Documentation

Familiarity with the OASIS item definitions and conventions can help occupational therapists identify and explain any apparent discrepancies in the documentation between previously recorded OASIS scores and scores or ratings obtained during an occupational therapy evaluation. Occupational therapists should not only understand these differences but also be able to translate findings accurately to both the occupational therapy evaluation and the relevant OASIS data items. If another discipline obtains an OASIS score that is inconsistent with the findings of the occupational therapy evaluation, the therapist should be able to communicate with the other clinician or manager, identify the appropriate score, and explain the rationale for the score. If an OASIS score is substantiated by occupational therapy evaluation but appears to be in conflict with the findings of a clinician from another discipline, the occupational therapist must be able to reference the OASIS conventions and explain why both the OASIS and the occupational therapy evaluation are accurate. Box 4.4 provides case examples describing actual and apparent discrepancies and communication by the occupational therapist to resolve the discrepancy.

> **Familiarity with the OASIS item definitions and conventions can help occupational therapists identify and explain any apparent discrepancies in the documentation between previously recorded OASIS scores and scores or ratings obtained during an occupational therapy evaluation.**

Priority Client Status Items to Integrate Into the Occupational Therapy Evaluation

HHQI and the OASIS have introduced several client status indicators that must be integrated into the occupational therapy evaluation process. These indicators are

Box 4.4. Resolving Discrepancies Between Occupational Therapy Evaluation Findings and OASIS Scoring

In some cases, occupational therapy practitioners working in home health find that a client's status on evaluation differs from that indicated by another professional's scores on the Outcome and Assessment Information Set (OASIS) for that client. The following two case examples describe two such instances and indicate how the occupational therapist handled each discrepancy.

Case Example 1: Improving OASIS Accuracy

Maria conducted an occupational therapy evaluation with **Mrs. T** 2 days after another discipline conducted the start-of-care (SOC) comprehensive assessment. Maria found that Mrs. T was unable to retrieve her clothes from her dresser or closet. The client also needed assistance to don and fasten her bra, to remove her socks or stockings, and to fasten and unfasten garments. She was able to don and doff the loose, pull-on garments her daughter had bought, but Mrs. T wanted to return to wearing the clothes she wore before her hospitalization, which included fasteners, and she definitely wanted to wear a bra.

After completing the evaluation, Maria noticed that the SOC OASIS had been scored to indicate that the patient was "able to dress upper [and lower] body without assistance if clothing and shoes are laid out or handed to the patient" (Centers for Medicare & Medicaid Services [CMS], 2015, Chapter 3, p. K-2). However, the *OASIS Guidance Manual* states that dressing is defined as "the patient's ability to dress upper body, including the ability to obtain, put on, and remove upper body clothing. Assess ability to put on whatever clothing is routinely worn" (CMS, 2015, Chapter 3, p. K-2). The definition of lower-body dressing is essentially identical.

Maria contacted the clinician who conducted the SOC assessment and informed the clinician that the occupational therapy evaluation indicated the patient's inability to retrieve clothing and to don, doff, and fasten clothes she usually wore, which would indicate a different score for both the upper- and lower-body dressing items consistent with a score of 2, "Someone must help the patient put on upper [and lower] body clothing" (CMS, 2015, Chapter 3, p. K-2). The clinician who conducted the SOC assessment realized that Maria's evaluation was based on more complete information about what the patient usually wore, so the clinician made the decision to change the dressing items scores before the OASIS was locked (i.e., finalized before transmission to the state Medicare agency).

Case Example 2: Applying OASIS Scores to All Aspects of Performance

Terry conducted an occupational therapy evaluation with **Mr. G** a week after another discipline conducted the SOC comprehensive assessment. Mr. G lived with his daughter, who worked from 8:00 a.m. to 5:00 p.m. Mr. G's priority was to bathe himself. His daughter had been taking time off from work since he came home. She had to help him get in and out of the shower and wash his lower legs and feet because he felt unsteady bending over in the shower. By the time he got out of the shower, he had no energy left to dry off or get dressed.

Mr. G's daughter needed to return to work soon, and he did not want to shower at night, which would be the only time his daughter would be able to assist him. Mr. G and his daughter both wanted Mr. G to be able to shower, shampoo, and dress by himself. He had also refused delivered meals, so he needed to be able to fix his own breakfast and lunch when his daughter returned to work. His daughter was concerned that he would skip meals or eat nothing but cereal and snack food, and she was worried about how this would affect his diabetes.

Terry's evaluation documentation identified the problems with the bathing and dressing routine and with meal preparation. The occupational therapy care plan included goals related to each of these needs. The clinical supervisor compared the supplement to the home health plan of care derived from Terry's evaluation with the SOC evaluation and found the following:

- The SOC OASIS upper- and lower-body bathing item scores indicated that Mr. G was "able to bathe in shower or tub with the intermittent assistance of another person (a) for intermittent supervision or encouragement or reminders, OR (b) to get in and out of the shower or tub, OR (c) for washing difficult to reach areas" (CMS, 2015, Chapter 3, p. K-6).
- The OASIS item for upper-body dressing items was scored "able to dress upper body without assistance if clothing is laid out or handed to the patient" (CMS, 2015, Chapter 3, p. K-2). The lower-body dressing item was scored similarly.
- The OASIS item for light meal preparation was scored to indicate that Mr. G was "able to independently plan and prepare all light meals for self or reheat delivered meals" (CMS, 2015, Chapter 3, p. K-18).
- Terry's supplemental care plan included goals and interventions related to bathing, dressing, and meal preparation.

(Continued)

> **Box 4.4. Resolving Discrepancies Between Occupational Therapy Evaluation Findings and OASIS Scoring** *(cont.)*
>
> If the OASIS scores indicated that Mr. G was independent in dressing and meal preparation, the clinical supervisor asked, why would Terry identify goals and interventions in these areas?
>
> Terry explained that Mr. G's self-care needs involved both assistance and energy. The activity of daily living goals focused on bathing, performing bathing transfers, and drying off independently. A second goal focused on completing the bathing–drying–dressing sequence in a timely fashion without fatigue. Terry noted that the OASIS scores were accurate but that they did not capture the breakdown in performance when Mr. G attempted to perform the tasks sequentially. The third goal focused on preparation of meals that would adhere to Mr. G's dietary requirements. Terry also explained that to manage his diabetes and accommodate his food preferences, the patient had to be able to prepare two meals a day while his daughter was at work.
>
> The OASIS scoring was accurate, and so was the occupational therapy evaluation. The issues the occupational therapist identified were important to the patient's overall health, safety, and functional abilities.

important not only because they are part of the OASIS data set but also because they have been found to be relevant to the health and well-being of the home health population. This section identifies some of these indicators, explains their scoring, and describes strategies within the scope of occupational therapy to accurately assess these indicators. Some of these indicators are mandated for assessment at multiple time points coinciding with comprehensive assessments conducted after the start of care.

Pain Assessment and Frequency of Pain

Two OASIS items pertain to pain (Chapter 3, Section E, Sensory Status). One item asks whether a standardized pain assessment has been used to gauge the client's perception of pain and its intensity. An occupational therapist completing the OASIS is responsible for determining and recording whether a standardized pain assessment has been performed, regardless of whether the assessment was performed by the occupational therapist or a clinician from another discipline.

The second item addressing frequency of pain asks whether the client's pain interferes with activity or movement. The item is based on both observation and the client's report. Item instructions from the *OASIS Guidance Manual* state,

> Pain interferes with activity when the pain results in the activity being performed less often than otherwise desired, requires the patient to have additional assistance in performing the activity, or causes the activity to take longer to complete. Include all activities (for example, sleeping, recreational activities, watching television), not just ADLs. . . . Pain that is well controlled with treatment may not interfere with activity or movement at all. (CMS, 2015, Chapter 3, p. E-6)

If a client experiences pain but it does not interfere with activity, the item is scored 0 (*no pain*). Several suggestions in Box 4.1 may be used to assess frequency of pain.

 Stop here! Go to Appendix D and read the section beginning "(M1242) Frequency of Pain Interfering with patient's activity or movement" on pages 238–239.

Wounds

Guidance by the National Pressure Ulcer Advisory Panel for assessing and staging pressure ulcers, stasis ulcers, and surgical wounds is incorporated into the *OASIS Guidance Manual*. The OASIS Integumentary Status (Chapter 3, Section F) items are designed so that clinicians of any skilled discipline (e.g., skilled nurse, occupational therapist, physical therapist, speech–language pathologist) can score the items accurately by following the instructions and considerations in the manual. Scoring of this indicator takes into account situations in which a wound cannot be directly observed because of the presence of a nonremovable dressing.

An important consideration is that some therapy-only clients may have early-stage pressure ulcers associated with limited mobility. Accurately recognizing a Stage I or II pressure ulcer can be critical to a client's health and well-being. Recognizing an early-stage pressure ulcer may also affect both occupational therapy intervention (e.g., positioning, pressure relief, activity) and the overall home health care plan by all disciplines.

 Stop here! Go to Appendix D and read the section "Pressure Ulcers" on pages 250–251.

Dyspnea

Dyspnea, or shortness of breath, is assessed as a function of activity. If a client uses supplemental oxygen continuously, dyspnea should be assessed with the oxygen in use. If a client uses supplemental oxygen intermittently, dyspnea should be assessed without the use of oxygen. The appropriate response item selected is based on how the client actually uses oxygen, not on how oxygen use is ordered or prescribed. This item does not reflect the reason the client experiences dyspnea, only that it is present.

The dyspnea item is scored primarily through observation. If a client is sedentary, the occupational therapist should prompt the client to engage in increasing levels of activity until dyspnea is present or until the client climbs stairs or walks more than 20 feet without experiencing dyspnea.

 Stop here! Go to Appendix D and read the section "G. Respiratory Status" on page 239.

Urinary Incontinence and Bowel Incontinence

Accurate scoring of the urinary incontinence and bowel incontinence items depends heavily on the therapist's use of sensory information (visual and olfactory) and on tactful questioning. The client is considered incontinent (score of 1) even if episodes of incontinence are occasional (e.g., when sneezing, some leaking). If the client depends on timed voiding, the score is 1. The *OASIS Guidance Manual* clarifies that "timed voiding is defined as scheduled toileting assistance or prompted voiding to manage incontinence based on identified patterns.

Timed voiding is a compensatory strategy; it does not cure incontinence" (CMS, 2015, Chapter 3, p. I-2). Night incontinence is also scored 1. The urinary incontinence item can be assessed sensitively in context while touring the home with the client.

 Stop here! Go to Appendix D and read the section "I. Elimination Status" on pages 240–241.

Depression Screening

The depression screening item (M1730, in Section J) is a measure of care process (defined in **Appendix D,** "OASIS Process Measure Item Guidance" section) and has two parts: (1) whether depression screening, a best-practice care process, has been used and, if so, (2) the results of the screening. The Patient Health Questionnaire–2 (PHQ–2; Kroenke, Spitzer, & Williams, 2003) is incorporated into the OASIS depression screening item, and agencies may choose to use the PHQ–2 for convenience. (The PHQ–2 is copyrighted by Pfizer, who has given permission for the PHQ–2 to be incorporated into OASIS.) CMS does not require HHAs to screen for depression, but doing so is considered best practice. If agency policy requires screening for depression, agencies may elect to use the PHQ–2 or a different standardized depression screen.

If a screening tool is required by the agency, occupational therapists should learn to conduct the screening and to score it accurately. Because engagement in activities may be negatively affected by depression, the results of such screenings have implications for occupational therapy goals and interventions, such as how education is delivered or how much time is allowed for learning new skills.

> Because engagement in activities may be negatively affected by depression, the results of such screenings have implications for occupational therapy goals and interventions, such as how education is delivered or how much time is allowed for learning new skills.

Medications and Medication Management

The OASIS items pertaining to medication include some items that measure whether certain care processes have been conducted and other items that measure the client's capacity to manage medications. All of these items have been formulated so they can be accurately assessed within the scope of the four professionals permitted to conduct the comprehensive assessment: (1) registered nurse, (2) occupational therapist, (3) physical therapist, and (4) speech–language pathologist.

An occupational therapist completing the OASIS is responsible for determining whether the care processes have been performed but not for performing the care processes. The HHA should have systems in place for the clinician responsible for the OASIS to determine whether each identified care process has been performed. Occupational therapists can complete a drug regimen review with assistance from designated staff (usually a nurse) or pharmacy software.

The *Framework* (AOTA, 2014) identifies medication routines (including administering and managing medications) as an IADL that is within the domain of occupational therapy. The OASIS items pertaining to medication management assess the client's ability to administer medications reliably and safely.

Inability to manage medication is associated with rehospitalization and poor health outcomes (Hubbard & McNeill, 2012). Occupational therapy practitioners' ability to analyze the various activities and components of medication management and to integrate these components into an effective, sustainable medication routine can benefit clients and agencies.

 Stop here! Go to Appendix D and read the section "L. Medications" (pp. 247–248) and the subsection "Medications" under the "OASIS Process Measure Item Guidance" section on pages 253–254.

Integrating Home Health Quality Initiative Priorities With Client Priorities

One of the challenges of the evaluation process is integrating client priorities with HHQI priorities. In some situations, clients identify needs or concerns that are congruent with or similar to issues that are scored for the OASIS and prioritized by HHQI. However, it is unlikely that clients will mention or even consider all of the areas addressed in the OASIS. How can an evaluation be client centered and also be consistent with HHQI priorities?

Occupational therapy practitioners can rely on their understanding of the domain of occupational therapy to answer this question. As noted previously, many of the OASIS items are scored in relation to clients' activities and abilities. The OASIS was designed not to be administered as a questionnaire but rather to be completed using information that is gathered during the course of the occupational profile and analysis of occupational performance and then integrated into the comprehensive assessment. **Appendix D** describes the regulation requiring integration into the comprehensive assessment.

 Stop here! Go to Appendix D and read the section "Incorporating OASIS Data Into the Comprehensive Assessment" on pages 226–227.

Information for many of the OASIS items can be obtained from responses to questions and observations while eliciting the occupational profile or touring the home.

As illustrated in Box 4.1, information for many of the OASIS items can be obtained from responses to questions and observations while eliciting the occupational profile or touring the home. For instance, it is much less intrusive to inquire about toileting or incontinence while interacting with the client in the bathroom or bedroom as part of the assessment than to ask blunt questions about continence while seated in the living room.

Letting clients and families know that the therapist will be addressing items relevant to home health services may make them more aware of or more comfortable with addressing issues they might otherwise overlook or avoid. For example, including specific, intentional queries about accessing routine and emergency assistance provides information about assistance, safety awareness, and specific telephone use skills. Raising the issue may also facilitate discussion about overall safety, which may concern clients or family members who may be reluctant to express worry about this area.

At times, citing "the rules" can be a helpful approach to initiate or normalize a topic that might otherwise be difficult to address. For example, many older adults are reluctant to acknowledge experiencing a fall. Direct probing about falls is unlikely to elicit an honest response. An occupational therapist may preface the topic by telling the client,

> One of the things we check on with everyone we see is falling. Even when people haven't had falls, they might give up things they want to do if those things start feeling risky. So we ask everyone if they've had any falls, and we check on some things that are associated with falling.

This explanation allows clients or family members to express concerns that might otherwise remain unspoken. For clients or family members who have never considered fall risk, this explanation exposes them to the issue and provides a foundation for more specific education.

The OASIS was designed to assess items known to be essential to the health and function of the home health population. What is assessed is more likely to be addressed. Conversely, what is never assessed may never be addressed. The assessment items included in the OASIS and the requirement to complete the OASIS means that agencies and practitioners are attending to client status indicators essential to staying at home safely and managing daily activities. With a focus on daily life activities, occupational therapy, perhaps more than any other home health discipline, is well equipped to integrate the assessment of clients' individual priorities with assessment of factors important to the health and well-being of the population served by home health.

Conclusion

In home health, the occupational therapy evaluation process not only informs occupational therapy intervention but may also inform agency data accuracy, health care quality efforts, and agency payment. These multiple uses of client data demand that occupational therapists attend to evaluation in relation not only to a specific client but also to HHA operations and to federally mandated initiatives.

The *Framework* offers practitioners a means to frame home health practice so that what occupational therapy addresses and the process occupational therapy practitioners use are communicated explicitly. The process begins with evaluation. The content and documentation of the evaluation process communicate what occupational therapy is to home health clients, drives intervention, and lays the groundwork for intervention. The evaluation comprises eliciting the occupational profile, conducting an analysis of occupational performance, and identifying outcome measures. In the home, the client's performance is conducted in the natural environment, providing rich data for the profile and opportunities to analyze performance through observation. The home environment also supports inquiry into the client's performance patterns.

Identifying goals and outcomes involves integrating the expertise of the therapist with the priorities and needs of the client. It is essential that this process be collaborative, yielding an understanding of expected outcomes that is shared by the client and the therapist.

Documentation communicates the substance of the evaluation process to other disciplines, regulators, and payers. The record of the evaluation must be accurate, must adhere to regulations, and must clearly identify the aspects of performance that affect the client's ability to manage day-to-day activities and stay in the home safely. The occupational therapist must choose appropriate parameters to document performance and the factors affecting performance because this record supports subsequent occupational therapy intervention.

The HHQI exists to promote quality care across the entire home health population. It encourages clinicians to identify and direct interventions to problems that are particularly relevant to the home health population. At times, occupational therapy practitioners may be expected to conduct required home health comprehensive assessments at specified time points within an episode of care. Comprehensive assessments include OASIS data items that are used as part of HHQI to monitor client status and to determine whether certain best practices have been used. Even when occupational therapy is not responsible for the CMS-required home health comprehensive assessment, accurate assessment of key aspects of a client's status is essential to support the agency's efforts to collect accurate client data. Data accuracy is important both for quality monitoring and for appropriate payment.

The interests of HHQI and the interests of clients intersect; clients need to be able to manage their health and daily activities to stay in their homes. With a focus on daily life activities, occupational therapy is well equipped to integrate the assessment of clients' individual priorities with assessment of factors important to the health and well-being of the population served by home health.

References

American Occupational Therapy Association. (2014). Occupational therapy practice framework: Domain and process (3rd ed.). *American Journal of Occupational Therapy, 68*(Suppl. 1), S1–S48. http://dx.doi.org/10.5014/ajot.2014.682006

American Occupational Therapy Association. (2015). Standards of practice for occupational therapy. *American Journal of Occupational Therapy, 69*(Suppl. 3), 6913410057. http://dx.doi.org/10.5014/ajot.2015.696S06

Amini, D. (2014). *Exploring the* Occupational Therapy Practice Framework: Domain and Process, *3rd edition short course* [Online course]. Bethesda, MD: AOTA Press.

Centers for Medicare & Medicaid Services. (2011a). *Part 409.44: Skilled services requirements.* Washington, DC: Author. Retrieved from http://www.gpo.gov/fdsys/pkg/CFR-2011-title42-vol2/pdf/CFR-2011-title42-vol2-sec409-44.pdf

Centers for Medicare & Medicaid Services. (2011b). *Part 484: Home health services.* Washington, DC: Author. Retrieved from http://www.gpo.gov/fdsys/pkg/CFR-2011-title42-vol5/pdf/CFR-2011-title42-vol5-part484.pdf

Centers for Medicare & Medicaid Services. (2012). *Outcome and Assessment Information Set (OASIS): Data set.* Retrieved from http://www.cms.gov/Medicare/Quality-Initiatives-Patient-Assessment-Instruments/OASIS/DataSet.html

Centers for Medicare & Medicaid Services. (2015). *OASIS–C1/ICD–10 version guidance manual.* Retrieved from http://www.cms.gov/Medicare/Quality-Initiatives-Patient-Assessment-Instruments/HomeHealthQualityInits/HHQIOASISUserManual.html

Health Care Financing Administration. (2000). Intermediary medical review guidelines for specific services: Change in level of assistance. In *Medicare Program Integrity Manual* (Chapter 6, § 7.3.4.1). Baltimore: Author.

Hubbard, T., & McNeill, N. (2012, October). *Improving medication adherence and reducing readmissions* (Issue Brief). Cambridge, MA: Network for Excellence in Health Innovation.

Kroenke, K., Spitzer, R. L., & Williams, J. B. (2003). The Patient Health Questionnaire–2: Validity of a two-item depression screener. *Medical Care, 41*, 1284–1294.

U.S. Department of Health and Human Services. (2012). *Report to Congress: Plan to implement a Medicare home health agency value-based purchasing program.* Washington, DC: Author. Retrieved from https://www.cms.gov/Medicare/Medicare-Fee-for-Service-Payment/HomeHealthPPS/Downloads/Stage-2-NPRM.pdf

CHAPTER 5

Home Health Plans of Care, Intervention, and Team Collaboration

Carol Siebert, MS, OTR/L, FAOTA

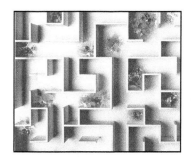

Learning Objectives

After completing this chapter, readers will be able to

- Delineate a process for identifying the need for occupational therapy and the outcomes of occupational therapy service provided as part of home health services;
- Identify pragmatic factors that must be considered in formulating an occupational therapy plan of care when providing home health services;
- Identify elements of a home health plan of care that fill the requirements of the Centers for Medicare & Medicaid Services;
- Identify three intervention implementation strategies used in home health practice; and
- Identify strategies to enhance interdisciplinary communication and coordination in home health care that contribute to coherent care planning.

Introduction

The occupational therapy process involves evaluation, intervention, and **outcomes.** Chapter 4 of this text and Self-Paced Clinical Course (SPCC) described the evaluation process in home health practice: eliciting the client's occupational profile, analyzing the client's occupational performance, and collaborating with the client to identify goals. The evaluation process produces a significant amount of information. What happens to all that information? This chapter describes the process of translating the evaluation findings into a plan for intervention and then into actual intervention.

The process of translating evaluation findings into intervention begins even before the evaluation concludes. Evaluation in home health produces a rich body of information about the client, the client's performance, the home environment, the caregivers, and the client's goals. Throughout the evaluation visit, the occupational therapist observes, asks questions, forms hypotheses about performance, and tests

Key Terms

- **home health certification and plan of care**
- **intervention implementation**
- **intervention plan**
- **intervention review**
- **modalities**
- **objective and measurable goals**
- **outcomes**
- **Person–Environment–Occupation Model**
- **plan of care**
- **pragmatic considerations**
- **procedures**
- **reassessment**
- **rehabilitation potential**
- **trajectory**

hypotheses by analyzing selected aspects of performance that either confirm these hypotheses or suggest alternative hypotheses about the factors contributing to the client's performance problems. Once all these data are collected, the therapist begins to envision likely outcomes of occupational therapy within the context of home health service delivery.

Envisioning the Outcomes of Occupational Therapy

For most clients, home health services are the last stage of postacute care. Other clients, who have been living in the community and have not had an inpatient stay immediately before receiving home health services, are called *community referrals*. Some community referrals need home health care to recover from an acute illness or injury and to regain function affected by the illness or injury, but others require home health during or after a period of deteriorating health or declining function with the expectation of stabilizing health and functional abilities. Regardless of which of the many paths led to a home health referral, it is essential to discern the **trajectory** of the client's health, participation, and caregiving needs to envision the client's future condition.

Envisioning the Trajectory

The future condition emerges as the occupational therapist elicits the occupational profile, forms hypotheses, and analyzes selected aspects of occupational performance. By eliciting information about prior as well as current performance, the therapist forms a picture of the client's occupational performance over time. This temporal picture typically focuses on performance of key activities important to the client but might include a broader perspective of occupational engagement over time.

Occupational therapists integrate what they know about the client's past performance with what they know about the client's current conditions to envision the trajectory.

A *trajectory* is "a path, progression, or line of development" (Merriam-Webster, 2015). Data about the client's past and current performance define a trajectory—the path from past to present and the likely course in the future. Occupational therapists integrate what they know about the client's past performance with what they know about the client's current conditions to envision the trajectory. Once envisioned, the therapist asks two questions about the trajectory:

1. Is this performance trajectory compatible with the client's goals?
2. Is this performance trajectory compatible with the client's ability to manage daily activities and remain at home safely?

If the envisioned performance trajectory is compatible with the client's goals and supports his or her ability to stay at home, it is unlikely that the client needs occupational therapy intervention. If the trajectory is not compatible with the client's goals and with managing safely at home, though, the therapist must consider two additional questions:

1. Could the trajectory be modified through occupational therapy intervention to be more compatible with the client's goals or more compatible with remaining safely at home?
2. What would the changed trajectory look like?

The answers to these questions suggest the outcomes that might be achievable through occupational therapy and the appropriate intervention approaches to achieve a more desirable trajectory.

Identifying Intervention Approaches

Occupational therapy approaches to intervention are conveyed by verbs such as *create, promote, establish, restore, maintain, modify,* and *prevent.* The occupational therapy practitioner selects intervention approaches on the basis of the findings of the evaluation, particularly the analysis of occupational performance, in the context of the current performance trajectory. By assessing and analyzing the factors contributing to performance problems, the occupational therapist can identify appropriate intervention approaches to address these problems and achieve the client's performance goals.

The **Person–Environment–Occupation (PEO) Model** (Law et al., 1996) is useful both for analyzing performance and for identifying appropriate intervention approaches. The PEO Model posits that occupational performance is a dynamic transaction among person, environment, and occupation (or activity). Greater compatibility (or fit) among these three components optimizes occupational performance. In simple terms, occupational performance exists at the intersection of a client's capabilities, the demands of the activity, and the attributes of the environment. Figure 5.1 conveys this relationship graphically.

Occupational therapy intervention is directed toward optimizing the intersection or fit among person, environment, and occupation. Occupational performance may be influenced by altering the client's capabilities, the environment, or the

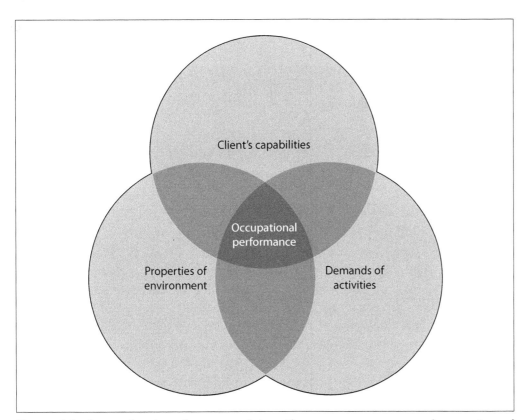

Figure 5.1. Occupational performance: Interaction among person, environment, and occupation.

Source. From "The Person–Environment–Occupation Model: A Transactive Approach to Occupational Performance," Figure 1b, by M. Law, B. A. Cooper, S. Strong, D. Stewart, P. Rigsby, & L. Letts, 1996, *Canadian Journal of Occupational Therapy, 63,* p. 15, copyright © 1996 by the Canadian Association of Occupational Therapists. Adapted by permission of SAGE Publications, Inc.

demands of a given activity, or through some combination of these efforts, but it is always directed toward optimizing the compatibility of the three components. The analysis of occupational performance, an understanding of the client's priorities and concerns, and awareness of the home health practice context guide the occupational therapist's decisions in selecting intervention approaches to achieve desired occupational performance. The approaches selected commonly involve

- Establishing or restoring performance skills, performance patterns, or client factors or modifying performance patterns (person);
- Modifying the environment (environment); or
- Modifying activity demands (occupation).

In some circumstances, the analysis of performance and consideration of the performance trajectory may support other approaches, including

- Maintenance of performance skills, performance patterns, or client factors (person);
- Prevention of deterioration of performance skills, performance patterns, or client factors (person);
- Maintenance of characteristics or aspects of the environment (environment);
- Creation or promotion of characteristics or aspects of the environment (environment); or
- Maintenance of activity demands (occupation).

In home health, intervention to create or promote, maintain, or prevent often involves establishing, restoring, or modifying performance patterns, environments, or activity demands, so more than one approach is often necessary to achieve a specific goal or outcome.

Synthesizing Trajectories and Intervention Approaches

Figure 5.2 illustrates four client performance trajectories and the conditional trajectories envisioned with occupational therapy intervention. In Figure 5.2a, the client has experienced a sudden, rapid decline in performance, perhaps as a result of a recent acute health event. The client has shown a small amount of improvement since the event, similar to that seen during inpatient postacute care. However, the improvement has not been sustained since the client was discharged to home, perhaps as a result of a different physical environment and different caregivers. The occupational therapist envisions that this client's future trajectory is unfavorable for performance of daily activities and for staying at home safely. The therapist reasons that home health occupational therapy intervention may improve performance. The therapist also determines that occupational therapy intervention can equip the client and caregivers to sustain the performance and even promote continued improvement after discharge from home health occupational therapy. In these circumstances, occupational therapy intervention is appropriate, with a likely focus on preventing further decline; restoring skills, client factors, and routines; and modifying environments and activity demands.

In Figure 5.2b, the client has a history of repeated decline and improvement in performance, likely associated with exacerbations and remissions of a chronic

In home health, intervention to create or promote, maintain, or prevent often involves establishing, restoring, or modifying performance patterns, environments, or activity demands, so more than one approach is often necessary to achieve a specific goal or outcome.

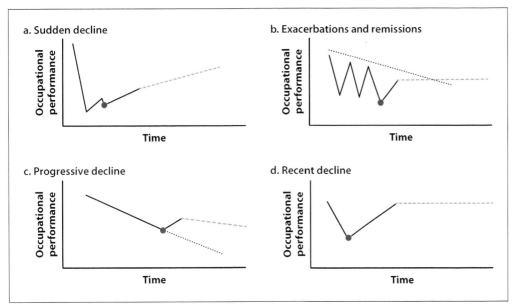

Figure 5.2. Trajectories in occupational performance over time.

Note. Dots represent the start of occupational therapy services, dashed lines represent the trajectory after client discharge from services, and dotted lines represent the expected trajectory without therapy.

condition. The occupational therapist notes that the client's current performance is likely associated with an exacerbation but also notes that the overall trajectory is one of decline, which suggests that future performance is likely to show continued overall decline in spite of spells of remission. The therapist recognizes that performance is likely to improve as the current exacerbation resolves. However, the therapist also determines that occupational therapy intervention may facilitate that improvement in performance while focusing on stabilizing performance even as the condition fluctuates in the future. In these circumstances, occupational therapy intervention is appropriate, with a likely focus on modifying the environment, performance patterns, and activity demands to restore and maintain safe, adequate performance in the home.

In Figure 5.2c, the client has experienced a long, slow decline in performance, perhaps associated with a progressive and chronic condition. Performance now requires assistance for adequacy and safety. The occupational therapist recognizes that without intervention, performance is likely to continue to decline and more intensive assistance will be needed, perhaps forcing a move to a care facility. The therapist determines that with occupational therapy intervention, performance may be slightly improved or can, at minimum, be stabilized to be safer for the client and to present less burden and risk for caregivers. In these circumstances, occupational therapy intervention is appropriate, with a likely focus on modifying activity demands, routines, and the environment; maintaining current performance levels; and preventing injury to client and to caregivers.

In Figure 5.2d, the client has experienced a recent decline in performance, perhaps associated with an illness or a surgical procedure. On the basis of the current, increased performance trajectory and the nature of the condition, the occupational therapist recognizes that performance is likely to return to previous levels when the illness or the effects of the procedure resolve and that future performance is likely to be comparable with past performance levels. In these circumstances, occupational therapy intervention is not appropriate at this time. On the basis of the client's specific conditions, it may be appropriate for the therapist to plan to reevaluate the client at a future point to verify that the anticipated improvement in performance is occurring consistent with the envisioned trajectory. If at that time the trajectory is altered or performance is not improving as expected, the therapist may determine that intervention is appropriate.

Envisioning Outcomes

After envisioning a changed future trajectory for the client and the intervention approaches that could produce a changed trajectory, the occupational therapist is ready to answer the question "What will the client and (if appropriate) the caregiver achieve through the provision of home health occupational therapy?"

The occupational therapist uses conditional reasoning to envision and communicate outcomes in terms of health, participation, or engagement in occupation.

What the client and caregiver can achieve constitute the outcomes of occupational therapy. The occupational therapist uses conditional reasoning to envision and communicate outcomes in terms of health, participation, or engagement in occupation (American Occupational Therapy Association [AOTA], 2014). Within the context of home health, the Centers for Medicare & Medicaid Services (CMS; Medicare.gov, 2014) has described home health outcomes for clients as getting better, regaining independence, and becoming as self-sufficient as possible.

Occupational therapists should be able to describe the envisioned outcomes of occupational therapy generally in no more than two to three sentences. Box 5.1 lists examples of outcome statements for three clients. Each of the examples in Box 5.1 paints a clear word picture relevant to a client's anticipated performance and ability to manage activities and remain safely at home.

Establishing a Shared Vision and Shared Expectation of Outcomes

The process of projecting a trajectory, determining whether intervention is needed and what intervention approaches are appropriate, and envisioning outcomes occurs while the occupational therapist is in the home during the evaluation visit. The therapist explains the conclusions of his or her reasoning to the client and caregiver (and significant others, if appropriate). This explanation addresses whether occupational therapy intervention is needed and how the intervention relates to the

---

Box 5.1. Examples of Home Health Occupational Therapy Outcome Statements

- Mrs. T will be able to remain at home and manage her personal care and simple home care activities. She will incorporate her medications and energy conservation strategies into her daily routines to manage her heart failure.
- Mr. S will remain at home but will begin attending an adult day program several times a week. His family caregivers will assist with his personal care using techniques to reduce his agitation, maintain his safety, and encourage his participation in ADLs, simple home management, and leisure activities he has previously enjoyed.
- Ms. C will return to managing her ADLs and IADLs independently, with modifications to her environment and her routines to reduce the risk of another injurious fall.

client's occupational performance goals and the goal of staying safely in the home. The explanation also includes a brief, general description of the kinds of interventions to be implemented on the basis of the intervention approaches identified. Most important, the occupational therapist describes what the client's life will be like in relation to his or her expressed goals or desires when the anticipated outcomes are achieved.

Communicating envisioned outcomes is likely the most challenging aspect of this interaction, but it is critical to establishing shared expectations. Sometimes occupational therapists feel uncomfortable discussing outcomes, citing uncertainty about the future or concerns about discouraging clients whose expressed desires exceed what is likely to be achieved by therapy. However, for the client to buy into and invest in the conditional future, the therapist must tactfully and sensitively convey how the intervention will lead to the expected trajectory and outcomes, thereby creating an expectation shared by both practitioner and client. This communication should be both hope affirming and realistic. During this discussion, the client and caregiver may ask questions or may refine the envisioned outcomes or priorities, but together client, caregiver, and therapist develop a shared expectation of what the occupational therapist will address and a shared vision of what occupational therapy intervention will achieve.

If the occupational therapist determines that occupational therapy intervention is not needed or not needed at this time, he or she should explain this determination in relation to the client's occupational performance goals. These explanations may be brief, but they inform the client's understanding and expectations of occupational therapy and influence all subsequent encounters with occupational therapy personnel.

Pragmatic Considerations in Developing an Intervention Plan

The ***intervention plan*** "directs the actions of occupational therapy practitioners" and "describes selected occupational therapy approaches and types of interventions to be used in reaching clients' identified outcomes" (AOTA, 2014, p. S15). Two **pragmatic considerations** that influence the occupational therapy intervention plan, related not to the client but rather to the practice setting, inform the therapist's clinical reasoning: (1) relevance to the practice context of the home and (2) the distinct value of occupational therapy in home health. Schell (2008) called clinical reasoning related to practice setting concerns *pragmatic reasoning*. Often this kind of reasoning is not made explicit but underlies the practitioner's decision making. This section makes these pragmatic factors explicit and describes their relevance to the formulation of the intervention plan.

Relevance to the Home Health Practice Context

The first pragmatic factor is that the intervention plan must be relevant to the home health practice setting: The client is in the home, with limited assistance and supports available. Home health practice presents the practitioner with the challenge of addressing occupations that are unlikely to be addressed in other settings and addressing these occupations in the actual environment in which they must be performed. These occupations represent some of the outcomes targeted by the Home Health Quality Initiative (HHQI) and thus address the agency's concern with quality

Two **pragmatic considerations** that influence the occupational therapy intervention plan, related not to the client but rather to the practice setting, inform the therapist's clinical reasoning: (1) relevance to the practice context of the home and (2) the distinct value of occupational therapy in home health.

improvement; **Appendix C, "Medicare as Quality Monitor"** (pp. 205–219), discusses the HHQI targeted outcomes in more detail.

**Stop here! Go to Appendix C and read the section
"Outcome Report" on pages 212–214.**

Occupations addressed in the home may include

- Activities of daily living (ADLs), including not only bathing, dressing, feeding and eating, toileting, grooming, and functional mobility but also bowel and bladder management and personal device care;
- Instrumental activities of daily living (IADLs), including meal preparation and cleanup, care of others, care of pets, communication management, health management and maintenance, safety and emergency maintenance, community mobility, and shopping;
- Rest and sleep, including identification of the need to rest and engagement in relaxation, sleep preparation, and activities resulting in going to sleep, staying asleep, and ensuring adequate sleep;
- Leisure, including exploration of and participation in activities that are intrinsically motivating and engaging to the client; and
- Social participation, including engagement in social pursuits with family and friends and in the community.

For Medicare to cover home health services, the client must be homebound, and home health services must be provided at the client's place of residence (see the definition of *homebound* in Box 3.1 in Chapter 3). However, the homebound requirement does not preclude addressing activities that occur away from the home. For example, aspects of shopping and community mobility are appropriately addressed in home health. For shopping, home health services may include identifying strategies for the client to shop if he or she is unable to leave the home or is able to leave only with assistance. For community mobility, services should include identifying strategies for the client to attend scheduled medical appointments, a key factor in avoiding hospitalization. These services may also include identifying or designing strategies for the client to get around in the community after home health care has ended.

Priorities in Setting Goals

It may be necessary not only to address but also to prioritize specific IADLs, such as being able to secure an entry door, call for assistance, retrieve prepared meals, or manage medications, over basic ADLs such as bathing. In home health, these IADLs may be the client's responsibility for all or part of the day, and the ability to manage these activities effectively has a more significant bearing on the client's immediate health and safety than does, for example, upper-body dressing. Similarly, the ADL goal of toileting independently may take precedence over other ADL goals, such as bathing or dressing, because the client, or the client and caregiver, has difficulty managing this activity, which occurs multiple times each day.

It may be necessary not only to address but also to prioritize specific IADLs, such as being able to secure an entry door, call for assistance, retrieve prepared meals, or manage medications, over basic ADLs such as bathing.

Selection of Intervention Approaches and Types of Intervention

The home health practice context also informs the selection of intervention approaches and, thus, the types of intervention selected. As discussed in Chapter 3 of this text and SPCC, the home health population consists primarily of older adults with chronic conditions. Intensive use of approaches to restore body functions, often using preparatory methods, is common in inpatient rehabilitation settings, especially settings in which clients with acute neurological and orthopedic conditions are treated. Home health, however, is not a rehabilitation setting. Home health clients and their families are concerned about clients' being able to regain and sustain the ability to manage safely in their homes. Policymakers and payers have prioritized similar concerns.

Given these characteristics and concerns, occupational therapists must carefully consider the likely benefit of restorative or remediation-oriented approaches and preparatory methods. In this population, therapists cannot assume that the client's body functions can be appreciably restored, that any restoration achieved will be sustainable, or that restoration of body functions will yield a favorable or sustainable effect on occupational performance. In many situations, interventions that modify the environment or the activity demands can produce a more timely, more effective, and more sustainable enhancement of occupational performance than interventions to restore body functions.

As discussed in Chapter 4, conducting the evaluation process in the home provides rich data regarding the environmental and activity demand aspects of performance as well as the roles and routines associated with the performance of any given activity. Assessment of selected aspects of performance does not pertain exclusively to assessing client abilities; it also pertains to assessing the environment and activity demands and the congruence or fit among the three. Box 5.2 offers some guiding questions occupational therapists can use in determining whether restorative approaches are appropriate for a given client's intervention plan.

Box 5.2. Questions to Guide Selection of Goals and Interventions to Restore Body Functions

- Is an improvement in this body function possible?
- If it is possible, how much improvement can reasonably be expected?
- How much time and effort will the client have to invest in a home program to achieve the expected improvement?
- Will an improvement in this body function make a meaningful difference in the client's performance of necessary or important activities? Will the anticipated improvement reestablish compatibility among the client's abilities, the demands of those activities, and the environment in which those activities occur?
- Will the expected improvement be something that lasts or that the client can sustain once discharged from occupational therapy? What will the client have to do, and for how long, to sustain the improvement? Given available information about the client and his or her circumstances, is this a reasonable expectation?
- Is the client open to interventions that match the demands of the problematic activities to his or her current abilities?
- Given other competing needs and available resources, what is the most effective and efficient intervention strategy to achieve a meaningful and sustainable participation outcome?

Physical Context Constraints

The physical practice context—the home—also informs the selection of intervention approaches and types of intervention. Therapy equipment found in clinic settings is not found in the home, and the logistics of transporting such items to the home makes use of most equipment incompatible with home health services. Although it may be ideal to have a mat table to establish or refine a specific transfer technique, in the home the only surfaces available may be a worn-out mattress and a too-low chair. These are, however, the surfaces the client encounters each time a transfer must occur, so addressing transfers must begin with the existing physical environment and the activity demands on the client (and, in many cases, the caregiver) rather than with a specific set of transfer skills that might be the starting point in other settings.

For occupational therapy practitioners who have come from settings in which ADLs take precedence over IADLs or in which restoring body functions or performance skills takes precedence over modifying activity demands or environments, constraints imposed by the physical context may necessitate a new way of thinking about what to address first. In home health, prioritizing the activities occupational therapy will address must be based on both the priorities of the client and the effect on the client's and caregiver's health, safety, and peace of mind.

Distinct Value of Occupational Therapy in Home Health

The second consideration when formulating the intervention plan is what the plan communicates about the contribution of occupational therapy. Confusion often exists about what occupational therapy addresses and what occupational therapists do in home health. To those reviewing the intervention plan, the goals and outcomes communicate what occupational therapy addresses, and the interventions or treatments communicate what occupational therapists do. The goals and interventions must reflect the domain and process of occupational therapy. Some overlap between occupational therapy and other disciplines may be appropriate in achieving client outcomes. Indeed, coordination among disciplines is essential. Any overlap, though, should be reflected in goals or interventions that are complementary to, not indistinguishable from, those of another discipline, and this issue should inform the therapist's overall consideration of the intervention plan even before specific goals are identified.

The value of occupational therapy should be apparent in the intervention plan. As discussed in Chapter 4, the priorities of payers and policymakers are converging with the priorities of clients and their families: that home health services should have a meaningful effect on a client's ability to manage at home and to stay at home safely. Put simply, home health services should make a meaningful difference compared with no services. By extension, occupational therapy services should make a meaningful difference compared with no occupational therapy. This issue is discussed in greater depth in Chapter 6 of this text and SPCC, but the occupational therapist is obligated to consider what the meaningful difference might be before formulating the plan to achieve that difference.

Interventions should be *evidence based:* "Evidence-based practice is the integration of best research evidence with clinical expertise and patient values" (Sackett et al., 1996, as cited in Institute of Medicine, 2001, p. 147). Far too few research studies have investigated the effectiveness of occupational therapy practice in home health, but practitioners have a duty to question the effectiveness of their interventions and to discard practices that have no evidence of effectiveness. *Effectiveness* means that the intervention produces the desired or expected result. Evidence does not have to be limited solely to the results of randomized controlled trials; research evidence may include evidence from the home health agency's (HHA's) Outcome-Based Quality Improvement (OBQI) efforts (see **Appendix C**). If the agency-specific OBQI reports show an improvement on a given outcome or outcomes after implementation of certain practices, the improved outcomes can be considered evidence of the effectiveness of those interventions with the agency's client population. Implementing evidence-based practice is both science and art as the practitioner integrates effective interventions with clinical expertise and the client's values.

> Implementing evidence-based practice is both science and art as the practitioner integrates effective interventions with clinical expertise and the client's values.

Stop here! Go to Appendix C and read the section "Outcome-Based Quality Improvement" on pages 209–219.

Home Health Intervention Plan and Plan of Care

In home health, the **plan of care** (POC) merges the intervention plans of all disciplines caring for a client. Some HHAs refer to the POC as "the 485," a CMS form that was originally provided for recording the **home health certification and plan of care.** The form is not required, but all elements of the form must be included in a document referred to as the *home health certification and POC* or *physician's POC.* Form 485 is shown in Exhibit 5.1.

Stop here! Go to Appendix A and read the section "Plan of Care" on pages 178–181.

Key aspects of the POC include the client's diagnoses relevant to home health care, the interventions to be provided, the frequency and duration of services, client goals listed by discipline, and the client's **rehabilitation potential.** *Rehabilitation potential* "addresses the patient's ability to attain the goals and an estimate of the time needed to achieve them. This information should be pertinent to [the] nature of the patient's condition and ability to respond" (CMS, 2002, pp. 25–26).

The HHA completes Form 485 (or its equivalent) and sends it to the client's physician for signature. As noted in Item 26, by signing the form the physician certifies that he or she has ordered or authorized the HHA to implement the POC and, for Medicare beneficiaries, that the client and the plan meet the eligibility criteria for the Medicare Home Health Benefit.

The home health certification and POC applies to the 60-day period coinciding with a payment episode of care. When occupational therapy services are initiated at the start of an episode, the occupational therapy POC may be included in the initial home health certification and POC the agency sends to the physician. When occupational therapy services are initiated at a time other than at the start of an episode, the HHA submits the occupational therapy POC to the physician as a supplement or

Exhibit 5.1. Home Health Certification and Plan of Care (Form 485)

Department of Health and Human Services Centers for Medicare & Medicaid Services		Form Approved OMB No. 0938-0357

HOME HEALTH CERTIFICATION AND PLAN OF CARE

1. Patient's HI Claim No.	2. Start Of Care Date	3. Certification Period From: To:	4. Medical Record No.	5. Provider No.

6. Patient's Name and Address	7. Provider's Name, Address and Telephone Number

8. Date of Birth	9. Sex ☐ M ☐ F	10. Medications: Dose/Frequency/Route (N)ew (C)hanged

11. ICD	Principal Diagnosis	Date	
12. ICD	Surgical Procedure	Date	
13. ICD	Other Pertinent Diagnoses	Date	

14. DME and Supplies	15. Safety Measures

16. Nutritional Req.	17. Allergies

18.A. Functional Limitations

1 ☐ Amputation	5 ☐ Paralysis	9 ☐ Legally Blind
2 ☐ Bowel/Bladder (Incontinance)	6 ☐ Endurance	A ☐ Dyspnea With Minimal Exertion
3 ☐ Contracture	7 ☐ Ambulation	B ☐ Other (Specify)
4 ☐ Hearing	8 ☐ Speech	

18.B. Activities Permitted

1 ☐ Complete Bedrest	6 ☐ Partial Weight Bearing	A ☐ Wheelchair
2 ☐ Bedrest BRP	7 ☐ Independent At Home	B ☐ Walker
3 ☐ Up As Tolerated	8 ☐ Crutches	C ☐ No Restrictions
4 ☐ Transfer Bed/Chair	9 ☐ Cane	D ☐ Other (Specify)
5 ☐ Exercises Prescribed		

19. Mental Status	1 ☐ Oriented	3 ☐ Forgetful	5 ☐ Disoriented	7 ☐ Agitated
	2 ☐ Comatose	4 ☐ Depressed	6 ☐ Lethargic	8 ☐ Other

20. Prognosis	1 ☐ Poor	2 ☐ Guarded	3 ☐ Fair	4 ☐ Good	5 ☐ Excellent

21. Orders for Discipline and Treatments (Specify Amount/Frequency/Duration)

22. Goals/Rehabilitation Potential/Discharge Plans

23. Nurse's Signature and Date of Verbal SOC Where Applicable:	25. Date of HHA Received Signed POT

24. Physician's Name and Address	26. I certify/recertify that this patient is confined to his/her home and needs intermittent skilled nursing care, physical therapy and/or speech therapy or continues to need occupational therapy. The patient is under my care, and I have authorized services on this plan of care and will periodically review the plan.
27. Attending Physician's Signature and Date Signed	28. Anyone who misrepresents, falsifies, or conceals essential information required for payment of Federal funds may be subject to fine, imprisonment, or civil penalty under applicable Federal laws.

Form CMS-485 (C-3) (12-14) (Formerly HCFA-485) (Print Aligned)

(Continued)

Exhibit 5.1. Home Health Certification and Plan of Care (Form 485) *(cont.)*

Privacy Act Statement
Sections 1812, 1814, 1815, 1816, 1861 and 1862 of the Social Security Act authorize collection of this information. The primary use of this information is to process and pay Medicare benefits to or on behalf of eligible individuals. Disclosure of this information may be made to: Peer Review Organizations and Quality Review Organizations in connection with their review of claims, or in connection with studies or other review activities, conducted pursuant to Part B of Title XI of the Social Security Act; State Licensing Boards for review of unethical practices or nonprofessional conduct; A congressional office from the record of an individual in response to an inquiry from the congressional office at the request of that individual.
Where the individual's identification number is his/her Social Security Number (SSN), collection of this information is authorized by Executive Order 9397. Furnishing the information on this form, including the SSN, is voluntary, but failure to do so may result in disapproval of the request for payment of Medicare benefits.
Paper Work Burden Statement
According to the Paperwork Reduction Act of 1995, no persons are required to respond to a collection of information unless it displays a valid OMB control number. The valid OMB control number for this information collection is 0938-0357. The time required to complete this information collection is estimated to average 15 minutes per response, including the time to review instructions, search existing data resources, gather the data needed, and complete and review the information collection. If you have any comments concerning the accuracy of the time estimate(s) or suggestions for improving this form, please write to: CMS, Mailstop N2-14-26, 7500 Security Boulevard, Baltimore, Maryland 21244-1850.

Source. Centers for Medicare & Medicaid Services (2014). In the public domain.
Note. BRP = bathroom privileges; CMS = Centers for Medicare & Medicaid Services; DME = durable medical equipment; HCFA = Health Care Financing Administration; HHA = home health agency; HI = health insurance; ICD = *International Classification of Diseases;* OMB = Office of Management and Budget; POT = plan of treatment; SOC = start of care.

addendum to the home health certification and POC. The supplemental POC must include the occupational therapy interventions, frequency and duration, goals, and rehabilitation potential for occupational therapy goals but may also include any of the other aspects (numbered items on Form 485) that support or pertain to the occupational therapy POC but are not identified on the initial home health certification and POC.

Occupational Therapy Intervention Plan in the Plan of Care

In occupational therapy, the intervention plan guides intervention. The intervention plan is the road map for the journey the occupational therapy practitioner and the client will take together. The journey's destination is defined by the outcomes that have been identified in collaboration with the client. Once a destination is determined, the stages along the journey can be identified. Similarly, once the outcomes of occupational therapy are identified, the specific elements of the intervention plan can be determined.

In home health, the specific elements of the plan must include the specific types of intervention to be used, the frequency of practitioner visits to the home, the duration of occupational therapy within the 60-day home health episode, and the specific goals to be addressed. Pragmatic factors influencing the intervention plan identified earlier in this chapter must be taken into account. Once those factors have been considered, the occupational therapy intervention plan must be formalized as part of the home health certification and POC.

The elements of intervention plans and intervention planning identified in the *Occupational Therapy Practice Framework: Domain and Process* (3rd ed.; AOTA, 2014) are not identical to the elements of the occupational therapy home health POC. Table 5.1 matches the steps in the occupational therapy intervention planning process with the corresponding elements of a home health occupational therapy POC and lists questions to guide the development of each element. The sections that follow describe each element of the occupational therapy home health POC in depth.

Table 5.1. Crosswalk: Elements of the Occupational Therapy Intervention Plan Matched With Those of the Occupational Therapy Home Health Plan of Care, With Guiding Questions

Element of the Occupational Therapy Intervention Plan[a]	Element of the Occupational Therapy Home Health Plan of Care	Guiding Questions
Objective and measurable goals with a time frame	Measurable goals[b] (implied time frame is by end of current certification period or when client is discharged from occupational therapy, if sooner)	What will performance look like, described so that anyone can observe the patient and determine whether the goal has been met?
Occupational therapy intervention approaches, based on theory and evidence	No specific plan of care element corresponds, but approaches are reflected in goals, rehabilitation potential, and treatments selected	What approaches are most effective to achieve the desired outcomes? What evidence exists to support effectiveness?
Mechanisms for service delivery • People providing intervention • Types of intervention • Frequency and duration of services	Orders for discipline and treatments (specify frequency, duration, amount[c])	What will occupational therapy do to achieve the goals? What types of intervention will be used? How many visits will be needed to achieve these goals? How will these visits be distributed (i.e., how often, and for how long)?
Discharge needs and plan	Discharge plan	What resources will be needed to support the client's performance and engagement after discharge? If appropriate, what caregiving will be needed to achieve goals or to sustain performance after discharge?
Outcome measures	Goals Rehabilitation potential	What will the client's life be like when the occupational therapy goals are met?
Recommendations or referral to others	Discharge plan Orders for discipline and treatments	What other services or supports outside of occupational therapy and not currently involved or provided are needed (or may be needed) to achieve the desired outcomes or to sustain the outcomes after discharge?
Rehabilitation potential	Rehabilitation potential	What is the client's ability to achieve the goals? In what time frame will the client achieve the goals?

[a]American Occupational Therapy Association (2014, p. S15).
[b]42 CFR [*Code of Federal Regulations*] § 409.44(c)(1)(iii) specifies that, for Medicare home health clients, occupational therapy goals must be measurable (Centers for Medicare & Medicaid Services, 2011b).
[c]*Amount* applies to modalities (e.g., heat, cold, sound, electrical stimulation).

Objective and Measurable Goals

The phrase ***objective and measurable goals*** may remind readers of their occupational therapy entry-level education, but the phrase has renewed significance in home health because these terms are used in the Medicare federal regulations regarding therapy POCs:

(i)   The patient's plan of care must describe a course of therapy treatment and therapy goals which are consistent with the evaluation of the patient's function. . .

(iii) Therapy treatment goals described in the plan of care must be *measurable* [italics added]. . .

(iv)   . . . The method used to assess a patient's function [includes] *objective* [italics added] measurements of function in accordance with accepted professional standards of clinical practice enabling comparison of successive measurements to determine the effectiveness of therapy goals. (CMS, 2011b, p. 336)

The phrase ***objective and measurable goals*** may remind readers of their occupational therapy entry-level education, but the phrase has renewed significance in home health because these terms are used in the Medicare federal regulations regarding therapy POCs.

Objective Goals

Goals are objective when the circumstances identified in the goal are perceptible and discernible to others and do not require others to know the thoughts or interpretations of the practitioner or the client. For example, "Mrs. J will learn energy conservation" is not objective because whether Mrs. J has learned something cannot be discerned by someone other than Mrs. J. How could this statement be transformed into an objective goal?

If Mrs. J implements energy-conserving strategies in her activities, these behaviors can be observed by others and would indicate that Mrs. J has learned something about energy conservation. So an objective goal could be "Mrs. J will demonstrate energy conservation strategies in her daily activities." A more specific objective goal would be "Mrs. J will use pacing and planned rests during her morning self-care routine." This goal identifies the specific energy-conserving techniques Mrs. J is expected to learn and demonstrate during a specific activity. Another objective goal might be "Mrs. J will use pacing and planned rests during her morning self-care routine without prompts or cues." Phrased this way, the goal indicates that Mrs. J has learned and incorporated the techniques to the point that she performs them independently and spontaneously (i.e., requires no assistance to recall or use the techniques). This goal is objective because it delineates observable behavior: pacing and planned rests in the absence of prompts or cues.

Measurable Goals

A goal is measurable when the circumstances identified in the goal are capable of being measured or appraised using one or more parameters that permit comparison with previous or subsequent circumstances. How can Mrs. J's goal be made measurable? For the goal to be measurable, the parameters for measurement should reveal whether she has learned and applied new knowledge. Mrs. J's baseline was that she was not familiar with energy conservation and never used energy-conserving strategies. An objective, measurable goal might be "Mrs. J will use pacing and planned rests during her morning self-care routine an average of 6 out of 7 days." Phrased this way, the goal both indicates that Mrs. J will learn and incorporate the techniques to the point that her performance is relatively consistent and allows Mrs. J and her occupational therapy practitioner to measure her progress toward this goal.

Objective and Measurable Goals Linked to Outcomes

Still another way to address the requirement for objective and measurable goals is to link the reason for learning energy conservation to the problem Mrs. J is experiencing: dyspnea. Framed this way, what is being measured is the dyspnea, not the techniques being used to minimize the dyspnea. So an objective goal might be "Mrs. J will not experience dyspnea during her morning routine by using pacing and planned rests." If Mrs. J's baseline is severe dyspnea limiting her ability to engage in her morning routine, it may not be reasonable to completely eliminate the dyspnea. In this case, an appropriate measurable goal might be "Mrs. J will not experience dyspnea rated greater than 2 (on a scale of 1 to 7) during her morning self-care routine." An important difference in these last two examples is that they relate the goal to an implied overall outcome that is prioritized by Home Health Compare

(HHC; http://www.medicare.gov/HomeHealthCompare/): performance that is less limited by dyspnea (and the underlying condition associated with the dyspnea).

Measuring Change in Performance

The means of measuring progress toward a goal should be appropriate to gauge the difference between baseline performance and the performance targeted by the goal. One of the many parameters for measuring aspects of performance is level of assistance but, as discussed in Chapter 4, in many situations level of assistance does not accurately capture the change in performance being sought. One of the enduring myths related to Medicare is that "potential for improvement" implies that performance must be less dependent on assistance from others to be considered improved. In home health, this is not the case. As noted in Chapter 3 and in the discussion of trajectories earlier in this chapter, for many clients who receive home health, health, participation, and engagement in occupation are on a declining trajectory that is not likely to be reversed by occupational therapy. Should such clients be ruled out as candidates for occupational therapy because they have no potential to improve? The answer is no.

In the development of OBQI, CMS (2010a) explicitly recognized that stabilization or "nonworsening" is a desirable outcome, especially for clients whose status would otherwise worsen in the absence of home health intervention. OBQI reports specifically include outcome data for clients whose performance has stabilized. Eleven of the 33 end-result outcomes reported in an agency's OBQI report are stabilization outcomes, and all are within the domain of occupational therapy (see **Appendix C**, Table C.1, p. 213). CMS expects HHAs to intervene to stabilize declining trajectories and worsening performance and expects occupational therapy to contribute to these efforts. From the perspective of CMS, and certainly from the perspective of clients and their caregivers, stabilized performance is an improvement over worsening performance.

It is essential that occupational therapists working in home health also recognize that stabilizing declining performance is an appropriate outcome of occupational therapy. In such situations, goals should convey that the intent is stabilization. One way to do this is to write an "in order to" goal. For example, Mr. M has a progressive condition resulting in increasing needs for assistance and increasing risk of injury to Mr. M and his caregivers during showering. An appropriate goal might read, "Caregivers will routinely perform safe bathing transfer techniques using transfer bench and transfer belt to stabilize assistance needs and reduce risk of injury." The term *routinely* implies that the caregivers will not only obtain the appropriate equipment and learn to use it but will also use the desired techniques and equipment on a consistent, predictable basis. This goal can be measured and compared with a baseline of no equipment and use of unsafe transfer techniques while showering.

Selecting Outcome Measures

The outcomes of greatest concern in the home health industry are those identified by the HHQI (described in **Appendix C**, pp. 206–209) and reported either on the HHC website (http://www.medicare.gov/HomeHealthCompare; see **Appendix C**, Box C.1, p. 208) or in the OBQI report (see **Appendix C**, "Outcome Report" section, pp. 212–214). Outcomes are reflected in the difference in client status from

In the development of OBQI, CMS explicitly recognized that stabilization or "nonworsening" is a desirable outcome, especially for clients whose status would otherwise worsen in the absence of home health intervention.

the start of home health care to discharge from home health care (further defined in **Appendix C,** "Outcome Definition" section, p. 209) as measured using relevant Outcome and Assessment Information Set (OASIS) items (the subject of **Appendix D**). However, the outcomes measured by OASIS may not be of greatest concern to the client. For some clients, outcomes may be gauged by personal measures of health, participation, and occupational engagement.

One additional factor to consider in formulating goals is the duration of the current episode and certification period. Because the home health POC applies to the current certification period, the goals identified for the current POC should be achievable within the period it covers.

Interventions: Procedures and Modalities

The *Framework* identifies the following intervention types: use of occupations and activities, preparatory methods and tasks, education and training, advocacy, and group interventions. However, these types of interventions are general. In the home health POC, more specific language should be included to identify the interventions that will be used to achieve the stated goals.

It might seem easiest to simply list any and all interventions that might be used to achieve the goals. However, the home health POC must be signed by a physician and, legally, is considered a physician's order. Thus, all interventions included in the POC have been ordered and must be carried out. Aside from legal considerations, the POC is the road map guiding the journey to outcomes. Just as one would not pack snowshoes for a trip to Florida, it makes no sense to clutter the POC by including interventions that do not contribute to the stated goals or the overall projected outcomes.

The home health Conditions of Participation (CoPs) state, "Orders for therapy services include the specific procedures and modalities to be used and the amount, frequency, and duration" (CMS, 2011c, § 484.18, p. 123; see **Appendix B,** p. 201). **Procedures** are "a manner of effecting change through the application of clinical skills and/or services that attempt to improve function. This . . . must include active interventions between the therapist and client" (CMS, 2011a, p. 41). **Modalities** are defined as "any physical agent applied to produce therapeutic changes to biologic tissue and include, but are not limited to, thermal, acoustic, light, mechanical, or electric energy" (CMS, 2011a, pp. 40–41).

The procedures and modalities should be consistent with both the goals and the intervention approaches selected. For example, if a client has a goal that involves his or her caregivers implementing a new technique or using a new device or item of equipment, then caregiver education or training would be an appropriate intervention. If a client has a goal that requires incorporation of a new technique to perform dressing, then ADL training in dressing would be an appropriate intervention for that client. In some cases, the verbs used to describe intervention approaches or procedures can be useful to identify interventions—for example, "modify home environment," "establish revised routines," or "modify activity demands." When restorative approaches are used to improve skills or client factors, the intervention should identify the purposeful activities or preparatory activities to be used.

As noted earlier, the scope of practice of occupational therapy will not be recognized if occupational therapy POCs do not articulate it. Interventions identified

Interventions identified in occupational therapy POCs using cryptic shorthand (e.g., "ther ex") or focusing almost exclusively on ADL training and exercise prevent clients and other clinicians from recognizing occupational therapy expertise related to performance patterns, context and environment, and activity and occupational demands.

in occupational therapy POCs using cryptic shorthand (e.g., "ther ex") or focusing almost exclusively on ADL training and exercise prevent clients and other clinicians from recognizing occupational therapy expertise related to performance patterns, context and environment, and activity and occupational demands. When identifying occupational therapy interventions in the POC, occupational therapists must reflect the necessity for occupational therapy services to achieve the stated goals.

Frequency and Duration of Services

The federal regulations governing HHAs specify that the POC state the frequency and duration of therapy services (CMS, 2011c, § 484.18). Frequency and duration communicate the dosing of occupational therapy services. In basic terms, frequency and duration answer the question "How much therapy will be needed to achieve these goals, and how often will it be provided?"

Research on the dosing of occupational therapy services in any setting is in its infancy. Until reliable evidence is available, the determination of frequency and duration in relation to outcomes in home health requires clinical reasoning that takes into account the client's current status, the goals and impact of the planned interventions, and the intensity of other services the client is receiving. Some aspects of intervention may have a predictable duration to achieve a desired goal. For example, if a client has sustained a fracture, the rate of healing can be anticipated, and the timing for various interventions or gains in performance is relatively predictable. Other issues are not as predictable; examples include the extent and rate of return of sensation, movement, or language after a stroke or the healing of wounds that may limit or complicate performance of ADLs.

When completing this aspect of the POC, the concept of trajectory is once again useful. The frequency and duration of occupational therapy services should be determined on the basis of the trajectory of the client's status and the magnitude of change represented by the goals. Some examples of such considerations include

- The changes, including those based on a change in activity demands, that the client or caregivers will have to learn and incorporate into existing habits and routines;
- The time required for the client or family to modify an environment or acquire an item of equipment; and
- The amount of practice between therapy sessions needed before the client can incorporate a newly acquired technique or skill.

In general, the frequency of intervention visits should taper as therapy progresses and the client's or caregiver's performance approaches the targeted goals. Tapering gradually reduces the client's dependence on the presence of a practitioner. Tapering also provides an increasingly longer window between therapy visits so that successively later visits in the episode provide increasing evidence of how the client or family will manage when occupational therapy is no longer involved. Although frequencies are most commonly defined on a per-week basis, it is also permissible and may be appropriate to write frequencies on an every-other-week or even a monthly basis. In some cases, allowing a significant passage of time between the next-to-last visit and the final visit, whether within one episode or spanning more than one episode, may be appropriate and may be particularly useful to gauge whether an expected postdischarge trajectory of stabilization is being established before the final occupational therapy visit. If the expected trajectory is in evidence, the discharge visit is completed. However, if the expected trajectory appears fragile or if unanticipated problems have arisen, the therapist then has the option to revise the plan either to provide limited intervention directed to the problems that have arisen or to monitor the client for a longer period before a newly projected final visit to allow the expected trajectory to be truly established.

Determining frequency and duration also requires an understanding of the difference between therapy visits and therapy interventions or services. The frequency and duration that must be included in the home health POC are based on occupational therapy practitioner visits to the home to deliver face-to-face interventions. Beyond face-to-face interventions, though, occupational therapy services to be provided may also include making referrals to other disciplines or to community services, coordinating provision of equipment with vendors, coordinating and collaborating with other disciplines within the HHA, and monitoring or coaching the client between therapy visits by telephone. These services can and should be identified in the POC, even though they may not be provided during the home visits.

Discharge Plan

Consideration of discharge needs and plans is an ongoing process that begins at evaluation and continues through to discharge. As the episode of care progresses, the occupational therapist uses conditional reasoning to continuously update and revise hypotheses about the postdischarge trajectory as the client or caregiver responds to therapy interventions. The therapist monitors needs for postdischarge services and resources and implements referrals so that services are in place when discharge occurs.

This discharge plan element of the POC should identify the criteria for discharge related to the occupational therapy goals outlined in the plan. It should also identify the supports and services anticipated to be needed at discharge and any plans to arrange for such services and supports during the course of intervention. In most cases, recommendations and referrals to other disciplines within the HHA as needed are included in the practitioner's efforts to plan for discharge needs and referrals.

Recommendations or referrals for other services may also be needed when the needs can be addressed by occupational therapy but cannot be addressed by home health occupational therapy—for example, when a client needs facilities or equipment that cannot be transported to the home or are not compatible with or available in the home environment. For clients who have improved sufficiently that they are no longer homebound and thus ineligible for continued home health services, but who still have needs that are most appropriately addressed by occupational therapy, a referral or recommendation to outpatient occupational therapy may be appropriate. Referrals are also appropriate when a client needs an evaluation or service, such as a driving evaluation or driver rehabilitation, that is not within the scope of home health practice but is necessary for effective discharge into the community. Anticipated referral to occupational therapy services after discharge from home health should be identified in the discharge plan. If the client continues

Anticipated referral to occupational therapy services after discharge from home health should be identified in the discharge plan.

to receive home health care, referrals for occupational therapy services outside the HHA must be coordinated by the agency through a contracted agreement and must be included explicitly in the POC.

Rehabilitation Potential

Although the term *rehabilitation potential* is used often in occupational therapy practice settings, it has different meanings. Seltzer and Charpentier (1983) identified three meanings of *rehabilitation potential:*

1. "Functions (such as walking) that were lost as a result of physical and/or psychological problems may be restored through rehabilitation" (p. 62).
2. "The patient has latent capabilities, e.g., a right-handed patient learning to write with his/her left hand after having a left hemispheric stroke" (p. 63).
3. "The potential [exists] for rehabilitation to result in no change in functioning (maintenance) or the slowing down of functional decline when the absence of rehabilitation treatment would be expected to result in more rapid decline in functioning" (p. 63).

The only "definition" provided by CMS (2002) is embedded in the instruction for completing this element of the POC:

> Rehabilitation potential addresses the patient's ability to attain the goals and an estimate of the time needed to achieve them. This information should be pertinent to the nature of the patient's condition and ability to respond. The words "Fair," or "Poor" alone, are not acceptable. Instead, descriptors must be added:

> **EXAMPLE:** Rehabilitation potential is good for partial return to previous level of care, but patient will probably not be able to perform ADL independently. (pp. 25–26)

In the author's experience, neither the CMS instruction nor Seltzer and Charpentier's (1983) definition are applied when this element of the POC is completed. Some agencies provide no definition but expect practitioners to estimate rehabilitation potential on the basis of the client's potential to achieve therapy goals. Some agencies estimate discipline-specific rehabilitation potentials according to each discipline's estimate of the client's potential to achieve that discipline's goals. One questions why any clinician would formulate goals that do not have good or excellent potential to be achieved. If no clear instruction is provided by the HHA, the therapist must make his or her meaning clear so that there is no question as to why occupational therapy is being provided or how likely the goals are to be achievable.

Physician Orders

Once the occupational therapist has developed the proposed POC, the next step is to obtain the physician's concurrence with the goals, interventions, and frequency needed to fulfill the therapy orders. This requirement is part of the home health CoPs (CMS, 2011c, § 484.18[c]; see **Appendix B,** p. 201). HHAs have different strategies and systems for securing therapy orders; most agencies use phone, secure email, or fax. Once the physician's concurrence is obtained, the POC is committed to appropriate forms and sent to the physician for hard-copy approval as evidenced by a signature.

Intervention Implementation

Intervention implementation is "ongoing actions taken to influence and support improved client performance and participation. Interventions are directed at identified outcomes. The client's response is monitored and documented" (AOTA, 2014, p. S10). In home health, some of these ongoing actions occur during client encounters or visits. However, face-to-face encounters are just one of three strategies for intervention available in home health practice. A second intervention strategy involves monitoring the client's progress between visits, most often by telephone, although in some circumstances monitoring may also be accomplished using other technologies such as secure email or phone- or Internet-based telehealth systems. These encounters may include monitoring but may also involve consultation, education, or advocacy. The third intervention strategy is homework for the client and, in some cases, the caregiver. Most practitioners are familiar with face-to-face intervention. Telephone and telemediated intervention and homework are described in more detail in the following sections.

Affecting Habitual Action vs. Isolated Performance

The three strategies are most effective when they are used together to achieve consistent, sustainable performance. One of the challenges of home visits is the time constraints of the visit. In some cases, such as those in which a client's routines are being modified significantly or a new routine is being established, it may be a challenge to address all aspects of the routine in a single visit because of time constraints. In other cases, the time of day a visit can be scheduled does not coincide with when an activity is usually performed or within the routine in which it usually occurs. In these circumstances, it is essential that the practitioner recognize that the performance witnessed is an artifact of the timing of the visit. For example, performance of personal care at a 1:00 p.m. visit may differ significantly from performance during the 7:00 a.m. morning routine of a client who has rheumatoid arthritis and experiences stiff, painful movement for most of the morning. Assessment of meal preparation during a visit may not reflect the level of fatigue experienced by a client with multiple sclerosis when meal preparation occurs after any activity other than rest. When possible, timing and duration of visits should be planned as much as possible so that the performance observed or elicited during the visit is consistent with or representative of the client's routine performance.

> It is essential that the practitioner recognize that the performance witnessed is an artifact of the timing of the visit.

Telephone and Other Telemediated Encounters

Telemediated encounters are consistent with the episodic nature of home health practice. Home visits are resource intensive. Supplementing home visits with telephone calls or other telemediated encounters allows the practitioner to monitor the client's condition, to resolve any misunderstandings about instructions given during the home visit, or to provide a booster to reinforce instructions or recommendations made at a previous visit.

Telemediated encounters can also optimize the value of the home visit. For example, during a home visit, a practitioner assesses a client's bathing progress and determines that the client needs a transfer bench. The practitioner provides the client and caregiver with information on obtaining an appropriate transfer bench. The client agrees, and a plan is established to have the transfer bench in the home in a week so that the therapist can train the client to use it. By making a phone call to the client a day or two before the planned visit, the practitioner can verify that the transfer bench has been obtained so the planned visit can proceed. If the bench has not been ordered or will not be delivered in time for the visit, the therapist can remind the client of the plan or revise the plan for the visit. This approach is more efficient and effective than arriving for the planned visit only to discover that the bench is not present.

A telemediated encounter may also prompt a change in the timing of an intended visit. In the example just given, the occupational therapist may decide to make a home visit a day or two later to accommodate the later-than-expected delivery of the bench. In other situations, a telemediated encounter may prompt the therapist to conduct a visit sooner than planned. For example, a client has agreed to carry out a home exercise program for her arm after a fracture. The occupational therapist calls the client a few days later to verify that the client is implementing the home program. The client reports that she has attempted to implement the program but that significant pain started after she did the exercises. This report prompts the therapist to arrange a home visit sooner than had otherwise been planned to reevaluate the exercises or to reinstruct the client.

Client and Caregiver Homework

An implied aspect of telemediated encounters is that progress toward goals depends on more than the interventions provided by the occupational therapist: It also depends on the actions of the client and the caregiver between the visit encounters. It is essential that the therapist communicate this expectation explicitly during the evaluation visit. Progress depends not only on what the practitioner does, but also on what the client does, especially between visits.

For clients or caregivers who do not want to fulfill this expectation, it may be helpful to do the math. Visits are a precious few minutes in the life of the client during the episode of care. A frequency of three visits a week represents less than 3 hours of the 100-plus hours per week that the client is awake. To achieve the goals important to the client (and the caregiver, if applicable), the third intervention strategy, homework, must be part of the plan. Assigning homework and monitoring the status of homework convey the message that both the client and the therapist are invested in the work and the progress that occurs between the visits.

Often homework involves *practice,* or repetition of an activity to improve or refine performance. If the client's performance requires the presence of an occupational therapy practitioner because of the activity's inherent risk or complexity, the client should perform the activity only when a therapist or assistant is present. If the practitioner's presence is not required, however, the client should practice such activities outside the home visit. For some clients, practice must be attended or supervised by a caregiver, such as a family member or an aide (preferably after receiving instruction from the practitioner about the desired level of performance and appropriate supervision). For other clients, practice is needed primarily to refine and establish consistency, so supervision may not be needed.

Intervention Review

Intervention review involves three aspects:

1. Reevaluating the plan and how it is implemented relative to achieving outcomes
2. Modifying the plan as needed
3. Determining the need for continuation or discontinuation of occupational therapy services and for referral to other services. (AOTA, 2014, p. S16)

To continue the metaphor of a home health episode of care as a journey, intervention review is the point at which one stops to check the map, determine whether the journey is proceeding as expected, and, if necessary, make course corrections to ensure the desired destination is reached. In some instances, a decision may be made to modify the destination, to select an alternative means to reach the destination, or even to terminate the trip entirely. Such changes might include progress occurring slower or faster than expected, unanticipated circumstances that influence progress, or new conditions that demand a revision in goals and outcomes. However, intervention review is, at some level, an iterative and ongoing process to ensure that interventions are appropriate and the course of intervention is on target to achieve desired outcomes.

> Intervention review is the point at which one stops to check the map, determine whether the journey is proceeding as expected, and, if necessary, make course corrections to ensure the desired destination is reached.

Periodic intervention review is mandated for Medicare Part A home health clients, although the regulation uses the term ***reassessment*** (CMS, 2014, § 40.2.1[b] [1][ii]; **Appendix A,** p. 185). A qualified occupational therapist (CMS, 2011c, § 484.32; see **Appendix B,** p. 202) must conduct a home visit for the purpose of reassessing the POC and progress toward achieving the therapy goals. The regulations mandate that these visits be made at least every 30 days (starting with the first occupational therapy visit). Specific requirements for reassessment also exist when more than a specific number of therapy visits (occupational therapy, physical therapy, and speech–language pathology combined) are anticipated.

It is important to recognize that both the description of intervention review in the *Standards of Practice for Occupational Therapy* (AOTA, 2015) and the federal requirement for reassessment focus on determining the continued suitability of the plan and the progress being made. Neither source suggests or implies that the intervention review include completely reevaluating the client. The federal regulation includes requirements for objective measurement, but these measurements apply to the measurement parameters identified by the goals.

So, for example, for a client who sustained a shoulder fracture and who has a goal of regaining affected extremity movement adequate to feed, dress, bathe, and wash and brush her hair, a measure could be range of motion (ROM) measurements in the affected joint, but a better measure would be adequacy of the movement to perform all of the identified activities. Obtaining repeated measures of ROM may convey progress but does not necessarily communicate function. Using activity-related motion as the measure conveys not only progress but also the functional implications. Specifically, if at baseline the client was unable to use the affected arm for any activity, a repeated measure may be stated as follows: "Improvement in using affected extremity to wash and dress lower body and to finger feed. Not yet able to feed with utensil, wash/brush hair, or wash/dress upper body using affected arm." This approach to measuring requires more words but paints a clearer picture for a reviewer to understand the improvement over baseline and the limitations that are still present.

One of the reasons for the Medicare-required reassessment is to justify the need for continued therapy. If progress toward goals is limited, the occupational therapist should consider revising the intervention plan or the goals. If meaningful progress is unlikely, then services should be terminated. These courses of action are consistent with those identified in the *Framework* (AOTA, 2014, p. S16).

Team Collaboration

Another enduring myth of home health is that of the lone clinician. For much of the history of home care, this myth had at least some legitimacy because clinicians could go about their territories untethered to smartphones, pagers, tablets, netbooks, or computers. Those days are past, however, and for as long as occupational therapy has been in home health, practitioners have been part of a home health team. In every agency, that team includes nurses, physical therapists, speech–language pathologists, social workers, and aides. The team also includes the physician who oversees the POC and supervisory and support staff. In some agencies, the team also includes dietitians, respiratory therapists, and nurse clinicians specializing in wound care or behavioral health. Of course, at the center of the team are the client and caregiver. The myth of the lone clinician is most definitely not a reality.

Team collaboration in home health encompasses many things. In this chapter, the term *team* pertains primarily to the members of the six home health disciplines—(1) nursing, (2) occupational therapy, (3) physical therapy, (4) speech–language pathology, (5) social work, and (6) home health aides—as well as the client and caregiver. Aspects of collaboration covered in the sections that follow include communication, coordination with aide services, coordination with nursing, and coherent care planning.

Communication

In home health, the number of ways team members can communicate seems to grow every year. Clinicians can tap a key or click on an icon and view documentation generated by a team member minutes or weeks earlier. Technology has made it possible for team members to quickly share information that once required phone calls, face-to-face encounters, or a trip to the records room in the office. Depending on the technology in use by a given agency, team members can use secure email, texting, or messaging systems integrated into documentation systems. *Secure* is the key word in this statement: Every agency should have policies in place regarding secure transmission of client information by both digital and analog technologies. Transmitting client information by nonsecure means (such as text or nonencrypted email from a personal smartphone or account) is a violation of federal and state patient privacy laws.

Today the challenge of communication is not that the clinician is alone. The challenge is that some clinicians choose to act like the mythical lone clinician and do not avail themselves of opportunities to communicate with their team members. Even with all of the available telecommunication technologies, home health occupational therapy practitioners must intentionally engage in communication with the team both by initiating communications with other team members and

Every agency should have policies in place regarding secure transmission of client information by both digital and analog technologies.

by receiving and responding to communications initiated by others. They must be aware of other clinicians with whom they share clients, remain current with the POCs developed for those clients by other disciplines, and stay apprised of clients' general status in reference to those POCs. The issue of communicating about other disciplines' POCs is addressed in the section "Coherent Care Planning."

Team Meetings and Case Conferences

Even with the various electronic technologies available for team communication, some communications are best accomplished in person. In home health, the most common example of in-person communication is the team meeting. In many agencies, team meetings or case conferences are held to discuss new or challenging clients. These meetings may be held on a regular basis or called only when the need arises. Often supervisory staff are present.

Team meetings and case conferences are both a responsibility and an opportunity. If a client receiving occupational therapy is to be discussed, the relevant occupational therapy practitioners have a professional responsibility to be present to report on the client's status and progress relative to occupational therapy and to acquire a better understanding of the client's status and progress relative to the domains of other disciplines. Communicating about a client within the care team in this manner promotes effective and efficient client care.

The opportunity aspect of such meetings is twofold. First, reporting on the client from the perspective of occupational therapy promotes greater understanding of the scope of occupational therapy among the members of the care team. Hearing about the client from the occupational therapy practitioner conveys far more than just reading occupational therapy documentation; hearing about the client and his or her needs or progress through the lens of occupational therapy promotes greater awareness and understanding of occupational therapy.

The second aspect of opportunity is to assist in solving other clinicians' problems, thereby increasing the demand for occupational therapy. During most case conferences or team meetings, some or even all of the meeting may be devoted to challenging clients and their needs. Even if not all of the clients discussed are receiving occupational therapy, engaging in the discussion is an opportunity to bring occupational therapy perspectives and solutions to problems other team members encounter. Engaging in this kind of problem solving may result in a new perspective or strategy that another team member opts to implement. In some cases, the result may be an occupational therapy referral being sought for the client or even other clients. Regardless of whether a referral is sought or a team member implements the advice of the occupational therapy practitioner, the result is increased understanding and appreciation of occupational therapy among the home health team. When occupational therapy is associated with solutions and effective interventions, the demand for occupational therapy referrals is likely to increase.

Joint or Overlapping Visits

Another mode for face-to-face communication is a joint or overlapping home visit with another discipline. Although this practice is not common because it requires additional planning and coordination, in some cases a planned covisit with a clinician from another discipline can enhance coordination of both disciplines' interventions. Covisits can also ensure that both clinicians, as well as the client and caregiver, share a common understanding of the client's needs and problems and of the plans and interventions for addressing those issues. For such an event to qualify as a visit, the client must be present, and elements of intervention must be identified in the POC for each of the disciplines involved. If a covisit involves two practitioners of the same discipline, it counts as only one visit, even if both practitioners deliver interventions.

Coordination With Aide Services

Aides are a critical part of the team. The primary service provided by home health aides is assistance with ADLs. One of the most common reasons for occupational therapy to be ordered is to address limitations in performance of ADLs. So coordination between occupational therapy and aide services to address a client's ADL performance is a natural collaboration, yet this collaboration can often require some facilitation. What are the keys to facilitating close collaboration between occupational therapy and home health aide services?

Aide Supervision

The first aspect influencing collaboration between occupational therapy and home health aide services is regulations that apply to the supervision of home health aide services. In federal regulations and in most state regulations, aide services are considered a part of nursing services. Home health aides are certified nursing assistants and are regulated by state boards of nursing. The federal regulations governing Medicare-certified HHAs specify that if nursing services are being provided (and are in the POC), a registered nurse must conduct the aide supervisory visits, which must occur at least every 14 days (CMS, 2011c, § 484.36). However, the regulations also state, "If the patient is not receiving skilled nursing care, but is receiving another skilled service (that is, physical therapy, occupational therapy, or speech–language pathology services), supervision may be provided by the appropriate therapist" (CMS, 2011c, § 484.36[d][1]).

Nowhere do the federal regulations define *appropriate therapist*. However, if occupational therapy is involved in the care of a client who is not receiving skilled nursing but who is receiving aide services, it seems difficult to justify why a clinician from any other therapy discipline would be more appropriate or qualified than an occupational therapist. The federal regulation specifies "appropriate therapist"; thus, the home health aide supervisory visits may be performed by an occupational therapist. The regulation does not permit aide supervisory visits by an occupational therapy (or physical therapy) assistant. In some states, nursing statutes require that any nursing personnel, including home health aides, always be supervised by nurses, even when skilled nursing services are not being provided. In these states, the stricter state requirement supersedes the federal regulation regarding supervision, meaning that an occupational therapist cannot conduct an aide supervisory visit.

Even in circumstances in which nursing must supervise the aide, it is always appropriate to coordinate the occupational therapy POC with the aide POC.

Aide Care Plan Coordination

Even in circumstances in which nursing must supervise the aide, it is always appropriate to coordinate the occupational therapy POC with the aide POC. This coordination benefits the client and the agency. Coordinating the aide POC so that intensity of assistance and frequency of service match the needs and the progress being made by the client ensures that the client is receiving consistent communication from agency staff and consistent expectations of performance. Coordination of the plans also ensures that aide personnel and resources are being used effectively to optimize client outcomes.

A second aspect of coordination between occupational therapy and aide services is coordination of discharge. Unless a client's circumstances dictate that long-term home health nursing will be needed as well as assistance with ADLs, there is no justification for aide services to continue beyond the client's discharge from occupational therapy. On the contrary, it should be common practice to discharge the client from home health aide services before discharge from occupational therapy. If a client needs long-term ADL assistance extending beyond home health care, it is appropriate to encourage the client or family to arrange alternative long-term assistance and then to discharge the client from home health aide services. It may also be appropriate for occupational therapy to provide training to any newly secured caregivers to ensure that the assistance they provide is compatible with the client's needs and abilities.

If a client has had an aide but has progressed so that assistance can be eliminated, the home health aide services should end to provide an opportunity for the occupational therapist to monitor the client's trajectory and ensure that the newly restored ADL performance is routinized and sustained before discharge from occupational therapy. Such an arrangement also provides an opportunity for further intervention by the occupational therapist if there is evidence that the newly independent performance is unstable or the trajectory is fragile.

Aide Support for the Therapy Plan of Care

A third aspect of coordination with the home health aide is for "assistance with activities that are directly supportive of skilled therapy services but do not require the skills of a therapist to be safely and effectively performed" (CMS, 2010b, § 409.45[b][1][iv]). Examples of this use of aides include coaching, prompting, or monitoring a client who is performing a home exercise program or coaching and cuing a client during practice of an activity that does not require a therapist to be present but that the client needs to refine. In some circumstances, unskilled support for skilled occupational therapy services may involve the client's performance of ADLs. For example, the client may experience fatigue at times while performing newly modified self-care routines, necessitating assistance by the aide, or the client may need prompts or reminders to incorporate new techniques or new equipment into existing routines.

Reasonable Expectations of Aides

A fourth aspect of coordinating with aide services focuses on keeping both the client's and the occupational therapy practitioner's expectations of aides reasonable. Some clients exhibit a desire or willingness to become more independent in ADLs when in the presence of the practitioner but expect or even demand more assistance than necessary when in the presence of the aide. When such situations persist or when the demands placed on the aide impede the client's progress toward goals, it may be appropriate for the therapist and the aide to conduct joint or overlapping visits. A face-to-face encounter among client, aide, and therapist can facilitate a shared understanding of what is expected of the client and of the aide. Such efforts may also facilitate strong relationships between occupational therapists and individual aides. When a joint visit is conducted, the therapist may provide education or training to the aide about roles and parameters for assistance that will maximize the client's progress, but the visit does not qualify as a therapy visit unless intervention is provided that involves the client.

Shared expectations also mean that occupational therapists must appreciate the time demands of an aide visit before attempting to incorporate newly introduced modifications or techniques into the aide POC. For example, a client who sustained a stroke may take half an hour or more to execute newly learned dressing techniques. It is unlikely that the time constraints on the aide visit will permit the aide to stand by for 30 minutes while the client attempts to dress without assistance. It may be feasible for the aide to provide distant monitoring of the client during this time while performing other related duties on the aide POC, such as preparing a meal, making the bed, or tidying the bathroom. However, if the client needs closer monitoring (e.g., because of safety concerns or fatigue) or the allotted duration of the visit still does not offer 30 minutes to monitor the client while dressing, the occupational therapist should reconsider whether distant monitoring by the aide is appropriate. Other options include refining performance to reduce the time demands before expecting to incorporate the dressing activity in the aide POC or introducing only part of the dressing task into the aide POC (e.g., upper-body dressing). More aspects of the task sequence can be added to the aide POC as performance improves and the time required decreases.

Coordination With Nursing

Coordination with nursing is an aspect of home health practice that is new to many occupational therapy practitioners who have worked in other settings. As in most other settings, coordination with other disciplines is focused primarily on other therapy disciplines, but coordination with nursing in home health is different from coordination with nursing in other settings.

Integrating Home Health Practice With Discipline-Specific Expertise

In almost every other setting involving nursing, the client is an inpatient, and assistance, including nursing care, is available 24 hours a day. In these settings, coordination with nursing involves notifying nursing about client behaviors or reported symptoms. If a nursing response is needed, a nurse is usually available immediately and on site. In home health, clients are considered medically stable enough to be at home, but their medical condition can change quickly. Family or other informal caregivers cannot always address routine care needs adequately or appropriately, which may produce urgent situations. Being a home health clinician means one is both a practitioner of one's discipline and a clinician of general home health skills and knowledge. Being a home health practitioner means acquiring some skills and knowledge that in other settings might be deemed within nursing's purview. Examples include familiarity with management of commonly prescribed medications, familiarity with normal or optimal clinical values for blood clotting (prothrombin time and international normalized ratio) or blood sugar (HbA1c), and a general understanding of wound-healing principles and best practices. Occupational

Being a home health clinician means one is both a practitioner of one's discipline and a clinician of general home health skills and knowledge.

therapy practitioners in home health have responsibilities that may require them to obtain additional skills and knowledge.

Coordinating Occupational Therapy and Nursing Interventions

In areas in which the domain of nursing and the domain of occupational therapy overlap, coordinating the goals and interventions of occupational therapy with those of nursing can optimize client outcomes. Most commonly, nursing addresses the clinical manifestations of a condition and promotes self-management, whereas occupational therapy addresses occupational performance, which also supports the client's effective self-management. For example,

- Nursing addresses self-catheterization and bowel management with a client who has a neurogenic bowel and bladder, and occupational therapy addresses the specific toileting access and hygiene needs as well as dressing and clothing adjustment so that the client can discontinue wearing incontinence products as bowel and bladder management become routinized.
- Nursing addresses diabetic diet, blood glucose monitoring, and medication teaching, and occupational therapy addresses incorporating both monitoring and medication administration into existing daily routines and incorporating dietary requirements into long-standing meal preparation and shopping habits.
- Psychiatric nursing addresses a client's depression through medication teaching and monitoring and focused counseling, and occupational therapy addresses the reestablishment of simple daily routines and incorporation of medication administration into those routines.

In each of these examples, the coordinated efforts of nursing and occupational therapy are likely to produce client outcomes that are more sustainable or more aligned with self-management than either discipline is likely to produce alone or through uncoordinated efforts. Coordination may include establishing regular communication with the nurse regarding client status and progress in the area in which the two disciplines overlap. Reinforcing instruction is another aspect of coordination. For example, asking a client whether she has checked her blood sugar or taken her medication reinforces the nurse's teaching and the importance of these activities. Reporting the client's response to the nurse can help the nurse gauge the client's learning and performance more accurately.

Coherent Care Planning

The examples of coordination among disciplines point to the theme of coherence in planning and implementing care. From the perspective of the federal regulations governing Medicare-certified HHAs, there must be a single home health POC. The contributions of each discipline are components of the plan, but the plan should convey a coherent picture of the client's current medical and functional status, the anticipated outcomes of home health services, the interventions to be provided by each discipline, and the intensity and duration of such interventions.

The way in which agency systems and documentation technologies have evolved, however, has made it easy to generate a POC but not necessarily a coherent POC. Checkboxes and pull-down menus embedded in evaluation documentation may map to specific POC elements. When all the boxes have been checked or menu items selected, a completed POC is generated. Using this process, even the POC contributions of a single discipline may lack coherence. When two or more disciplines are involved, care must be taken to ensure that the resulting POC is coherent and coordinated.

Reviewers (Medicare surveyors, accreditation surveyors, insurance or Medicare claims reviewers, and others) of a single client's POC may encounter five or more goals for each discipline, dozens of interventions, and confusing and contradictory determinations of functional limitations, activities permitted, and rehabilitation potential. Because they have no direct contact with either the client or the clinicians, reviewers depend on the POC to convey a clear picture of the client's status, anticipated outcomes of home health, and interventions to be implemented. If the POC is incoherent, it is also unlikely that the client has a clear idea of what the outcomes of home health will be, what is expected of him or her, and how the activities of the various practitioners visiting his or her home fit together.

Ideally, a coherent POC identifies a set of outcomes that both the client and the full team are committed to achieving. Discipline-specific interventions make complementary contributions toward achieving those shared goals. Interventions and frequencies are based on providing the right discipline with the right intervention at the right dosage at the right time. This is the ideal. Current reality is not congruent with this ideal, but regardless of the limitations of technologies, policies, or other factors, occupational therapy practitioners and other team members who value client-centered care, who embrace collaboration, and who strive for coherence can produce POCs and interventions that achieve meaningful outcomes for their clients and value for payers and agencies.

Communicating with other disciplines and participating in team or case conferences not only facilitate ongoing communication about clients' needs, as required in the CoPs (CMS, 2011c, § 484.14[g]; see **Appendix B,** p. 200), but also support the establishment of coordinated practice patterns. For example, if a discussion between a nurse and an occupational therapist at a case conference results in successful collaboration to achieve a client's heart failure self-management, it is likely that that particular nurse and occupational therapist will seek to collaborate again when either or both encounter a client with similar needs. Through case conferences, team meetings, and in-services, collaboration can grow from an ad hoc effort to formalized practice patterns implemented across the agency and even the home health industry.

> An understanding of the occupational therapy POC as a component—ideally an integrated component—of the home health POC should inform the therapist's reasoning as the occupational therapy POC is formulated.

An occupational therapist alone cannot enforce coherent care planning, but an understanding of the occupational therapy POC as a component—ideally an integrated component—of the home health POC should inform the therapist's reasoning as the occupational therapy POC is formulated. Occupational therapy practitioners' understanding of the goals, priorities, and concerns of the client contributes to coherence. Practitioners apply the skills of activity analysis and activity synthesis to the implementation of the POC, helping colleagues from other disciplines appreciate the client's tolerance for change and capacity for new learning in addition to the client's priorities. Discussing client capacities and expectations within the team facilitates a shared understanding and makes it more likely that team members will consider the impact of their own contributions to the POC both on the client and on the effectiveness of their colleagues' contributions.

Conclusion

The occupational therapy intervention process includes intervention planning, intervention implementation, and intervention review. Intervention planning begins during the occupational therapy evaluation visit. Drawing on the occupational profile and the analysis of selected aspects of performance, the occupational therapist identifies the trajectory of the client's performance and envisions a more favorable trajectory that could be achieved through occupational therapy intervention. This conditional future trajectory translates to possible outcomes of occupational therapy. The occupational therapist communicates this conditional future trajectory and the likely intervention approaches to achieve it with the client (and caregiver) to establish a shared vision and a shared expectation of outcomes and intervention.

Intervention planning is informed by an understanding of occupational performance and by two pragmatic factors: (1) the relevance of the goals and interventions to home health practice context and (2) the need to communicate occupational therapy services and expertise to others who are involved with the intervention plan. Goals and outcomes should reflect the effect of occupational therapy on the client's ability to manage at home and, when appropriate, should be linked to the outcomes prioritized by the HHQI. The occupational therapy intervention plan is part of the home health certification and POC. The home health POC specifies objective and measurable goals, interventions, frequency and duration of services, rehabilitation potential, and discharge plan, most of which correspond to steps or aspects of occupational therapy intervention planning (AOTA, 2014).

Intervention implementation strategies include home visits and the activities conducted during the visit, telemediated encounters that may occur between home visits, and homework activities performed by clients and caregivers between therapy encounters to promote progress toward goals. Whenever possible, intervention should be timed (by frequency and by scheduling) to promote and establish changes in performance patterns, rather than isolated instances of performance, to achieve sustainable occupational performance outcomes.

Intervention review involves taking stock of the POC and of the effects of intervention to date and, if necessary, modifying the goals or POC to adjust for unexpected changes. For Medicare beneficiaries, federal regulations mandate intervention reviews, called *therapy reassessments,* at specified time points or time frames.

Effective, efficient home health service delivery depends on a coherent POC with services that are complementary and coordinated. Occupational therapy practitioners can promote coherent POCs by communicating and coordinating with other disciplines while consistently addressing occupational performance and delivering effective interventions within the domain of occupational therapy.

References

American Occupational Therapy Association. (2014). Occupational therapy practice framework: Domain and process (3rd ed.). *American Journal of Occupational Therapy, 68*(Suppl. 1), S1–S48. http://dx.doi.org/10.5014/ajot.2014.682006

American Occupational Therapy Association. (2015). Standards of practice for occupational therapy. *American Journal of Occupational Therapy, 69*(Suppl. 3), 6913410057. http://dx.doi.org/10.5014/ajot.2015.696S06

Centers for Medicare & Medicaid Services. (2002, March 18). *Medicare program integrity manual* (Transmittal 23, Chapter 6, Exhibit 31). Baltimore: Author. Retrieved from http://www.cms.gov/Regulations-and-Guidance/Guidance/Transmittals/downloads/R23PIM.pdf

Centers for Medicare & Medicaid Services. (2010a). *Outcome-Based Quality Improvement (OBQI) manual.* Baltimore: Author. Retrieved from https://www.cms.gov/HomeHealthQualityInits/Downloads/HHQIOBQIManual.pdf

Centers for Medicare & Medicaid Services. (2010b). *Part 409.45: Aide services requirements.* Washington, DC: Author. Retrieved from http://www.gpo.gov/fdsys/pkg/CFR-2010-title42-vol2/pdf/CFR-2010-title42-vol2-sec409-45.pdf

Centers for Medicare & Medicaid Services. (2011a). Appendix B—Guidance to surveyors: Home Health Agencies. In *State operations manual* (Publication No. 100-7). Baltimore: Author. Retrieved from https://www.cms.gov/Regulations-and-Guidance/Guidance/Manuals/downloads/som107ap_b_hha.pdf

Centers for Medicare & Medicaid Services. (2011b). *Part 409.44: Skilled services requirements.* Washington, DC: Author. Retrieved from http://www.gpo.gov/fdsys/pkg/CFR-2011-title42-vol2/pdf/CFR-2011-title42-vol2-sec409-44.pdf

Centers for Medicare & Medicaid Services. (2011c). *Part 484: Home health services.* Washington, DC: Author. Retrieved from http://www.gpo.gov/fdsys/pkg/CFR-2011-title42-vol5/pdf/CFR-2011-title42-vol5-part484.pdf

Centers for Medicare & Medicaid Services. (2014). *Medicare benefit policy manual: Chapter 7—Home health services.* Retrieved from https://www.cms.gov/Regulations-and-Guidance/Guidance/Manuals/downloads//bp102c07.pdf

Institute of Medicine. (2001). *Crossing the quality chasm: A new health system for the 21st century.* Washington, DC: National Academy Press.

Law, M., Cooper, B. A., Strong, S., Stewart, D., Rigsby, P., & Letts, L. (1996). The Person–Environment–Occupation Model: A transactive approach to occupational performance. *Canadian Journal of Occupational Therapy, 63,* 9–23.

Medicare.gov. (2014). *What's home health care and what should I expect?* Retrieved from http://www.medicare.gov/what-medicare-covers/home-health-care/home-health-care-what-is-it-what-to-expect.html

Merriam-Webster. (2015). *Trajectory.* Retrieved from http://www.merriam-webster.com/dictionary/trajectory

Sackett, D. L., Straus, S. E., Richardson, W. S., Rosenberg, W., & Haynes, R. B. (2000). *Evidence-based medicine: How to practice and teach EBM* (2nd ed.). London: Churchill Livingstone.

Schell, B. A. B. (2008). Pragmatic reasoning. In B. A. B. Schell & J. W. Schell (Eds.), *Clinical and professional reasoning in occupational therapy* (pp. 169–187). Baltimore: Lippincott Williams & Wilkins.

Seltzer, G. B., & Charpentier, M. O. (1983). Maximizing independence for the elderly: The social worker in the rehabilitation center. *Journal of Gerontological Social Work, 5,* 61–79. http://dx.doi.org/10.1300/J083V05N01_04

CHAPTER 6

Sustainable Outcomes in Home Health

Carol Siebert, MS, OTR/L, FAOTA

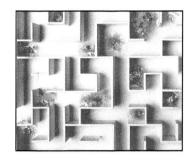

Learning Objectives

After completing this chapter, readers will be able to

- Identify sustainable outcomes in home health occupational therapy practice;
- Recognize the significance of self-management in relationship to other desired home health outcomes;
- Identify advantages and limitations of outcomes measured as end results in home health practice; and
- Recognize the relationship between trajectory and sustainable outcomes in home health practice.

Key Terms

- **end-result outcome**
- **outcomes**
- **self-management**
- **sustainable**

Introduction

An **outcome** is "something that follows as a result or consequence" (Merriam-Webster, 2015a). The term *outcome* has prominence in the lexicon of health care practice in general and in occupational therapy practice in particular. During much of the second half of the 20th century, health care practice focused primarily on problems and processes. Health care policies aligned with and reinforced this focus, with payment systems based on problems identified using *International Classification of Diseases* codes (National Center for Health Statistics & Centers for Medicare & Medicaid Services, 2015) and processes identified using *CPT®* (*Current Procedural Terminology®*) codes (American Medical Association, 2013).

Two important stakeholders began to emphasize the concept of health care outcomes: payers and clients. For payers, particularly the Medicare program, outcomes gained increasing attention as the costs of health care continued to grow. Evidence showed that the quantity and type of treatments being provided often had little to do with the results. For clients, *outcomes*—how they would live and function after a procedure or treatment—had been of primary interest all along.

In the late 20th century, technology made it possible to amass and analyze large quantities of data relating to health care procedures and costs, particularly data pertaining to the care of Medicare beneficiaries. Policy ideas caught up with consumer goals in part through intense analysis of research and data. This analysis revealed a health care system that was much like the American auto industry in the 1970s: Procedures were highly refined and specialized but often produced avoidable mistakes, and the results required frequent and intensive attention and care (repair). This examination caused a shift in how quality was defined in health care. It began to be understood that quality encompassed both *outputs* (treatments or procedures) and *outcomes* (results).

In many fields, *quality* has come to mean "doing the right things right" (Clark, 1995; McManus, Haggerty, & Murman, 2005; Pennsylvania State University, 2006). In health care, the Agency for Healthcare Research and Quality further refined this concept of *quality* as "getting the right care to the right patient at the right time—every time" ("What Is Health Care Quality and Who Decides?," 2009, para. 4). Health outcomes have come to mean

> the impact healthcare activities have on people—on their symptoms, ability to do what they want to do, and ultimately on whether they live or die. Health outcomes include whether a given disease process gets better or worse, what the costs of care are, and how satisfied clients are with the care they receive. It focuses not on *what is done* for clients but *what results* from what is done. (My Health Outcomes, 2015, para. 1)

Outcomes From the Client's Perspective

As noted earlier, outcomes have always been of concern to clients and to their families. The questions that clients or family members most often ask about outcomes are familiar: "Will I be able to stay at home?" "Will she be able to cook again?" "Will he be able to stay by himself?" In many respects, the paradigm shift toward outcomes has aligned the priorities of payers and policymakers with the priorities of clients and their families around two key questions: (1) What will the result of care be and (2) will the result matter and make a difference? This perspective aligns well with occupational therapy's purpose.

The paradigm shift toward outcomes has aligned the priorities of payers and policymakers with the priorities of clients and their families around two key questions: (1) What will the result of care be and (2) will the result matter and make a difference?

Identifying Client Expectations

Clients may not always be clear in envisioning and communicating their outcome expectations, so occupational therapy practitioners must be vigilant in seeking to identify and understand their desires. Some clients assume that the professionals providing care are aware of their expectations and desires.

Clients who have moved through acute and postacute care settings may need help to understand the unique goals of home health. They may expect that home health in general, and occupational therapy in particular, is more of the same care they have already received, but provided in the home. Often clients experience inpatient interventions focused on stabilizing or remediating impairments and come to assume that resolution of impairments will restore a prior level of health or participation (Wallenbert & Jonsson, 2005). Clients with frequent or prolonged inpatient experiences may have learned to medicalize their expectations, using the language of impairment and remediation as a proxy for expectations of health and engagement. For these clients, the explicit outcome expectation is resolution of impairments, but the implicit expectation may be sustaining important roles and regaining important occupations.

It is important for all home health clinicians to appreciate clients' expectations regarding impairments. For occupational therapy practitioners in home health, however, such awareness is not enough. It is essential that occupational therapy practitioners also uncover clients' expectations, both explicit and implicit, associated with health and participation. Identifying client expectations and desires is consistent with the domain of occupational therapy: "achieving health, well-being, and participation in life through engagement in occupation" (American Occupational Therapy Association [AOTA], 2014, p. S2). Home health provides the ideal environment for addressing clients' expectations of participation and health. No other home health team member addresses what the client expects daily life to be like when he or she is discharged from home health, so the home health occupational therapy practitioner has uniquely important opportunities and duties.

The occupational therapy practitioner has the sensitivity and clinical reasoning skills to recognize and respond to comments or questions from clients that communicate expectations. Sometimes these communications allude to roles, routines, and rituals important to the client. Box 6.1 provides a case example in which

Box 6.1. Use of a Client's Cues in Selecting Desired Outcomes

Mrs. C was a 78-year-old widow who had sustained a stroke 1 month previously. She was referred for home health care after 3 weeks of rehabilitation therapy in a skilled nursing facility. When she returned home, her extended family provided round-the-clock assistance and supervision. She could ambulate short distances with a hemi walker and close supervision, but otherwise she used a wheelchair, which she could not propel on the carpets in her home. She could approximate a gross grasp with her dominant right hand but had limited control of movement throughout the right upper extremity. Various female family members assisted her with personal care.

During the evaluation visit, the occupational therapist asked Mrs. C about her goals. Mrs. C responded, "I need my arm to work." The therapist asked Mrs. C what it would mean if her arm were working better. Mrs. C responded, "I need my arm because I'm sick of pizza." The therapist was puzzled initially but asked Mrs. C why she was sick of pizza. Mrs. C sighed and said,

> My daughters think cooking is putting something in the micro. Or they call out for pizza. Even that therapist in rehab wanted to make a pizza. That's not cooking. And if I can't get my arm to work, I'm going to be stuck with pizza or those microwave things for good.

The therapist looked around the kitchen—the room where Mrs. C was clearly most comfortable. Cupboards were full of jams and preserves Mrs. C had prepared. Her refrigerator was covered with recipes—some handwritten, some torn from magazines—all yellowed and dog-eared. The therapist replied,

> I can't make any guarantees about your arm. But I can see—you are a cook! It might take doing some things differently, but I think we can say goodbye to pizza and microwave meals. Can we agree that we're going to work on you being able to make your own meals in this kitchen?

For Mrs. C, having her arm work was not just about her arm; she associated being able to use her arm with being able to cook. For Mrs. C, cooking was not just meal preparation but rather an activity with history and meaning. She associated the loss of function in her arm with the loss of an occupation that engaged her and mattered to her. The therapist recognized that Mrs. C associated her arm function with something else—her aversion to pizza. Even though this association did not initially make sense to the therapist, the therapist chose to follow this lead to understand what it meant to the client. Mrs. C was someone who cooked, not someone who operated a microwave oven or assembled (or ordered) a pizza. Limited function in her arm likely affected many or even most of her routine activities, but the impact that most distressed her was being unable to cook. How Mrs. C gauged the effectiveness of occupational therapy was not likely to be range of motion or grip strength or even independence in meal preparation. She would gauge its effectiveness by her ability to resume cooking.

an occupational therapist takes cues from the client's expressed expectations to identify desired participation outcomes.

Promoting Client Self-Management

An outcome home health clients often desire is to "take care of myself," which often means being able to stay in the home with only the assistance necessary for safety and health. This "taking care" may involve any number of different activities and routines, although it is often focused on personal care. However, for people with chronic health conditions, an important aspect of taking care of themselves is health management and maintenance. This important instrumental activity of daily living (IADL) is well within the domain of occupational therapy (AOTA, 2014).

Self-management refers to simultaneous management of one's health or health conditions and of the role demands and emotional challenges of living with a health condition (Institute of Medicine, 2004). Managing one's own condition effectively means being able to "monitor one's condition and to effect the . . . responses necessary to maintain a satisfactory quality of life" (Barlow, Wright, Sheasby, Turner, & Hainsworth, 2002, p. 178). Self-management is often a key aspect of health management and maintenance, and practitioners should emphasize to clients that self-management is critical to achieving their goals.

For most clients, managing health conditions includes managing medication, or administering the right medication at the right dose at the right time, on a routine basis. Depending on the specific chronic conditions a client has, self-management may also include monitoring blood glucose levels, engaging in appropriately paced physical activity, adhering to specific dietary recommendations, managing supplemental oxygen, and performing daily monitoring of blood pressure or weight. Self-management means not simply performing these activities, but performing them on a routine basis so that they are integrated with other daily activities. Self-management may also necessitate altering existing activities and routines to accommodate precautions or restrictions associated with a chronic condition. Additionally, management of the condition involves monitoring one's own body and responding in a timely fashion to signs or symptoms that might indicate a worsening of the condition.

For some clients, self-management itself is an explicitly desired outcome of home health intervention. For other clients, the outcomes they desire depend on effective self-management. In either case, occupational therapy intervention may be integral to enabling clients to master specific self-management tasks (especially to achieve an optimal balance between capabilities and activity demands), incorporate self-management tasks into daily routines, and adjust existing daily activities and routines to accommodate precautions or restrictions. Addressing self-management through the lens of performance patterns, rather than simply demonstrating isolated skills or tasks, makes an important contribution to the outcome of optimal health and participation.

Sustainable Outcomes in Home Health Occupational Therapy

Outcomes are a key aspect of the occupational therapy process (AOTA, 2014). As stated in Chapter 5, the occupational therapy process is a journey taken with a client; it has a starting point and a destination. As with any other journey,

Self-management refers to simultaneous management of one's health or health conditions and of the role demands and emotional challenges of living with a health condition.

a destination is selected and the journey itself is oriented to and informed by the destination: The journey is about the destination. Although achievement of outcomes may signal the end of the occupational therapy process, desired outcomes, identified early in that process, inform or orient every other aspect of the process. In home health, outcomes drive the home health episode in which the occupational therapy process occurs.

From the occupational therapist's first contact with a client, conditional reasoning focused on outcomes begins with the end in mind (Covey, 2004). Outcomes are conceived not merely as end points or discharge indicators, but as trajectories in which home health occupational therapy intervention has made a positive difference. When outcomes drive intervention, specific goals and interventions are selected and resources are aligned for the contribution they make to the outcomes being sought. The occupational therapist has conducted an evaluation, has applied comprehensive clinical reasoning, and has formed a picture of what the client will look like on discharge and beyond—before any intervention is initiated. But practitioners must consider the sustainability of outcomes.

Sustainability and Outcomes

The term **sustainable** has a traditional meaning and a more contemporary meaning; both are applicable to occupational therapy outcomes and to home health practice. The traditional meaning is "capable of being sustained" (Merriam-Webster, 2015c); *sustain* means "keep up" or "prolong" (Merriam-Webster, 2015b). The more contemporary meaning of *sustainable* includes consideration of the resources required to support sustainability, specifically the social, economic, and natural resources required (Slaper & Hall, 2011). This meaning changes *sustainability* from a metric of the possible to a metric of the practical: Are the resources required to achieve the result worth the result achieved? Are the resources required to sustain the result reasonable?

What does sustainability mean in home health practice? The decision about whether occupational therapy is needed and, if so, what services are needed should be based not on whether occupational therapy can do something, but on what result occupational therapy can achieve, whether the result is meaningful, whether the resources needed to achieve the result are reasonable, and whether the resources to sustain the result are reasonable and available. Although these considerations may seem daunting, they are no different from those one must analyze before undertaking any journey, particularly a journey in which the goal is to remain at the destination.

Outcomes and the Home Health Context

The occupational therapy process and the outcomes achieved through occupational therapy exist within the context of home health care. Under the Medicare home health benefit and for most other insurers, home health services must be delivered in the client's place of residence, and the client must be homebound (see the section "Assessment Considerations for Homebound Status" in **Appendix A, "Medicare as Payer,"** pp. 178–179). Because the client seldom leaves the home and because intervention must be delivered at home, the outcomes selected are associated with participation within the home.

> This meaning changes *sustainability* from a metric of the possible to a metric of the practical: Are the resources required to achieve the result worth the result achieved? Are the resources required to sustain the result reasonable?

As noted in Chapter 3, the population served by home health agencies (HHAs) comprises primarily older adults who are homebound, often have multiple chronic health conditions, and may be at risk of being unable to stay in their homes and manage daily activities. The needs, priorities, and concerns of any given client drive the selection of outcomes for that client, but the home health context also informs the selection of outcomes.

Providing services in the home demands that the practitioner attend to the client's management of daily activities essential to being able to stay at home safely. These activities go beyond personal care or activities of daily living (ADLs), and even beyond IADLs such as meal preparation or laundry. Many tasks that most people take for granted are challenges or risks for clients receiving home health services. These tasks may include taking care of pets, taking care of others, retrieving mail, paying bills, managing medications and other health-related tasks, securing the home, managing illumination and ventilation, entering and exiting the home, and entering and exiting vehicles. In most cases, clients experience challenges or risks during these activities because the demands of the activities exceed the capabilities of the client. As noted in Chapter 5, focusing intervention at the intersection of client capabilities, the demands of the activity, and the characteristics of the environment can result in reduced risk and reengagement in activities essential to staying in the home.

The Medicare Perspective: End-Result Outcomes

Home health led much of the paradigm shift to a focus on outcomes among Medicare-driven practice settings. The Outcome and Assessment Information Set (OASIS) was developed and mandated to capture outcome data, guide quality improvement, configure the payment algorithm, and capture process data (see **Appendix D, "Outcome Assessment Information Set [OASIS],"** for an overview of OASIS). *Outcome* is thus a key term in the home health lexicon (see the section "Outcome Definition" in **Appendix C, "Medicare as Quality Monitor,"** p. 209).

A common method for measuring outcomes is to identify the change in status from when the intervention begins to when the intervention ends. The difference in status is the *outcome*, specifically an ***end-result outcome.*** Most of the outcomes measured on Home Health Compare and in agency-level Outcome-Based Quality Improvement (OBQI) reports are end-result outcomes (see the section "Outcome Report" in **Appendix C,** pp. 212–214). *End-result outcomes* reflect the difference in client status (clinical or functional) between the start of home health care and discharge (or transfer) from home health care. The measures used are OASIS item scores, and each end-result outcome is based on the difference between start-of-care (SOC) and discharge scores for a given OASIS item. For example, a client scores 3 (*continuous assistance*) on the OASIS bathing item at SOC and 2 (*intermittent assistance*) on the same item at discharge. Lower numbers are associated with less assistance, so the outcome in bathing is that the client improved, or became less dependent, in bathing.

Exhibit C.1 in **Appendix C** shows how this outcome is reported in aggregate for an HHA. For the current reporting period, the agency had 262 patients who were eligible to improve in bathing (SOC OASIS bathing score > 0). Of those eligible to improve, 156 patients (59.5%) actually improved in bathing.

End-result outcomes reflect the difference in client status (clinical or functional) between the start of home health care and discharge (or transfer) from home health care.

Focusing on outcomes solely from the perspective of end results has some limitations. One limitation is that an end-result outcome provides information only on the difference in status or performance between evaluation and discharge based on some predefined means of measuring status or performance. Such an outcome does not measure whether the difference is meaningful or acceptable to the client. So, for example, a change in bathing score from 3 to 2 may be meaningful to the practitioner and to the agency but not to the client or family. If the client's expectation was that intervention would result in being able to bathe in private without assistance, the client may not view the end result of 2 as a positive or desired outcome. Similarly, for the family member providing or paying for assistance, a change from continuous assistance to intermittent assistance does not reduce the amount of time the family member must be present or the hired aide must be paid to assist the client with bathing. For the client discussed in Box 6.1, improvement in bathing may not be meaningful or even relevant unless she also achieves her desired outcome, being able to cook.

Another limitation is that end-result outcomes provide no information about future status. In the previous example, the score of 2 on bathing is based on the client's ability on the day of discharge from home health as determined by the clinician conducting the discharge. Even though the difference in scores indicates that the client has improved in bathing, it cannot be assumed that the client's future performance will be consistent with the performance on the day of discharge.

Beyond End-Result Outcomes: Trajectories as Outcomes

At this time, measures obtained by a clinician during a visit are the only means HHAs have to measure end-result outcomes. However, clients and policymakers expect an end-result outcome to provide some indication of future status. Projecting a trajectory leading to an expected future status is well within the knowledge and expertise of occupational therapists.

Trajectories were discussed in Chapters 4 and 5 of this text and Self-Paced Clinical Course to identify past and expected future changes in a client's health and participation over time. Trajectories offer another way to understand outcomes that goes beyond end results. When selecting outcomes, occupational therapists must consider both the anticipated end-result outcomes (i.e., aspects of the client's health and participation at the time of discharge) and the client's health and participation in the weeks and months after discharge. This conditional reasoning is essential to ensure that the interventions selected produce truly sustainable outcomes.

The occupational therapist may base intervention on a trajectory that extends beyond home health discharge and supports the client's expectation of resuming community engagement. For example, if a client is currently dependent on other people to grocery shop and desires to resume this activity, interventions may be targeted that support this outcome, even though achievement of the outcome may occur after home health occupational therapy has ended. Similarly, for any essential task that is being managed by another person on a temporary basis, the occupational therapist should consider how the client's health and participation will be affected when this temporary assistance is no longer available. In some cases, the client may expect to resume the task and end the temporary assistance, which may be an achievable goal. In other cases, resuming the task independently may not be a feasible outcome, but the assistance is clearly temporary. In the latter

The occupational therapist may base intervention on a trajectory that extends beyond home health discharge and supports the client's expectation of resuming community engagement.

circumstance, occupational therapy intervention, often with the collaboration of social work or other disciplines, can assist in identifying and securing longer term resources that match the client's abilities and meet the client's needs.

Box 6.2 describes four scenarios in which the same end-result outcome is achieved, but the trajectories—and results for the client—are different. The difference in trajectories is based in part on a difference in interventions provided, but the difference in interventions is based on a different conceptualization of outcomes. In Scenarios 1 and 2, the interventions were focused on the end result of home health intervention. In these scenarios, there was no consideration of the sustainability of the outcome—whether it could be sustained and what resources were required to make it sustainable. In Scenario 3, intervention was intended to sustain the outcome, but whether the resources to achieve sustainability were actually available was not considered.

In Scenario 4, the desired outcome and sustainability were addressed at the time occupational therapy was initiated; implementation of intervention was aligned with the desired outcome and directed toward sustainability. Unlike the first three scenarios, the end-result outcome in Scenario 4 was congruent with and predictive of the client's future performance trajectory.

Conclusion: Occupational Therapy Is About OuTcomes

Home health was one of the first health care settings to experience public reporting of agency-level performance on the basis of client outcomes when the Home Health Compare website went live in 2003 (see the section "Empowerment of Consumers Through Public Disclosure," **Appendix C,** pp. 207–208). As the volume of data from multiple settings has grown and as the data have been scrutinized, the focus has grown not only on quality but also on value. Both clients and policymakers are seeking optimal value for health care dollars spent. Public sentiment and public policy are converging in the expectation that health care interventions should deliver results that are meaningful and sustainable.

In home health, those results can be translated to the desires that clients so often express: to stay at home, to manage being at home, and to stay out of the hospital or care facility. *Staying at home* and *managing at home* mean being able to manage daily demands effectively with minimal risk. *Staying out of the hospital or care facility* means managing one's health and health conditions. *Delivering value* means applying expertise and delivering interventions that achieve these results not for a day, not for 60 days, and not from admission through discharge, but that the client and caregivers can sustain after home health care has ended.

The outcomes associated with value—the outcomes being sought by clients, by policymakers, and by payers—are dependent on the client's engagement in a variety of occupations, engagement that is often jeopardized in home health clients. The domain of occupational therapy—what occupational therapy addresses—is "achieving health, well-being, and participation in life through engagement in occupation" (AOTA, 2014, p. S2). What occupational therapy brings is a perspective and an expertise essential to the home health enterprise. The difference between occupational therapy being an ancillary service and occupational therapy being an essential service in home health does not depend on a change in policy; rather, it depends on occupational therapy providing the outcomes and the value that clients and payers are seeking now. Occupational therapy is about OuTcomes.

Box 6.2. Four Scenarios With the Same End-Result Outcome but Different Trajectories

The desired end-result outcome for **Mrs. R,** a patient living alone, was improvement in bathing from moderate to minimal assistance as noted in a change in Outcome and Assessment Information Set (OASIS) score from 3 to 2. Nursing and a home health aide were initially ordered, and after 2 weeks nursing obtained an order for occupational therapy to address Mrs. R's activity of daily living (ADL) needs.

Scenario 1: Intervention Provided Until Occupational Therapy End Result Is Reached

Occupational therapy intervention was directed to advancing Mrs. R's bathing abilities. The home health aide continued to provide the same intensity of assistance even as the occupational therapist noted gains in Mrs. R's abilities. Her gains in ability plateaued at the point at which she needed no assistance with the bathing task but needed assistance with the transfer, even with a transfer bench.

When no further improvement seemed possible, the occupational therapist informed the nurse that Mrs. R needed minimal assistance only for bathing, specifically with the transfer, consistent with an OASIS score of 2. Occupational therapy discharged, and nursing and aide services continued. The client continued to receive moderate assistance from the aide, however, and when nursing discharged and the home health episode ended, the nurse scored the client as 3 on the OASIS item. The client and family were unable to afford or provide assistance at this level, so with no aide assistance available, Mrs. R stopped attempting to shower in the tub and was instead forced to sponge bathe from a basin.

Scenario 2: Intervention Coordinated Until Episode End Result Is Reached

Occupational therapy intervention was directed to advancing Mrs. R's bathing abilities. The occupational therapist coordinated with the nurse to modify the aide care plan as Mrs. R's bathing ability improved. Aide and occupational therapy visit frequencies were tapered. Mrs. R's gains in ability plateaued at the point at which she needed no assistance with the bathing task but needed assistance with the transfer, even with a transfer bench.

Aide services ended when nursing discharged, and occupational therapy discharged the next day. The occupational therapist scored Mrs. R as 2 on the OASIS bathing item because she continued to need assistance with the bathing transfer. However, Mrs. R and her family were unable to afford or provide assistance at this level, so Mrs. R stopped attempting to shower in the tub and was instead forced to sponge bathe from a basin.

Scenario 3: Intervention Coordinated Until End Result Achieved, With Efforts to Sustain Result

The occupational therapist coordinated with the nurse to modify the aide care plan as Mrs. R's bathing ability improved. Aide and occupational therapy visit frequencies were tapered. Reassessment indicated that Mrs. R would continue to need assistance with the bathing transfer, even with a transfer bench. The occupational therapist contacted the family member who had been the main point of contact and provided a handout on how to assist with a bathing transfer. The therapist emphasized that Mrs. R had to have assistance with the transfer to bathe safely.

Aide services ended when nursing discharged, and occupational therapy discharged the next day. The occupational therapist scored Mrs. R as 2 on the OASIS bathing item because she continued to need assistance with the bathing transfer. Once or twice a month, a family member made a special trip to Mrs. R's house to assist with the bathing transfer, but for all other bathing, Mrs. R performed sponge bathing from a basin.

Scenario 4: Intervention Based on Achieving a Sustainable Outcome

The occupational therapist discussed desired outcomes regarding bathing with Mrs. R and her family before establishing goals. Mrs. R wanted to bathe in the shower. Two family members were assisting with meal preparation, transportation, and errands but could not spend more time assisting with ADLs. The family could not afford to hire assistance.

Everyone agreed on a goal of optimizing Mrs. R's bathing ability through solutions that did not increase the time commitment required from family members. The occupational therapist coordinated the aide care plan with Mrs. R's increasing abilities so that her performance was refined at each aide visit. Reassessment by the occupational therapist indicated that Mrs. R would need continued assistance during the bathing transfer, even with a transfer bench.

The occupational therapist discussed an option for Mrs. R to bathe while her family members were already in the home assisting with instrumental activities of daily living and received tentative agreement. Aide services were suspended. On two different days, a family member was present during Mrs. R's transfer to the shower and then resumed meal preparation while she bathed. Mrs. R and her family members agreed to continue this effort. Aide services were discharged, and the occupational therapist suspended visits for 2 weeks to allow Mrs. R and her family to adjust to this change in routine. Nursing discharged during this time.

At the end of 2 weeks, Mrs. R and her family members reported that the arrangement was workable. Occupational therapy discharged, scoring Mrs. R at 2 on the OASIS bathing item. Months later, Mrs. R and her family members were continuing the arrangement, and Mrs. R continued to shower in the tub using the transfer bench.

References

American Medical Association. (2013). *CPT™ 2014.* Chicago: American Medical Association Press.

American Occupational Therapy Association. (2014). Occupational therapy practice framework: Domain and process (3rd ed.). *American Journal of Occupational Therapy, 68* (Suppl. 1), S1–S48. http://dx.doi.org/10.5014/ajot.2014.682006

Barlow, J., Wright, C., Sheasby, J., Turner, A., & Hainsworth, J. (2002). Self-management approaches for people with chronic conditions: A review. *Patient Education and Counseling, 48,* 177–187.

Clark, T. J. (1995, December). Doing the right things right. *Department of Defense Finance and Accounting Service Newsletter,* pp. 12–13.

Covey, S. R. (2004). *The 7 habits of highly effective people.* New York: Free Press.

Institute of Medicine. (2004). *First annual Crossing the Quality Chasm Summit: A focus on communities.* Washington, DC: National Academies Press.

McManus, H., Haggerty, A., & Murman, E. (2005, August). *Lean engineering: Doing the right thing right.* Paper presented at the First International Conference on Innovation and Integration in Aerospace Science, Belfast, Northern Ireland.

Merriam-Webster. (2015a). *Outcome.* Retrieved from http://www.merriam-webster.com/dictionary/outcome

Merriam-Webster. (2015b). *Sustain.* Retrieved from http://www.merriam-webster.com/dictionary/sustain

Merriam-Webster. (2015c). *Sustainable.* Retrieved from http://www.merriam-webster.com/dictionary/sustainable

My Health Outcomes. (2015). *Basic concepts of health outcomes.* Retrieved from http://myhealth outcomes.com/faqs/3000

National Center for Health Statistics & Centers for Medicare & Medicaid Services. (2015). *International classification of diseases, 10th revision, clinical modification.* Hyattsville, MD: National Center for Health Statistics.

Pennsylvania State University, Office of Planning and Institutional Assessment. (2006). Doing the right things right: Enhanced effectiveness and cost savings. *Innovation Insights Series No. 6.* Retrieved from http://www.opia.psu.edu/sites/default/files/insights006.pdf

Slaper, T. F., & Hall, T. J. (2011, Spring). The triple bottom line: What is it and how does it work? *Indiana Business Review,* pp. 4–8. Retrieved from http://www.ibrc.indiana.edu/ibr/2011/spring/pdfs/article2.pdf

Wallenbert, I., & Jonsson, H. (2005). Waiting to get better: A dilemma regarding habits in daily occupations after stroke. *American Journal of Occupational Therapy, 59,* 218–224. http://dx.doi.org/10.5014/ajot.59.2.218

What is health care quality and who decides? Hearings before the Subcommittee on Health Care of the Senate Committee on Finance, 111th Cong., testimony of Carolyn M. Clancy. (2009). Retrieved from http://www.hhs.gov/asl/testify/2009/03/t20090318b.html

CHAPTER 7

Community Resources and Living Life to Its Fullest

Ann O'Sullivan, OTR/L, LSW, FAOTA

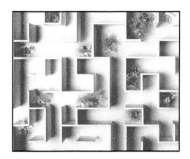

Learning Objectives

After completing this chapter, readers will be able to

- Identify challenges faced by clients and family caregivers after the home health episode ends;
- Recognize the significance of self-management in the ongoing well-being of clients and family caregivers;
- Recognize the critical role of family caregivers and challenges they face in assisting a person in the community;
- Recognize the role of the occupational therapy practitioner in facilitating the transition from home health care to self- and family management, including client reengagement with the community and assistance with caregiver needs; and
- Identify resources to help clients and family caregivers reengage and participate in their communities after the home health episode.

Key Terms

- **caregiver assessment**
- **family (informal) caregiver** *or* **caregiver** (Essential Term— see definition in the "Introduction" to this text and SPCC)
- **reengagement**
- **self-management**

Home health care can be critical in helping clients develop or regain functional skills within the context of their home environment. It is, however, a short-term service. This chapter describes the roles and needs of clients and family caregivers and suggests strategies to support their participation in meaningful life roles after the home health episode has ended.

What Happens After Home Health Finishes?

Occupational therapists use the process of evaluation, intervention, and targeting of outcomes to promote the client's end goal of achieving health, well-being, and participation in life through engagement in occupation (American Occupational Therapy Association [AOTA], 2014). Occupational therapy practitioners who work in home health can contribute to the achievement of this goal most effectively by helping clients and caregivers develop plans and identify resources for when the home health episode is finished and normal life, or a new version of it, resumes. The goal is for clients to be able to sustain the gains made during the episode of care and to reintegrate into their lives and communities.

Elements of **reengagement** include sustaining optimism about recovery, focusing on abilities, and feeling empowered to achieve personal goals, including resuming meaningful roles, enjoying social relationships and leisure activities, carrying out necessary health-related activities, feeling hopeful about life, and regaining as much independence as possible (Heart and Stroke Foundation of Ontario, 2013). Successful reintegration may require both exploration of new options and reconsideration of past and current ones.

An important element in the success of planning for life after the home health episode (which is referred to as the *ongoing plan* in this chapter) is the engagement of **family (informal) caregivers.** A *family caregiver* may be an unpaid relative, partner, friend, or neighbor who provides essential assistance to an adult or child who has an acute or chronic illness or disability or is frail or cognitively impaired. The caregiver may provide or manage some or all of the care, part-time or full-time, and may or may not live with the care recipient. Not every client needs or has a family caregiver, and not every family member is a caregiver. The resources, strategies, and suggestions in this chapter also apply to a client who does not have a caregiver.

When home health discharges the client, the caregiver may have increased responsibilities as advocate, coordinator, and provider of assistance. Before the home health episode ends, occupational therapy practitioners can help the client and caregiver plan for follow-up with physicians and therapists, learn about assuming responsibilities for tasks done by agency staff (e.g., medication management, supply ordering), consider whether privately hired help is needed and available, learn about community resources, organize care (e.g., scheduling), and consider how friends and family can help. These activities will make the transition to self- and family care management smoother and create an opportunity to problem solve proactively during a noncrisis time (United Hospital Fund [UHF], 2010).

What Can Be Done During the Episode to Support Living Life to the Fullest?

The core strategy for having clients and caregivers actively involved in the client's care is to create a culture of collaboration.

The core strategy for having clients and caregivers actively involved in the client's care is to create a culture of collaboration (Collaboration for Homecare Advances in Management and Practice [CHAMP], 2009b). Client and caregiver involvement is a key element in many positive outcomes. To promote the active engagement of clients and caregivers, occupational therapy practitioners should help them become informed, effective partners in developing and implementing individualized care plans that support **self-management** (CHAMP, 2009a). Practitioners can help identify tools, support groups, and outside services to complement the services of home care staff and to build and reinforce the care management skills of clients and their caregivers.

Achieving the active involvement of clients and caregivers in care management requires some specific skills and actions on the part of occupational therapy practitioners. A mind-set shift from "discharge" to "continuous care management" is needed. Rather than focus solely on the period when the client is directly in their care, practitioners must communicate across sites and collaborate in a partnership with other clinicians, clients, and caregivers in forming a common plan for treatment and an ongoing plan for the future. Occupational therapy practitioners can initiate ongoing planning well before the end of the home health episode and help the client and caregiver find needed resources to develop and implement the ongoing plan and manage their well-being on their own (Coleman & Fox, 2004).

Promoting Client Self-Management After Home Health Ends

A key concept in continued health and well-being is that of self-management (see the discussion of self-management as an outcome in Chapter 6). *Self-management* can be thought of as the series of ongoing decisions and actions people take that affect their health. Nine in 10 Americans ages 65 or older have at least one chronic health condition, and 77% have multiple chronic conditions (Family Caregiver Alliance, 2010). The health care system in general is more equipped to deal with acute conditions than with chronic conditions, but home care organizations serve many older adults who have multiple chronic conditions. Eight percent of Medicare beneficiaries use home health services each year, and people with chronic conditions account for 98% of home health visits (CHAMP, 2009a).

The aims of health promotion for people with disabilities are to reduce secondary conditions (e.g., obesity, hypertension, pressure sores), to enable them to maintain functional independence, to provide opportunities for leisure and enjoyment, and to enhance overall quality of life by reducing environmental barriers to good health (Rimmer, 2010). Until recently, health promotion activities have been neglected. Rimmer (2010) defined health promotion for people with disabilities as consisting of four parts: (1) promotion of healthy lifestyles and a healthy environment, (2) prevention of health complications (medical secondary conditions) and further disabling conditions, (3) preparation of people with disabilities to understand and monitor their own health and health care needs, and (4) promotion of opportunities for participation in commonly held life activities.

People with chronic conditions self-manage their care every day. They decide what to eat, whether to exercise, and whether and when they will take medications. The critical question is whether they actually make changes that have been recommended to improve their health-related behaviors and clinical outcomes (Bodenheimer, MacGregor, & Sharifi, 2005). *Self-efficacy* is a person's level of confidence that he or she can carry out a behavior necessary to reach a desired goal (Bandura, 1994), and it is an important component of any self-management program for health change.

Self-management support necessitates a fundamental shift in the client–provider relationship to an emphasis on building a partnership between them, with shared responsibility for making and carrying out health-related decisions (Bodenheimer et al., 2005). In home health, particularly, this partnership also includes the family caregiver to maximize potential for success. What do occupational therapy practitioners do during the home health episode to set the client and caregiver up for successful self-management after discharge?

> Self-management support necessitates a fundamental shift in the client–provider relationship to an emphasis on building a partnership between them, with shared responsibility for making and carrying out health-related decisions.

Promoting Client Reengagement

Since 1948, the World Health Organization (WHO) has defined *health* as "a state of complete physical, mental and social well-being and not merely the absence of disease or infirmity" (p. 100). Health-related quality of life is strongly influenced by a person's ability to participate in life (Office of Disease Prevention and Health Promotion, 2011). Supporting health and participation in life through engagement in occupation is the broad, overarching outcome of the occupational therapy intervention process (AOTA, 2014). Active engagement in occupation promotes, facilitates, and maintains health and participation.

Motivation for engagement stems from ongoing cyclical and routine participation in the everyday activities and special events that make life meaningful and worthwhile. Participation in home and community occupations involves physical, cognitive, and social activities that are the natural foundation of health and well-being. When this foundation of activity and participation is undermined by chronic illness or disability, the habits and routines that motivate and perpetuate performance and participation are compromised (Stevens-Ratchford, 2005). Occupational therapy practitioners recognize the core significance of participation in activities, habits, and routines in clients' and caregivers' quality of life.

Home health clients and caregivers often need assistance from occupational therapy practitioners in identifying remaining strengths and developing new foci and connections to adapt to changed abilities and to resume or reengage in meaningful activities of daily living (ADLs), community interests, and life roles. Reengagement, which includes a return to mainstream family and active community living and continued contributions to one's social groups and family life, is a component of the continuum of care. Reengagement in participation is considered a pivotal outcome of successful rehabilitation (Merry-Lambert & Nichol, 2009). For an individual experiencing a change in function, participation may require some adaptation of task performance, structure and support, or environmental modification, all aspects of the domain of occupational therapy. The planning and problem-solving process can be key in occupational therapy treatment.

The client's and caregiver's ongoing plan for reengagement may include addressing health issues (including prevention); identifying personal goals around family, vocational, or community involvement; addressing barriers to and facilitators for achieving goals; incorporating caregiver respite if needed; and identifying the needs of both client and caregiver for psychosocial support (e.g., stress management, problem solving, relationship changes; Heart and Stroke Foundation of Ontario, 2013).

Several factors have been identified that influence a client's successful reengagement. Clients' process of grieving for their prior life, the strength of their coping techniques before the acute episode, and their beliefs about personal responsibility all play a role in their success in reengagement. Other factors that may drive the process include their prior medical background, insurance coverage, personal support network, and ability to control the various elements of their situation (Glazer, 2005).

Role of the Family Caregiver

The Centers for Medicare & Medicaid Services (CMS) issues home health agencies' (HHAs') Patient-Related Characteristics Report, based on Outcome and Assessment Information Set (OASIS) data, which shows client attributes or circumstances that are likely to affect health status; one such circumstance is the presence of a caregiver (see the section "Outcome Report" in **Appendix C, "Medicare as Quality Monitor,"** pp. 212–214). According to national reference data reported in 2010, almost 65% of home health clients live with others, and about 80% of these caregivers are available around the clock (CMS, 2010). Caregivers of home health clients provide assistance with ADLs to 68% of clients, assistance with instrumental activities of daily living (IADLs) to 87%, medication management for 58%, and supervision or other safety help to 52%. The data clearly illustrate the important roles caregivers play in the lives of home health clients (CMS, 2010).

Transitions from one care setting to another are particularly risky (Coleman & Williams, 2007). Substantial evidence has shown that client safety can be compromised by miscommunication and failure to adequately prepare the people at the new setting to meet client needs. When the receiving "provider" is an untrained and fearful family member, the risks are multiplied. In the transition that occurs at the end of a home health episode, the client's continued health and well-being depend on the caregiver. That person must be willing and able to handle the client's complex health, financial, legal, and social needs (UHF, 2008). Engaging caregivers as early as possible in the home health episode supports both a useful and workable discharge plan and an ongoing plan for community reengagement.

Functional item scores on the OASIS are based in part on intensity of caregiving—that is, whether hands-on care, supervision, or no assistance is needed— rather than on resources needed (e.g., adaptive equipment; see the section "OASIS Occupational Performance Items and Scoring Conventions" in Chapter 4 of this text and Self-Paced Clinical Course [SPCC]). Thus, by using the OASIS to document client functional status, home health practitioners have already identified the client's need for paid or unpaid assistance, and the next step is to ensure the sustainability of that caregiving, in collaboration with the client, caregiver, and any needed outside resources (the subject of Chapter 6 of this text and SPCC).

Health care professionals have traditionally evaluated the needs of clients but not generally the needs of the caregiver, except to identify that person as a resource in discharge planning. This lack of attention to caregivers is changing, however, and professionals are increasingly transitioning the care responsibilities for very sick or disabled clients to family caregivers when the home health episode ends (UHF, 2008). Most caregivers already have a variety of occupations in their lives and do not actively seek out the occupation of caregiving; instead, it is thrust upon them, and usually they have little or no preparation (Reinhard, Levine, & Samis, 2012). Caregivers become not only an essential element of the health care system but also the first line of support for their ill or disabled relative or friend. Caregivers often experience a loss of independence and inadequate time to manage their multiple roles and responsibilities, which can change or diminish their participation in their previous occupations, roles, and routines (Moghimi, 2007).

Caregivers can make or break occupational therapy interventions. Reinforcement and buy-in by family caregivers are required to achieve success not only in client self-care but also in financial management, community mobility, home modification, fall prevention, time management, coping skills, and adjustment to disability. Occupational therapy practitioners train family members to provide appropriate assistance, implement strategies for maintaining gains achieved, and follow up on recommendations for adaptive equipment, home modification, and assistive technology. When a client lacks insight into his or her decline in function or is not ready to accept changes in daily tasks or the home environment, the caregiver may offer the only pathway to long-term adjustment and remediation of functional loss

Substantial evidence has shown that client safety can be compromised by miscommunication and failure to adequately prepare the people at the new setting to meet client needs.

(Bookwalter & Siskowski, 2010). The success of most care plans, from hospital discharge to everyday care in the home, often rests on the caregiver's shoulders (Feinberg, Wolkwitz, & Goldstein, 2006). Therefore, caregivers are a critical part of the treatment team and the ongoing well-being of the client. To engage and support caregivers, occupational therapy practitioners first need to understand them.

As discussed in Chapter 2, one of the primary barriers to understanding and addressing caregiver needs is the lack of recognition of caregivers as a type of client. Although most home health care services are based on an evaluation of the individual client, not the client–caregiver dyad, caregivers make important contributions to ensuring quality, safety, and adherence to client preferences, and their role needs to be recognized and supported. The occupational therapy evaluation should include identification of the caregiver's strengths and limitations to develop a realistic ongoing plan that ensures that both the client's well-being and the caregiver's capacities and needs are considered and addressed (UHF, 2008).

Caregiver Assessment

According to Feinberg (2008), *caregiver assessment*

> is a systematic process of gathering information to describe a caregiving situation. It identifies the particular problems, needs, resources, and strengths of the family caregiver and approaches issues from the caregiver's perspective and culture to help maintain her or his well-being. (p. 38)

The goal of caregiver assessment is to increase the occupational therapy practitioner's awareness of caregiving demands and detect any issues so that interventions can quickly be put into place to prevent adverse outcomes.

The goal of caregiver assessment is to increase the occupational therapy practitioner's awareness of caregiving demands and detect any issues so that interventions can quickly be put into place to prevent adverse outcomes. The assessment also helps the practitioner and caregiver to develop a better understanding of the rewarding aspects of the caregiving role and to help build on and strengthen these aspects (Moghimi, 2007).

In home health care, the caregiver assessment may be performed by one team member and the information made available to the rest of the team, or sections can be performed by relevant disciplines. Ideally, it should take place early enough in the home health episode to be useful in the discharge plan (UHF, 2008). Elements of a thorough caregiver assessment are listed in Table 7.1.

During the assessment, the practitioner may identify areas in which the client and caregiver will be collaborative with each other and areas in which they have competing interests. Areas of concern include who provides care, where the client and caregiver live, and how money is spent on care. The client and caregiver may not agree on how much time or assistance the caregiver can realistically provide. In cases in which conflicts are present that might compromise the client's or caregiver's well-being, a social work referral may be appropriate.

The *Occupational Therapy Practice Framework: Domain and Process* (3rd ed.; AOTA, 2014, p. S3) includes the caregiver as a client of occupational therapy and calls for caregiving to be addressed in the occupational profile and intervention plan. The *Framework* also includes care of others (including selecting and supervising paid and unpaid caregivers) as an important IADL to be addressed by occupational therapy. Practitioners' lack of recognition that they need to assess caregivers and integrate them into the plan of care is a key barrier to a successful occupational therapy

Table 7.1. Elements of the Caregiver Assessment

Category	Elements
General	What are the caregiver's background, age, education, employment, other family responsibilities, and living arrangements?
	What is the caregiver's perception of the care recipient's health and functional status?
	How long has the caregiver been providing care?
	What are the caregiver's greatest worries about caregiving?
	What are the caregiver's values and preferences regarding caregiving (e.g., distasteful tasks, willingness to accept help)?
	What is the impact of caregiving on the caregiver's emotional status and finances and on other family members?
	What is the caregiver's current level of knowledge, skills, and ability to perform necessary caregiving tasks?
	What resources are currently being used, and what resources is the caregiver interested in obtaining?
Physical status	How is the caregiver's health?
	Do the activity demands match the caregiver's physical abilities?
Time	Does the caregiver live with the client? If not, how long does it take him or her to reach the client's home? How often does the caregiver need to visit the client's home?
	Does the caregiver work?
	Does the caregiver have children or a spouse?
	Does the caregiver assist more than one person?
	How does the caregiver get time off from providing care (i.e., respite)?
Relationship between caregiver and client	How can the relationship between caregiver and client be characterized?
	What is the caregiver's relationship to the client?
	How are other family members and friends involved?
	What is the client's response to accepting help?
	Do the client, caregiver, and others involved agree on goals and a course of care?
Environment	Does the environment support client and caregiver safety?
	How far away do the caregiver and other helpers live?
	Will the environment be adaptable to meet future client and caregiver needs?
Other issues	Is the caregiver willing to provide the needed assistance?
	Are some tasks unacceptable to the caregiver?
	Has the caregiver been trained to do tasks safely and effectively?

intervention. Practitioners must understand the caregiving process itself and its effects and risks, as well as the clinical and communication skills needed to conduct an assessment (Feinberg et al., 2006).

Addressing Family Caregiver Needs

Occupational therapy practitioners can address common caregiver issues of life imbalance, stress, depression, and need for training in task performance. Practitioners can also support caregivers who experience sudden or long-term changes in their lifestyle and priorities and assist those at risk for negative health consequences (AOTA, 2007).

Occupational therapy practitioners bring broad expertise to intervene with family caregivers to facilitate caregiving and promote better health because of their unique knowledge and skills in addressing the physical, psychosocial, cognitive, sensory, and contextual elements that affect participation and engagement in everyday life activities. Specific areas of occupational therapy interventions with family caregivers include the following:

- ADL and IADL assistance and task adaptation and simplification
- Medication management

- Continence management
- Vision and visual perception
- Communication
- Cognitive strategies
- Adaptive equipment
- Body mechanics, safe mobility, and fall recovery
- Energy conservation
- Home modification
- Home and community accessibility
- Community mobility and transportation
- Community participation and engagement
- Resources for ongoing needs
- Psychosocial support
- Empowerment and self-efficacy.

Occupational therapy practitioners can support family caregivers in balancing personal needs and caregiving responsibilities by providing information on community programs, respite care, and educational opportunities and by linking caregivers to these programs (Heart and Stroke Foundation of Ontario, 2013).

Home health occupational therapy practitioners have unique access to clients' homes, families, and daily lives, and they are trained to develop a comprehensive view of clients' needs, wants, and resources. With this information, practitioners can use their insight and expertise to identify and address challenges faced by people who want to stay in their homes and communities after a home health episode (CHAMP, 2009b). To be most effective, practitioners need to understand clients' and caregivers' values and care preferences (Family Caregiver Alliance, 2000), recognize all family members' rights to make their own life choices (even if others disagree), and make every effort to incorporate evidence-based strategies into their existing routines.

Several challenges common in work with clients and caregivers involve constraints on the occupational therapy practitioner's role. Practitioners must balance competing priorities within a short time frame, recognizing that families have unmet emotional and training needs that health benefits are not designed to address. For instance, the occupational therapist may recognize that the caregiver is experiencing life imbalance because of his or her caregiving responsibilities. Although this imbalance can be addressed in the context of identifying ways to reduce the client's need for assistance, the practitioner may have to limit the time spent addressing this issue with the caregiver because payers require clinical time to be focused on the client. Practitioners may face conflicting professional roles as client advocates and service gatekeepers (Hokenstad, Hart, Gould, Halper, & Levine, 2006). For example, a practitioner may identify an unmet caregiver need but, because of reimbursement limitations or agency pressures, may feel prevented from addressing it. Overall, by engaging the client and caregiver in the development of an ongoing plan, starting early in the episode, practitioners can prioritize and maximize the effectiveness of the intervention.

The *Framework* guides occupational therapy practitioners to look at several aspects of all client situations, including activity demands, client factors,

To be most effective, practitioners need to understand clients' and caregivers' values and care preferences, recognize all family members' rights to make their own life choices (even if others disagree), and make every effort to incorporate evidence-based strategies into their existing routines.

performance skills and patterns, and context or physical environment (AOTA, 2014). The extent of overlap between client factors and family caregiver factors may determine a client's ability to reengage with and reintegrate into the community. The ability to problem solve, possession of needed skills, and availability of needed assistance are all factors that affect both client and caregiver. Occupational therapy practitioners can help identify existing strengths and areas for intervention to maximize skills and minimize obstacles to performance and engagement for the client and caregiver.

Connecting Clients and Caregivers With Community Resources

Occupational therapy practitioners can facilitate client reengagement by assisting clients and caregivers in initiating connections to community resources and the financial means to obtain them. In fact, an important factor in preparing a client for rehabilitation and community reengagement is the ability of health care providers to answer questions about available community services (Glazer, 2005). Many older people and their families do not fully understand the services that are available to help them in their communities, and finding out about these services and how to access them is a critical first step.

The many demands placed on clinicians working in HHAs sometimes take priority over helping clients and family caregivers find and obtain available resources. Agencies may reserve social work services, often key to knowledge about community resources, for their most difficult clients (Hokenstad et al., 2006). Unfortunately, because gaining access to community resources can be such an important step in client reengagement and caregiver support, failure to address this step before discharge from home health may negatively affect clients' long-term outcomes. Occupational therapy practitioners can familiarize themselves with resources in the community, match them to clients' and caregivers' identified needs and goals, and assist them in making connections and problem solving access difficulties. Knowing about services (and about how to learn more) and knowing how to help clients and caregivers overcome barriers are key to creating these important linkages.

A great deal of variation exists from area to area regarding available services. The first step is to know how to find out what resources exist. Area Agencies on Aging (AAAs) are a primary resource for learning about services and supports in the community for older adults and people with disabilities. Some AAAs are state run and some are private nonprofits, but all have a core of services, including information and referral. Every state has some kind of resource with information on services for older adults that can be identified at http://www.eldercare.gov. The U.S. Administration on Aging (which merged into the Administration for Community Living in 2012) has, over the past several years, supported the transition of AAAs into Aging and Disability Resource Centers (ADRCs) to broaden them as a resource for younger adults with disabilities as part of the No Wrong Door System and make service access simpler (Administration for Community Living, 2015). Thus, those seeking resources for a younger adult with a disability can also get needed information through an ADRC.

States have created a "211" system for information and referral. In the same way people can dial 411 for directory assistance, they can dial 211 to learn about community resources across the age span. The call is free, and each state system has developed a database of services and supports across regions. Access information for local programs can be found at http://www.211.org.

An enormous range of services and supports may be available to people in the community. Although variation exists among communities, some basic resources, described in the sections that follow, are likely to be available in most places.

Help in the Home

Many types of assistance beyond skilled care may be available to people in the home. Such assistance may include personal care, homemaking assistance, meal preparation, assistance with errands, companionship, reminders, and escorts to appointments or activities. These services may be available through agencies, privately hired individuals, or volunteer programs. Clients and caregivers with the resources to pay privately for assistance often find more options available to them than those whose care is funded through Medicaid programs, which may not cover certain services and whose funding is subject to state and federal budget constraints. The U.S. Department of Veterans Affairs (VA) also assists eligible veterans in their homes. When a client depends on a caregiver for assistance, it is prudent to use available resources as part of a backup strategy to have ready should the caregiver be unavailable (e.g., during appointments, when ill).

> When a client depends on a caregiver for assistance, it is prudent to use available resources as part of a backup strategy to have ready should the caregiver be unavailable (e.g., during appointments, when ill).

Respite Services

Respite services give family caregivers a break from their caregiving responsibilities. The National Family Caregiver Support Program defines *respite* broadly to include a break from any aspect of caregiving responsibilities (e.g., calling a client with a reminder to take medications so the caregiver does not have to make this phone call; Lewin Group, 2002). Some state-funded programs include respite components, but these programs may be limited or have waiting lists for services. Faith communities and other volunteer organizations may have people available who can help a caregiver take a break. Nonmedical home care agencies, private individuals, and the VA all may be resources for caregiver respite. Students, particularly those in schools of health care, may be available to provide relatively low-cost care.

Caregivers may need encouragement to allow someone else to provide care, and clients may need encouragement to accept it. Practitioners can provide alternative caregivers with clear information about the client's routines, preferences, communication and behavioral strategies, and interests to help set the stage for success. Caregivers often make their own self-care a low priority, and they may need guidance and support in finding some life balance. They can be encouraged to identify ways to take a break, such as meditation, exercise, yardwork, or other activities that bring satisfaction and have meaning to them.

Adult Day Programs

Adult day programs offer a safe environment in which adults can spend time with other adults and participate in activities, meals, and socialization. In general, participants return to their homes at night. Different programs accommodate different needs, so it is important for participants and family members to get a sense of the fit between person and program.

Transportation

Even while a client is homebound, occupational therapy practitioners in home health can help determine whether a client is able to drive safely, requires evaluation for adaptations or restrictions, or needs help preparing for a formal driving assessment. Although Medicare Part A rules require a person receiving home health services to be homebound (see Chapter 3), practitioners can address how the client will travel to community-based activities after discharge. Clients who are unable to continue with previous modes of transportation may need assistance in identifying alternatives so they can continue to engage in important activities. In some areas, transportation is readily available through formal or volunteer programs; in other areas, options are very limited. ADRCs can help identify resources, which might include faith communities or local service clubs. Some groups, such as the American Cancer Society, have volunteers who help transport people to treatments.

Meals

Lack of money, transportation, cognitive skills, or mobility may restrict a person's ability to obtain groceries and prepare safe and adequate meals. In addition, loss of ability to participate in meaningful occupations related to eating (e.g., cooking, socializing) may diminish a person's interest in eating. When occupational therapy practitioners determine that a client is not safe preparing his or her own meals, they can identify community resources, such as friends, family, neighbors, and faith communities, who may be willing to prepare and deliver meals. Meals on Wheels is a program funded through the Older Americans Act of 1965 (Pub. L. 89–73) that serves homebound people who are unable to get meals another way. In addition to reducing the risks of a person cooking unsafely and ensuring access to a nutritious meal, this program also offers social contact with the person delivering the meal. The program has no financial eligibility guidelines, but the Older Americans Act requires providers to request a donation from people receiving the meals. Meals may also be available to younger adults with disabilities and to caregivers who cannot leave the home because of their caregiving responsibilities.

Congregate dining sites offer an opportunity for older adults to enjoy a mealtime experience with other adults in the community. Such sites may be coordinated by AAAs or other community groups, such as faith communities or local elders groups. For those who cannot afford food, food security programs may be available; AAAs or ADRCs are a good initial contact point to find out what is available and how to connect with it.

Self-Management Resources

Self-management of chronic conditions, as discussed earlier, is an important component of ongoing well-being and the ability to participate in meaningful occupations. With increased federal, state, and grant support, many communities have evidence-based programs available to teach people the necessary skills for self-management (Lorig et al., 2001). Some programs are geared to a specific condition, such as Gateway to Wellness for people with multiple sclerosis (Neufeld & Kniepmann, 2001). Condition-based support groups offer an important opportunity for people to share related health experiences. People may also use resources such as gyms, exercise classes, or tai chi to support their own self-management.

Condition-based support groups offer an important opportunity for people to share related health experiences.

Health and Wellness Resources

Wellness can be defined as a multidimensional state of positive health characterized by quality of life and a sense of well-being (Corbin & Pangrazi, 2001). Health and wellness resources can be valuable for both clients and caregivers. Senior centers, community recreation and adult education programs, YMCAs and YWCAs, and social clubs may have opportunities for clients and caregivers to reap physical, mental, emotional, and social benefits from participation in activities. Some programs offer assistance with transportation. Other viable options include classes or individual sessions from a business or private provider in yoga, personal training, or other area of interest. Caregiver support groups can be an important resource for family caregiver wellness; the AAA can be a starting point for learning what is available.

Education Options

Staying engaged in learning about both familiar and new things can be an important factor in healthy aging (Harvard Medical School, 2010; Landau et al., 2012). Community adult education programs often have a variety of low- or no-cost classes available on a range of topics. Senior college programs are aimed specifically at older adults. For those able to travel, Road Scholar (formerly Elderhostel) may be an option. An ever-growing number of web-based educational programs are available as well that may meet the needs of clients and caregivers who are unable to leave the home.

Social Opportunities

Social opportunities are important for both clients and caregivers, either together or apart. Senior centers, community programs, and interest groups such as book clubs or bridge groups offer opportunities to socialize. Technology also offers many opportunities to stay socially engaged through email, social networking, video chat, and online discussion or support groups. Occupational therapy practitioners can help clients and family caregivers with problem solving the logistics of maintaining or developing social opportunities that are appropriate for changed physical or cognitive abilities. Helping them develop self-efficacy around this issue also gives them tools to use in the future as their situation evolves.

Geriatric Care Managers

Geriatric care managers are professionals, generally paid for privately, who assist older adults and families by assessing their situation and linking them with appropriate help. If a client is expected to have ongoing care coordination needs after home health discharge, hiring a geriatric care manager is an option to consider. Care management can be especially useful when family members are not nearby, when the primary caregiver is overwhelmed by the care recipient's needs or other life demands, or when an objective third party's input is needed.

Work and Volunteer Options

Work and volunteer occupations offer important opportunities for participation and engagement. They may provide socialization, fulfillment, and perhaps additional financial resources. Subsidized volunteer programs, such as Foster Grandparents, offer a small stipend to volunteers with low incomes. Programs through the United Way or RSVP can help match community needs with the skills and interests that clients have spent a lifetime developing.

Conclusion

Occupational therapy practitioners working in home health have both a responsibility and an opportunity to help clients resume engagement in meaningful activities in their communities after home health ends, and they have unique skills to support this effort. For many clients, the assistance of a caregiver can be pivotal in the success of the ongoing plan. Despite not being recognized as clients in their own right, caregivers should receive assessment and services to address their needs as part of the home health intervention.

A critical factor in a client's reintegration into the community is awareness of and access to resources in the community. Such resources may provide help with necessary tasks and options for engagement in meaningful activities for both clients and caregivers. Occupational therapy practitioners in home health should be mindful of the types of services, supports, and options that are available in the community and help clients and family caregivers make connections to access these resources to improve long-term outcomes for both.

Despite not being recognized as clients in their own right, caregivers should receive assessment and services to address their needs as part of the home health intervention.

References

Administration for Community Living. (2015). *Aging and Disability Resource Centers Program/ No Wrong Door System.* Washington, DC: U.S. Department of Health and Human Services. Retrieved from http://www.acl.gov/Programs/CIP/OCASD/ADRC/index.aspx

American Occupational Therapy Association. (2007). AOTA's statement on family caregivers. *American Journal of Occupational Therapy, 61,* 710. http://dx.doi.org/10.5014/ajot.61.6.710

American Occupational Therapy Association. (2014). Occupational therapy practice framework: Domain and process (3rd ed.). *American Journal of Occupational Therapy, 68*(Suppl. 1), S1–S48. http://dx.doi.org/10.5014/ajot.2014.682006

Bandura, A. (1994). Self-efficacy. In V. S. Ramachandran (Ed.), *Encyclopedia of human behavior* (Vol. 4, pp. 71–81). New York: Academic Press.

Bodenheimer, T., MacGregor, K., & Sharifi, C. (2005). *Helping patients manage their chronic conditions.* Oakland: California Health Care Foundation. Retrieved from http://www.chcf. org/publications/2005/06/helping-patients-manage-their-chronic-conditions

Bookwalter, R., & Siskowski, C. (2010). *Family caregiver: Doing double duty* (Continuing Education Course OT 268). McLean, VA: Gannett Education.

Centers for Medicare & Medicaid Services. (2010). *Outcome-Based Quality Improvement (OBQI) manual.* Baltimore: Author. Retrieved from http://www.cms.gov/Medicare/Quality-Initiatives-Patient-Assessment-Instruments/HomeHealthQualityInits/downloads/ HHQIOBQIManual.pdf

Coleman, E., & Fox, P. (2004). One patient, many places: Managing health care transitions, Part II: Practitioner skills and patient and caregiver preparation. *Annals of Long-Term Care, 12*(10), 34–39.

Coleman, E., & Williams, M. (2007). Executing high-quality care transitions: A call to do it right. *Journal of Hospital Medicine, 2,* 287–290. http://dx.doi.org/10.1002/jhm.276

Collaboration for Homecare Advances in Management and Practice. (2009a). *Care coordination, management and transitions* (Series C, Rep. 2). New York: Visiting Nurse Service of New York, Center for Homecare Policy & Research. Retrieved from http://www.champ-program.org/static/CHAMP-%20Care%20Coordination%20Management%20and%20 Transitions.pdf

Collaboration for Homecare Advances in Management and Practice. (2009b). *Framework for geriatric home health care* (Series C, Rep. 1). New York: Visiting Nurse Service of New York, Center for Home Care Policy & Research. Retrieved from http://www.champ-program. org/static/CHAMP-Overall%20Brief.pdf

Corbin, C. B., & Pangrazi, R. P. (2001). Toward a uniform definition of wellness: A commentary. *President's Council on Physical Fitness and Sports Research Digest, 3*(15), 1–8. Retrieved from https://www.presidentschallenge.org/informed/digest/docs/200112digest.pdf

Family Caregiver Alliance. (2000). *Helping families make everyday care choices* (Fact Sheet). San Francisco: National Center on Caregiving. Retrieved from https://caregiver.org/helping-families-make-everyday-care-choices

Family Caregiver Alliance. (2010). *Health care reform and family caregivers.* San Francisco: National Center on Caregiving. Retrieved from https://caregiver.org/sites/caregiver.org/files/pdfs/HCR%20provisions%20for%20caregivers-2010.pdf

Feinberg, L. F. (2008). Caregiver assessment. *American Journal of Nursing, 108*(9, Suppl.), 38–39. http://dx.doi.org/10.1097/01.NAJ.0000336412.75742.6e

Feinberg, L. F., Wolkwitz, K., & Goldstein, C. (2006). *Ahead of the curve: Emerging trends and practices in family caregiver support.* Washington, DC: AARP. Retrieved from http://assets.aarp.org/rgcenter/il/2006_09_caregiver.pdf

Glazer, D. (2005). *A physical therapist's perspective of community integration.* Birmingham, AL: National Center on Health, Physical Activity and Disability. Retrieved from http://www.nchpad.org/57/424/Physical~Therapist~s~Perspective~of~Community~Integration

Harvard Medical School. (2010). *Living better, living longer: The secrets of healthy aging.* Boston: Harvard Health.

Heart and Stroke Foundation of Ontario. (2013). *A guide for stroke caregivers.* Ottawa: Author.

Hokenstad, A., Hart, A., Gould, D., Halper, D., & Levine, C. (2006). Closing the home care case: Clinicians' perspectives on family caregiving. *Home Health Care Management and Practice, 17,* 388–397. http://dx.doi.org/10.1177/1084822305275504

Landau, S. M., Marks, S. M., Mormino, E. C., Rabinovici, G. D., Oh, H., O'Neil, J. P., . . . Jaqust, W. J. (2012). Association of lifetime cognitive engagement and low β-amyloid deposition. *Archives of Neurology, 69,* 623–629.

Lewin Group. (2002). *The National Family Caregiver Support Program resource guide.* Washington, DC: Administration on Aging, U.S. Department of Health and Human Services.

Lorig, K. R., Ritter, P., Stewart, A. L., Sobel, D. S., Brown, B. W., Jr., Bandura, A., . . . Holman, H. R. (2001). Chronic disease self-management program: 2-year health status and health care utilization outcomes. *Medical Care, 39,* 1217–1223.

Merry-Lambert, L., & Nichol, L. (2009, October). *A client-centered approach to community re-engagement.* Paper presented at the Occupational Therapy Research and Innovation Symposium, Winnipeg, Manitoba.

Moghimi, C. (2007). Issues in caregiving: The role of occupational therapy in caregiver training. *Topics in Geriatric Rehabilitation, 23,* 269–279. http://dx.doi.org/10.1097/01.TGR.0000284770.39958.79

Neufeld, P., & Kniepmann, K. (2001). Gateway to Wellness: An occupational therapy collaboration with the National Multiple Sclerosis Society. *Occupational Therapy in Health Care, 13*(3–4), 67–83. http://dx.doi.org/10.1080/J003v13n03_07

Office of Disease Prevention and Health Promotion. (2011, June 29). *Health-related quality of life and well-being.* Washington, DC: U.S. Department of Health and Human Services. Retrieved from http://www.healthypeople.gov/2020/topics-objectives/topic/health-related-quality-of-life-well-being

Older Americans Act of 1965, Pub. L. 89–73, 79 Stat. 218, 42 U.S.C. § 3001 et seq.

Reinhard, S. C., Levine, C., & Samis, S. (2012). *Home alone: Family caregivers providing complex chronic care.* Washington, DC: AARP Public Policy Institute. Retrieved from http://www.aarp.org/home-family/caregiving/info-10-2012/home-alone-family-caregivers-providing-complex-chronic-care.html

Rimmer, J. (2010). *Health promotion for people with disabilities: The emerging paradigm shift from disability prevention to prevention of secondary conditions.* Birmingham, AL: National Center on Health, Physical Activity and Disability. Retrieved from http://www.nchpad.org/123/996/Health~Promotion~for~People~With~Disabilities~~The~Emerging~Paradigm~Shift~From~Disability~Prevention~to~Prevention~of~Secondary~Conditions

Stevens-Ratchford, R. (2005). Occupational engagement: Motivation for older adult participation. *Topics in Geriatric Rehabilitation, 21,* 171–181.

United Hospital Fund. (2008). *Assessing family caregivers: A guide for health care providers.* New York: Author. Retrieved from http://nextstepincare.org/uploads/File/Guides/Provider/Assessing_Family_Caregivers.pdf

United Hospital Fund. (2010). *When home care ends: A family caregiver's guide.* Retrieved from http://nextstepincare.org/uploads/File/Guides/Home_Care/When_HC_Ends/When_Home_Care_Ends.pdf

World Health Organization. (1948). *Preamble to the Constitution of the World Health Organization as adopted by the International Health Conference, New York, 19–22 June, 1946; signed on 22 July 1946 by the representatives of 61 States (Official Records of the World Health Organization, no. 2, p. 100) and entered into force on 7 April 1948.* Retrieved from http://www.who.int/about/definition/en/print.html

Section III: Home Health and the Occupational Therapy Profession

INTRODUCTION TO

"Home Health and the Occupational Therapy Profession"

Karen Vance, BSOT

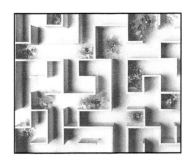

To this point, this text and Self-Paced Clinical Course has provided guidance for successful occupational therapy practice in the home health setting. The chapter in this section—Chapter 8, "Home Health Occupational Therapy Practitioners and the Occupational Therapy Profession"—addresses how occupational therapy practitioners in home health can be successful in this practice setting, how occupational therapy educators and researchers can support the profession's growth and success in this practice area, and how home health administrators and managers can recruit and retain occupational therapy practitioners who use best practices.

Chapter 8 begins by providing information about qualifications and competencies required to practice occupational therapy in home health. This chapter then discusses the many traditional and nontraditional roles available for occupational therapy practitioners choosing to pursue a career in this practice setting and implications for education and research. Guidance on practitioner preparation and professional development, including elements of a mentoring program, is provided. Finally, this chapter addresses misperceptions about occupational therapy by some in the home health industry.

In sum, Chapter 8 provides guidance and structure for both the home health agency as an employer and occupational therapy practitioners to ensure the most appropriate utilization of occupational therapy services in home health. Using this guidance and structure to full advantage can help practitioners elevate their practice and exceed the expectations of all stakeholders and, most important, the occupational therapy profession itself.

CHAPTER 8

Home Health Occupational Therapy Practitioners and the Occupational Therapy Profession

Tina Shadley, OTR/L, and
Carol Siebert, MS, OTR/L, FAOTA

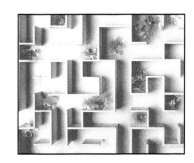

Learning Objectives

After completing this chapter, readers will be able to
- Identify the qualifications and competencies necessary for a home health occupational therapy practitioner;
- Recognize roles in home health agencies and in the home health industry available for occupational therapists and occupational therapy assistants on the basis of qualifications;
- Identify ways that occupational therapy education, research, and practitioner preparation and professional development can sustain occupational therapy's stake in home health;
- Recognize the benefits of a mentoring program to support the professional development of practitioners in home health; and
- Identify misperceptions about the extent of occupational therapy's role in the home health industry.

Introduction

Between 2005 and 2009, the number of Medicare-certified home health agencies (HHAs) grew by 28.7% (National Association for Home Care & Hospice, 2010). During that same interval, the number of Medicare beneficiaries receiving home health per year grew by 10.3% (Centers for Medicare & Medicaid Services [CMS], 2010a). These numbers suggest that the number of occupational therapy practitioners working in home health should also have grown during the same interval. Yet studies of the occupational therapy workforce have not supported this contention. In 2010, a study conducted by the American Occupational Therapy Association (AOTA; 2010b) indicated that 5.8% of the occupational therapy workforce was working in home health. A similar study conducted in 2006 indicated that 6.9% of the workforce worked in home health (AOTA, 2006). Taken together, the workforce study results suggest that the proportion of occupational therapy practitioners working in home health is declining, even as industry data suggest a growing demand for personnel.

Key Terms

- **clinician** (Essential Term—see definition in the "Introduction" to this text and SPCC)
- **Conditions of Participation**
- **entry level**
- **home health competencies**
- **mentoring**
- **occupational therapy competencies**
- **precepting**
- **qualified occupational therapist**
- **qualified occupational therapy assistant**

This apparent discrepancy between growing demand and declining practitioner supply is both puzzling and troubling. The Home Health Quality Initiative has prioritized outcomes associated with function that include not only the more obvious functional outcome indicators (e.g., being able to bathe or get to the toilet) but also outcome indicators that are more subtle but still relevant to performance (e.g., activity affected by dyspnea, pain with activity, management of medications; CMS, 2010b, 2014a). This initiative's emphasis on routine, daily activities suggests a need for more occupational therapy practitioners, not fewer. Within the occupational therapy profession and among HHAs, the significant shortage of occupational therapy practitioners in home care is generally recognized. Our experience over several years of staffing the AOTA exhibit at National Association for Home Care & Hospice annual conferences indicates that HHA administrators and managers are actively seeking strategies to successfully recruit and retain occupational therapy practitioners.

The occupational therapy profession has a significant stake in home health care. Historically, occupational therapy has been underused in home health care (Cisneros, 2008). With the aging of the population and growing longevity, it is reasonable to expect that the home health population will increase. With this increase will come a growing demand for home health services to sustain functional abilities, self-management, and the ability to live safely at home. Occupational therapy brings unique knowledge and critical expertise to meet this demand. It is critical to the future of the profession that occupational therapy's presence in this practice setting continue to grow and that occupational therapy's contribution to home health care be recognized and depended on.

Individual occupational therapy practitioners working in home health also have a stake. In much of the home health literature and in trade publications, the term **_clinician_** continues to be used synonymously with _nurse_ (in this text and Self-Paced Clinical Course [SPCC], _clinician_ refers to all health care professionals inclusively and is not discipline specific). The home health industry has only recently begun to recognize both the presence and the contributions of the therapy disciplines—occupational therapy, physical therapy, and speech–language pathology—to home health care. For home health to be a setting in which occupational therapy practitioners establish careers, both practitioners and HHA administrators must update their perceptions of occupational therapy in this practice setting. Occupational therapy practitioners who want to work long term in this practice setting—to establish a home health career—have a critical stake not only in their own success but also in the success of the clients they serve and of the agency and industry in which they work.

> Occupational therapy practitioners who want to work long term in this practice setting—to establish a home health career—have a critical stake not only in their own success but also in the success of the clients they serve and of the agency and industry in which they work.

This chapter addresses aspects of being successful and established in home health occupational therapy practice. It is written for three audiences: (1) occupational therapy practitioners working or interested in working in home health who want to be successful in this practice setting, (2) occupational therapy educators and scientists who want to support the profession's growth and success in this practice area, and (3) home health administrators and managers who want to successfully recruit and retain occupational therapy practitioners who want to be professionally challenged and fulfilled.

Qualifications to Work in Home Health

Occupational therapists and occupational therapy assistants must meet specific personnel qualifications to work in home health. For Medicare-certified HHAs, the personnel qualifications are specified in federal regulations as part of the HHA **Conditions of Participation** (CoPs) in the *Code of Federal Regulations* (CFR), Title 42, Part 484 (CMS, 2011). When the CoPs, the *Medicare Benefit Policy Manual* (CMS, 2014b), or other documents refer to a *qualified therapist* or *qualified therapy assistant,* they mean therapists (or assistants) who meet the qualifications stated in the CoPs.

Occupational Therapist Qualifications in the Federal Regulations

The qualifications in the CoPs were revised and updated in the first decade of this century to be consistent with current education, professional credentialing, and state regulation of occupational therapy (see the section "Personnel Qualifications" in **Appendix B, "Medicare as Regulator,"** pp. 198–200). Section 484.4 (CMS, 2011, p. 115) states that a ***qualified occupational therapist*** is a person who meets all of the following criteria:

(1) Is licensed or otherwise regulated, if applicable, as an occupational therapist by the State in which practicing, unless licensure does not apply;

(2) Graduated after successful completion of an occupational therapist education program accredited by the Accreditation Council for Occupational Therapy Education (ACOTE) of the American Occupational Therapy Association, Inc. (AOTA), or successor organizations of ACOTE; and

(3) Is eligible to take, or has successfully completed the entry-level certification examination for occupational therapists developed and administered by the National Board for Certification in Occupational Therapy, Inc. (NBCOT).

The same qualifications apply to occupational therapists educated outside the United States, with one difference; they must have graduated from an occupational therapy program accredited by ACOTE, a successor organization of ACOTE, the World Federation of Occupational Therapists, or a credentialing body approved by AOTA.

These qualifications specify that an occupational therapist is a qualified occupational therapist in home health if he or she has been educated by an ACOTE-accredited program, has passed or is eligible to take the certification examination administered by the NBCOT, and is licensed or otherwise regulated by the state in which he or she is practicing. The CoPs do not require a qualified occupational therapist to have work experience before working in home health.

Occupational Therapy Assistant Qualifications in the Federal Regulations

Section 484.4 (CMS, 2011, p. 116) states that a **qualified occupational therapy assistant** is a person who meets all of the following criteria:

(1) Is licensed, unless licensure does not apply, or otherwise regulated, if applicable, as an occupational therapy assistant by the State in which practicing.

(2) Graduated after successful completion of an occupational therapy assistant education program accredited by the Accreditation Council for Occupational Therapy Education (ACOTE) of the American Occupational Therapy Association, Inc. (AOTA) or its successor organizations.

(3) Is eligible to take or successfully completed the entry-level certification examination for occupational therapy assistants developed and administered by the National Board for Certification in Occupational Therapy, Inc. (NBCOT).

These qualifications specify that an occupational therapy assistant is a qualified occupational therapy assistant in home health if he or she has been educated by an ACOTE-accredited program, has passed or is eligible to take the certification examination administered by NBCOT, and is licensed or otherwise regulated by the state in which he or she is practicing. Again, the CoPs do not require a qualified occupational therapy assistant to have work experience before working in home health.

State Licensure and State Regulation

In addition to the qualifications specified in the CoPs, the state or territory may establish additional qualifications. If a state requires licensure or registration of occupational therapists or occupational therapy assistants, then to provide home health services the therapist or assistant must hold a license from or be listed in the registry of the state in which the client lives. If an HHA's service territory crosses state boundaries, therapists and assistants must hold a license or be registered in every state in which they provide services.

Any therapist or assistant planning to work in home health, and any HHA hiring occupational therapy practitioners, should consult with the state agency that regulates occupational therapy to identify any additional requirements.

In addition to licensure or registration, the occupational therapy practice acts or regulations of some states specify additional requirements for an occupational therapist or occupational therapy assistant to work in home health. Any therapist or assistant planning to work in home health, and any HHA hiring occupational therapy practitioners, should consult with the state agency that regulates occupational therapy to identify any additional requirements. The two most common state-imposed requirements are (1) work experience before working in home health and (2) caseload size or supervision intensity applicable to the therapist–assistant supervisory relationship.

Competencies for Home Health Practice

To be successful in home health practice, an occupational therapy practitioner must demonstrate two different but related classes of competencies: **home health competencies** and **occupational therapy competencies.** The sections that follow explore these two types of competencies.

Home Health Clinician Competencies

Home health competencies are those that any home health clinician (again, *clinician* refers to all health care professionals inclusively) must demonstrate, regardless of discipline. Home health practice demands a set of clinician competencies that differ in many ways from competencies necessary in other practice settings. Providing services to clients in their homes demands skills, knowledge, and behavior that differ from those required in a traditional inpatient or outpatient care setting. For a seasoned home health clinician or manager, these aspects of home health practice may seem so familiar and common that they may not be recognized as competencies, but they are essential to effective and successful practice in home health. Table 8.1 lists examples of home health competencies and the aspects (knowledge, skill or ability, critical and ethical reasoning, interpersonal skills) associated with each.

Table 8.1. **Examples of Home Health Clinician Competencies**

Competency	Aspect of Competency
Logistical	
Locate client residence	Skill
Navigate to client residence efficiently	Skill or ability
Identify, maintain, and transport supplies and materials needed for evaluation and intervention	Critical reasoning Skill or ability
Adhere to and implement universal precautions	Knowledge Skill or ability
Manage and complete documentation according to the requirements of the documentation system and agency policy	Knowledge Critical reasoning Skill or ability
Manage dual roles as professional and guest in the home	Knowledge Critical and ethical reasoning Interpersonal skills Ability
Health monitoring and responding	
Monitor vital signs	Knowledge Skill or ability
Monitor for signs and report those indicating an adverse change in condition	Knowledge Critical reasoning Interpersonal skills Ability
Monitor client response and adherence to home health interventions	Knowledge Critical reasoning
Respond to adverse changes in client condition	Knowledge Critical reasoning Skill
Monitor circumstances in and around the home that may affect client health, safety, and well-being	Knowledge Critical reasoning Interpersonal skills
Related to regulatory and payment requirements	
Conduct comprehensive assessment, including collection of OASIS data and completion of drug regimen review[a]	Knowledge Critical reasoning Interpersonal skills Skill or ability
Supervise home health aide, conduct aide supervisory visits, and manage aide care plan[a]	Knowledge Critical reasoning Interpersonal skills Skill or ability
Monitor and appraise homebound status	Knowledge Critical reasoning
Communicate effectively with other disciplines through designated modes of communication and coordination	Knowledge Interpersonal skills Critical reasoning

Note. OASIS = Outcome and Assessment Information Set.
[a]Competency pertinent to registered nurses and therapists only; related tasks may not be delegated to practical nurses or therapy assistants.

Unlike other practice settings, clients' homes have no crash carts, response teams, or defibrillators. Monitoring clients is a responsibility that all home health clinicians must carry out during client encounters, as is responding to any conditions detected by such monitoring that may affect the client's safety, health, or well-being. Monitoring may include specific tasks, such as checking vital signs, but it also includes eliciting reports of any new symptoms, monitoring for signs that a condition is deteriorating or improving, and noting the client's response to or implementation of prior instruction.

Regulatory and payer coverage requirements are the basis of agency policies and procedures and can be found in **Appendix A, "Medicare as Payer,"** and **Appendix B, "Medicare as Regulator."** (Chapter 1 of this text and SPCC describes the responsibility of occupational therapy practitioners in following these requirements.) Regulation and accreditation require that HHAs establish competencies for all clinicians; *establishing competencies* includes both identifying necessary competencies and verifying that clinicians demonstrate competency.

Occupational Therapy Competencies

Occupational therapy competencies are "knowledge, performance skills, interpersonal abilities, critical reasoning, and ethical reasoning skills necessary to perform current and future roles and responsibilities within the profession" (AOTA, 2015, p. 1). Occupational therapy competencies for home health include competencies supporting generalist occupational therapy practice and competencies specific to occupational therapy practice in this setting. Generalist competencies are relevant across multiple practice settings and populations, such as the ability to elicit an occupational profile, analyze selected aspects of occupational performance, and collaborate with a client to identify desired outcomes and goals.

Occupational therapy competencies more specific to home health practice include knowledge competencies, such as knowledge of conditions and impairments prevalent in the home health setting; critical reasoning competencies, such as identifying the appropriate durable medical equipment compatible with the client's abilities and the constraints of the home environment; skills, such as operating a floor-based lift safely and correctly; and interpersonal skills, such as effectively teaching a low-literacy caregiver how to operate a lift to transfer the client safely. Table 8.2 provides examples of home health occupational therapy competencies, including those relevant to both therapists and assistants and those relevant to therapists only and to assistants only; required competencies may vary among agencies to meet the needs of the agency and the specific home health population served.

Roles of Home Health Occupational Therapy Practitioners

The most obvious role is that of clinician on the home health clinical team. However, other roles are also available that constitute career opportunities for occupational therapy practitioners in home health.

Occupational therapists and occupational therapy assistants, depending on their qualifications, may hold a variety of roles in home health. The most obvious role is that of clinician on the home health clinical team. However, other roles are also available that constitute career opportunities for occupational therapy practitioners in home health. These roles are described briefly in the following sections.

Clinician

Clinician is the role held by most occupational therapists and occupational therapy assistants working in home health; much of this text and SPCC is written for those in that role. The role of clinician has several different aspects: provider of a skilled service, member of a clinical team, and, in many cases, clinical educator.

Table 8.2. Examples of Home Health Occupational Therapy Competencies

Type of Practitioner	Competency[a]
Occupational therapist, occupational therapy assistant	**Knowledge competencies** • Mastery of the occupational therapy process as it is applied in home health • Integration of relevant evidence, literature, and epidemiological data related to home health clinician responsibilities and the home health population • Integration into practice of current professional guidance regarding practice and legislative, legal, and regulatory issues • Ability to anticipate what new knowledge is necessary to meet the needs of the home health population **Critical reasoning competencies** • Use of deductive and inductive reasoning in making decisions specific to roles and responsibilities • Problem-solving skills necessary to carry out responsibilities • Ability to analyze occupational performance as influenced by environmental factors, including the physical, social, and cultural environment • Ability to reflect on one's own practice • Management and synthesis of information from a variety of sources in support of making decisions • Application of evidence, research findings, and outcome data in making decisions • Ability to assess previous assumptions against new evidence and revise decision making accordingly **Interpersonal skill competencies** • Use of effective communication methods that match the abilities, personal factors, learning styles, and therapeutic needs of clients, caregivers, clinical team members, and administrative staff • Effective interaction with people from diverse backgrounds • Use of feedback from clients, supervisors, and colleagues to modify professional behavior • Collaboration with clients and professionals to attain optimal client outcomes • Ability to develop, sustain, and refine team relationships to meet identified outcomes **Performance competencies** • Practice grounded in the occupational therapy process • Therapeutic use of self, therapeutic use of occupations and activities, use of the consultation process, and provision of client education to bring about change and achieve outcomes • Integration of current practice techniques and technologies • Selection and implementation of interventions on the basis of current best evidence, clinical experience, and client values and preferences • Ability to update performance on the basis of current evidence with consideration given to client desires and clinician judgment • Implementation of quality improvement processes that prevent practice error and optimize client outcomes **Ethical practice competencies** • Understanding of and adherence to the current version of the *Occupational Therapy Code of Ethics* (AOTA, 2015a), other relevant codes of ethics, and applicable laws and regulations • Use of ethical principles and the occupational therapy profession's core values to understand complex situations • Integrity to make and defend decisions on the basis of ethical reasoning • Integration of varying perspectives in the ethics of clinical practice
Home health occupational therapist	• Evaluation of clients in the home to identify aspects of the domain of occupational therapy contributing to limitations in performance or risks to safety • Collaboration with clients and caregivers to identify goals and outcomes • Formulation of the occupational therapy intervention plan as part of the home health plan of care to effectively and efficiently achieve identified goals • Reassessment of the intervention plan intermittently and at required time points to gauge progress, identify and respond to unanticipated changes in client status, and revise goals or plan as needed in response to such changes • Accurate identification of when goals are met or when occupational therapy services are no longer necessary for the client to meet his or her goals • Delegation of responsibilities to occupational therapy assistants on the basis of current and anticipated client status and the demonstrated competencies of the occupational therapy assistant • Active engagement in the process of supervising occupational therapy assistants, including assessment and development of the assistant's competencies
Home health occupational therapy assistant	• Performance of standardized assessments as delegated by the supervising occupational therapist • Provision of timely feedback to the supervising occupational therapist regarding implementation of the occupational therapy intervention plan and any unanticipated changes in the client's status • Informing the supervising occupational therapist of any needs to develop competencies • Active engagement in the supervision process

Note. AOTA = American Occupational Therapy Association.
[a]Competency categories are from AOTA (2015b).

Provider of a Skilled Service

Medicare regulations and coverage policies refer to *skilled occupational therapy* (see "§ 40.2, Skilled Therapy Services," in **Appendix A,** p. 183). Occupational therapy is one of four skilled services provided in home health. A home health occupational therapist is a professional who brings a high level of expertise and knowledge to the HHA to evaluate and address the needs of home health clients in relation to their desired occupations. For this population, those occupations most often pertain to being able to manage in the home, being able to live safely at home, and being able to incorporate management of various health conditions. A home health occupational therapy assistant brings important expertise and knowledge to provide interventions related to these needs.

Clinical Team Member

The home health occupational therapy practitioner is also a member of the clinical team providing services to home health clients served by the agency. Although client encounters typically occur one-on-one with the practitioner, any given client may be receiving services from multiple disciplines. The occupational therapy practitioner is part of the clinical team and is responsible for coordinating with the other team members to optimize the care and the outcomes achieved for any given client.

There is a second aspect of being part of the home health clinical team: Not all clients receive occupational therapy services, but being a part of the team also means being available to consult with other team members to problem solve, to advise, and thus to optimize the care provided to all agency clients. In some cases, such consultation may identify the need for a referral to occupational therapy services. In other cases, consultation may offer another clinician valuable insights or perspectives that he or she can then pursue with a client even though the client is not receiving occupational therapy as a skilled service.

Clinical Educator

The role of clinical educator is often overlooked in home health. Whenever more than one occupational therapy practitioner is working at an HHA, the opportunity exists to educate and to be educated by occupational therapy colleagues. When occupational therapy assistants are part of the team, education is an essential part of the supervisory relationship, and that education can be mutual.

Home health occupational therapy practitioners may also opt for the role of fieldwork educator for occupational therapy students doing their fieldwork placements. Fieldwork educators expose students to and prepare them for the home health practice setting. Being a fieldwork educator also provides practitioners the opportunity to learn about new theories or practices from students and the chance to discuss and problem solve client situations with someone else over the course of the day, an experience typically not available in home health practice.

Other Roles and Career Opportunities

Careers for occupational therapy practitioners in home health are not limited to the role of clinician. As the home health industry grows, new roles and positions are continually being created. Many of these career opportunities are ideally suited to occupational therapy practitioners who have worked as clinicians in home health but who seek either new challenges or a broader span of responsibility and influence.

Only a very few positions in home health (e.g., clinical director) are mandated by regulation to be filled by a specific discipline, so occupational therapy practitioners may be qualified for positions other than clinician within an HHA or in the home health industry. Although currently relatively few occupational therapy practitioners are in most of these roles, familiarity with them may provide readers with a new perspective on and new horizons for establishing a career in home health occupational therapy. The following sections describe several such positions or roles.

Therapy Manager

Many HHAs elect to create a therapy manager position to manage the therapists on the clinical team. The responsibilities of this position vary. In some agencies, the therapist in this role provides overall administrative supervision of the agency's therapists; in others, the position may include additional management and administrative responsibilities. Typically, the position does not include discipline-specific or clinical supervision. Nothing in the CoPs dictates the qualifications of a clinical or therapy manager, and there is no prohibition on occupational therapy practitioners holding such a position. Occupational therapy practitioners in this role assume greater responsibility within the agency and have a greater opportunity to influence agency decisions. Some agencies may create a clinical manager position similar to a therapy manager position in which the manager oversees a team of clinicians, including not only therapists but also nurses, aides, and social workers; this model for managing clinicians is less common.

Quality Improvement Coordinator

Many HHAs have a designated quality improvement coordinator. Although in many agencies this role is assumed by a nurse, there is no federal requirement for the position and, thus, no requirement for a specific discipline to hold the position. The quality improvement coordinator's role is directed toward identifying areas for improvement across the agency, identifying practices to produce improvement, coordinating implementation efforts, and evaluating the effectiveness of such efforts. Typically, the quality improvement coordinator works with all clinical teams and all disciplines as well as with administrative and support staff. Occupational therapy practitioners with an interest in improving and refining practice at the agency level may find this position an attractive career option.

> The quality improvement coordinator's role is directed toward identifying areas for improvement across the agency, identifying practices to produce improvement, coordinating implementation efforts, and evaluating the effectiveness of such efforts.

Administrator or Executive

The number and titles of administrative and executive positions in home health vary across agencies and according to the size of the organization. Often, such positions require additional education in health or business administration or a similar field. Occupational therapy practitioners with an interest in the financial or operations aspects of home health who have the appropriate qualifications may find career opportunities in such positions. Combining the knowledge and experience of a home health clinician with expertise in operations management, financial management, or organizational leadership offers an attractive career path to occupational therapy practitioners with the necessary qualifications.

Consultant

In the home health industry, a wide variety of organizations provide resources and services to HHAs. Examples include software vendors and organizations providing resources and services related to regulatory compliance, financial management, quality improvement, and development of specialty product lines, among others. Occupational therapy practitioners who have worked as clinicians in home health may find career opportunities with these entities, which are external to HHAs but whose services support and influence agency operations. One particular area in which a stronger occupational therapy presence is needed is in the development of documentation software to ensure that the templates that shape occupational therapy documentation are consistent with the domain and expertise of occupational therapy. Seeking a role with any of these consultative entities provides home health occupational therapy practitioners who have the necessary qualifications an opportunity to influence the home health industry.

Issues for Occupational Therapy Education

One of the enduring perceptions of occupational therapy practice in home health is that it is not **entry-level** practice—that any occupational therapy practitioner intending to work in home health must first have experience in other settings before working in home health. In some states, this notion has been codified in the occupational therapy practice act or in the associated regulation. In these states, occupational therapy practitioners must have 1 or 2 years of practice in other practice venues before working in home health. In all other jurisdictions, however, no such requirement exists.

As the population served by home health continues to grow, and as health care continues to shift toward community-based care rather than inpatient care, home health care will likely become the leading service setting for clients needing time-limited skilled care. This shift mirrors health care patterns in many other countries, where health care delivered in the home is the dominant means of health service delivery for certain populations. For occupational therapy to be an integral aspect of home health care, it is essential that practitioners, educators, and administrators recognize that home health practice is an appropriate practice setting for entry-level practitioners.

Home health practice must be addressed and taught as part of entry-level occupational therapy and occupational therapy assistant education. Educational curricula must reflect the growing presence of home health services, rather than inpatient services, in the lives of older adults and people with chronic health conditions. Including content on home health may be a challenge for faculty who are not familiar with home health practice, but they can call on experienced home health practitioners as course consultants and guest lecturers if necessary. Case examples and course assignments referencing home health must be as common as those referencing practice in inpatient settings or outpatient clinics. Occupational therapy students' awareness of home health practice must begin as early as possible in their academic careers.

Fieldwork experiences in home health must expand. One of the most powerful ways for students to become aware of home health practice is to observe and participate in the practice through a Level I fieldwork experience. Such an experience

Educational curricula must reflect the growing presence of home health services, rather than inpatient services, in the lives of older adults and people with chronic health conditions.

has a powerful effect not only on students who participate but also on those students' classmates as they share experiences formally in course work and informally in casual conversation. Supervising a Level I fieldwork student requires only a limited time commitment from home health occupational therapists and agencies, particularly because travel time between clients is an ideal opportunity to discuss and debrief.

Supervising a Level II fieldwork student in home health requires a more significant commitment from a home health occupational therapy practitioner and agency. Ideally, this fieldwork experience should be offered only when at least one occupational therapist is available other than the designated clinical educator so the student has the opportunity to observe and learn from more than one practitioner and another practitioner is always available when the designated clinical educator is out. It is neither practical nor advisable for a Level II fieldwork student to conduct home visits independently, but fieldwork educators have a variety of options for adjusting the intensity of supervision while still being on site in the home.

For educational programs, embracing home health fieldwork creates the need for a larger and more varied pool of fieldwork sites and fieldwork educators. For home health practitioners, being a fieldwork educator is an opportunity to develop and refine skills, to challenge their own knowledge, and to contribute to the growth and knowledge of an entry-level practitioner. For HHAs, the decision to serve as a fieldwork site builds relationships with academic programs and ultimately increases the availability of occupational therapy practitioners prepared for and excited about working in home health.

Issues for Occupational Therapy Research

Occupational therapy in home health is practice in the natural environment. Yet there is a paucity of assessments, intervention protocols, and outcome studies specific to occupational therapy practice in home health. Most assessments developed for the home have been developed by occupational therapists in other countries; unfortunately, they are based on service delivery systems, regulations, and payers that are not compatible with home health service delivery in the United States. As expectations of evidence-based practice increase, the scarcity of home health–specific assessment tools creates a dilemma for home health practitioners, who must decide whether to use or adapt assessments and protocols not designed or standardized for use in the home or, alternatively, to assess and provide intervention using their best judgment and experience but without the benefit of evidence-based tools. There is a need for assessments that are both standardized for use in the home and compatible with the portability and infection control demands of home health practice and the documentation requirements and conventions of the U.S. home health industry.

For the same reasons that occupational therapy education must embrace home health practice, occupational therapy scientists must also embrace the home, and specifically home health service delivery, as a venue for research. Data are already available for some types of research. Use of the Outcome and Assessment Information Set (OASIS) since 2000 has yielded rich data about the clinical and functional status of millions of clients through the course of their home health care. The databank may be accessed by qualified scientists to conduct research. At the time of this writing, no occupational therapy scientists have accessed the OASIS database for outcomes research.

Outcomes are a growing priority for HHAs. Scientists interested in partnering with HHAs and developing occupational therapy protocols that are compatible with home health service delivery and documentation can help identify the contribution occupational therapy is making or could make to important client outcomes.

Issues for Practitioner Preparation and Professional Development

Whether recent graduates or experienced, occupational therapy practitioners require a unique constellation of knowledge, expertise, and reasoning to provide effective home health practice skills. The sections that follow describe practitioner preparation for entry-level practice in home health and professional development opportunities through **mentoring** programs, networking, and continuing professional education (CPE).

Preparation for Entry-Level Practice

In occupational therapy, the term *entry level* is most often used to refer to the generalist competencies associated with having recently graduated from an educational program, including fieldwork, and having passed a credentialing examination. As noted earlier, it is an enduring myth that occupational therapy practitioners must have other work experience before working in home health. With the exception of the few states that require such work experience, no federal regulation or Medicare requirement for experience exists. Indeed, there are strong reasons why a recent graduate may be an asset to an HHA.

The entry point for practice as an occupational therapist requires a master's degree, so completion of a degree at this level implies a level of maturity beyond what might be expected from a recent college undergraduate. While in school, students learn about and experience fieldwork in both traditional and emerging practice settings. During their academic career, most recent graduates become proficient in using the Internet to find both evidence and evidence-based practice resources to support their clinical reasoning. Recent graduates also tend to respond to technologies more readily than those whose practice experience has been dominated by face-to-face, in-the-same-room communication and intervention and pen-and-paper documentation. As home health service delivery models and technologies evolve and the demand for best, effective practices continues to grow, recent graduates bring an easily overlooked set of skills and experiences to HHAs.

Entry level in home health does not apply only to recent graduates. Practitioners with experience in other practice settings or with other populations are also entry level in home health in regard to the home health regulatory and payment context and the service delivery model. Even practitioners who have worked in other Medicare-dominated settings, such as skilled nursing facilities, or who have worked with older adults in rehabilitation settings are not likely to have established competencies related to supporting client self-management and working with family caregivers. Agency managers have reported to us that home health is attractive to therapy practitioners who have been away from practice for an interval (e.g., to raise children) and who want to return to practice on a flexible or part-time schedule. Returning or reentering practitioners are also entry level (AOTA, 2010a) and need

In occupational therapy, the term *entry level* is most often used to refer to the generalist competencies associated with having recently graduated from an educational program, including fieldwork, and having passed a credentialing examination.

to develop competencies related to the occupational therapy needs of the home health population and to service delivery in the home health regulatory and payment environment.

It is reasonable for an occupational therapy practitioner with recent home health experience to take on a full caseload after receiving orientation regarding agency-specific policies and procedures. It is not reasonable for a practitioner new to home health—who is entry level in home health—to take on a full client caseload and to function effectively in home health without adequate support. Regardless of whether an agency has one occupational therapy practitioner or many, the agency must have in place a system to develop, assess, and refine practitioners' knowledge and competencies for home health practice.

Development of Mentoring Programs

Mentoring is a journey, an interactive process that occurs between professionals with differing levels of experience and knowledge. It is an ancient concept; in Homer's *Odyssey*, Odysseus entrusted the education and guidance of his son, Telemachus, to a wise and learned man named Mentor (Cahill & Blanchard, 2000). Mentoring involves a relationship in which the mentor, who is usually more experienced, works closely with a mentee for the purpose of teaching, guiding, supporting, and facilitating professional growth and development (Milner & Bossers, 2004).

In a clinic situation, it is natural and convenient for peers of the same discipline to observe one another and share expertise through impromptu conversations. When service is provided in the home, however, these natural opportunities for observation and conversation do not exist or occur only rarely. Mentoring formalizes this kind of learning within the context of a relationship that has benefits for both the mentee and the mentor.

In **precepting,** a more experienced clinician orients and guides a less experienced clinician who is new to the agency. In response to the nursing shortage and to interest newly graduated nurses in embarking on a home health career, HHAs developed precepting programs to improve recruitment and retention of nurses being precepted and to provide recognition and satisfaction to nurses serving as preceptors (Carnigan, Baker, Demers, & Samar, 2007; O'Neil, 2008). For HHAs that already employ one or more experienced occupational therapy practitioners, establishing an occupational therapy preceptorship program can be a means to recruit and support entry-level occupational therapy practitioners and to recognize the expertise of the practitioners serving as preceptors.

When an occupational therapist is the only occupational therapist at an HHA, there is no opportunity for precepting—yet. Nonetheless, an occupational therapist in this situation still needs support to develop, assess, and advance his or her home health knowledge and competencies. Mentoring offers an opportunity for professional development for the occupational therapist being mentored.

The following sections outline elements of a mentoring program for home health occupational therapy practitioners. For lone occupational therapists in an agency or for practitioners working for a staffing agency or subcontracted to an HHA, seeking a home health mentor outside the agency supports the practitioner's professional development and the stakeholders' expectation of competent personnel. Agencies seeking to hire and retain additional occupational therapy

> For lone occupational therapists in an agency or for practitioners working for a staffing agency or subcontracted to an HHA, seeking a home health mentor outside the agency supports the practitioner's professional development and the stakeholders' expectation of competent personnel.

practitioners can develop a precepting program based on this mentoring program. For Level II fieldwork, the mentoring program can be adapted to meet the needs of the agency, the fieldwork educator, and the student practitioner.

Identifying the Need for a Mentoring Program

For a prospective or current home health occupational therapy practitioner, certain questions can assist in identifying the need for mentoring:

- When I have a professional question, is there someone from whom I can obtain an accurate and reliable answer?
- Are professional growth opportunities accessible?
- Do my available opportunities for professional growth meet my needs?

A negative answer to any of these questions indicates that the practitioner will benefit from mentoring. An HHA manager may also pose similar questions to occupational therapy staff or prospective staff to determine whether an occupational therapy precepting program is needed.

Structuring the Mentoring Program

Whether the mentoring program involves a mentoring agreement between two occupational therapy practitioners, a formal precepting program, or a student fieldwork experience, a format and structure must be established. Mentorship is about relationship and collaboration between people with a shared, defined outcome in mind. When structure is provided and responsibilities are identified for both the mentor and the mentee, then parties have an equal sense of control, responsibility, and accountability.

If a mentoring program is between two occupational therapy practitioners, mentor and mentee should create and sign a memorandum of agreement that includes the specifics of the commitment, such as starting and ending dates and the dates and times when meetings will occur. If the program is incorporated into a precepting program within an HHA or modified for a student fieldwork experience, the content of the memorandum of agreement may be incorporated into other specific forms or agreements used by the agency for such arrangements. Exhibit 8.1 provides a template for a memorandum of agreement between mentor and mentee.

Communication Options and Frequency

Encounters may be face-to-face or may be mediated by technology such as phone calls, email, or videoconferencing or a mix of communication methods. A mentoring program does not have to be totally structured, but the frequency of interaction should be defined. If the program is adapted for precepting a new employee or structuring a student fieldwork experience, more structure is appropriate to be consistent with agency new-employee timelines or the duration of the fieldwork experience.

Content

The overall goal of the program is to support the development of knowledge, skills, and competencies of the mentee or new home health occupational therapy practitioner. If the mentee is an occupational therapy practitioner who is new to home

Exhibit 8.1. Memorandum of Agreement for a Mentoring Program

Mentor Program Agreement

This agreement is between the following individuals:

_____ from _____

Mentee   Agency

and

_____ from _____

Mentor   Agency

The mentorship program will consist of at least _____ hours of one-on-one interaction between mentor and mentee through face-to-face and/or technology-mediated encounters. Each participant may elect to submit this activity as evidence of continuing professional development or education activities where such activity is recognized by credentialing or licensing authorities.

This mentorship program will begin on _____ [date] and end on _____ [date].

The mentor and mentee will keep track of their own contact hours using an activity report log.

Measurable goals for learning objectives for the mentee and plan of instruction by the mentor will be documented in a plan of action.

Both parties will complete a mentorship pretest and posttest. Also, at the end of the program, both parties will complete an evaluation.

Both parties attest to the fact that this is not a part of a supervisory plan or fieldwork experience. Both parties also agree that this program will be separate from and will not interfere with expectations from either employer.

Neither party is liable for the actions of the other party.

_____   _____

Mentee   Date

_____   _____

Mentor   Date

---

health or who seeks to strengthen his or her knowledge and competencies, the selection of content may be more flexible depending on the existing knowledge and competencies of the mentee. If the program exists to precept new occupational therapy employees, then the content may be more fixed and may incorporate aspects of agency procedures and processes. If the program is adapted to structure a student fieldwork experience, the content may be adapted to ensure the outcome of generalist entry-level competencies. A pretest–posttest questionnaire can be used to identify specific content areas that may need more attention or to measure outcomes such as a change in the mentee's confidence or competencies. Exhibit 8.2 provides an example of a confidence self-assessment questionnaire that can be used to compare the confidence level of the mentee at the beginning of the mentoring program with his or her confidence level when the program is completed.

The content of the mentoring program should be based on the student's or practitioner's level of experience, the type of agency, and the location of the agency to ensure that the content is consistent with state occupational therapy regulations. The order in which topics are covered during a mentoring program should be based on the needs and priorities of the mentee. In a precepting program, the order in which topics are addressed can be adapted to coincide with the agency's

The content of the mentoring program should be based on the student's or practitioner's level of experience, the type of agency, and the location of the agency to ensure that the content is consistent with state occupational therapy regulations.

Exhibit 8.2. Confidence Self-Assessment Questionnaire

_____ Pretest _____ Posttest					
Name: _____ Date: _____					
Please answer the following questions on the basis of your knowledge and experience working as an occupational therapist in home health. Circle the number that best defines your current confidence level.					
	Confidence				
	Least				Most
Local Peer Support					
I have good peer support from local occupational therapists.	1	2	3	4	5
Resources					
I usually know where to turn for professional resources when I encounter a new challenge or question related to my home health responsibilities.	1	2	3	4	5
Skilled Occupational Therapy Services					
I feel confident in providing and documenting occupational therapy services to my home health patient population.	1	2	3	4	5
Referrals					
I am effective in team conferences in reporting on clients, collaborating and problem solving, and securing appropriate occupational therapy referrals.	1	2	3	4	5
Quality Assurance: Outcomes					
I understand the outcome and process improvement goals my agency is working on and how they relate to services I provide.	1	2	3	4	5
Home Health Aides					
I am confident in supervising or working with home health aides.	1	2	3	4	5
Informal Presentations					
If I was asked to do an in-service for my agency, I would be able to easily identify an important and relevant topic and could easily identify and gather information for the presentation.	1	2	3	4	5
Familiarity With the _Framework_					
I am familiar with the _Occupational Therapy Practice Framework: Domain and Process._[a]	1	2	3	4	5
Application of the _Framework_					
I implement the _Framework_ to evaluate, plan, and implement intervention and achieve meaningful outcomes for my home health clients.	1	2	3	4	5
Job Satisfaction					
I feel very satisfied working in home health and at my agency.	1	2	3	4	5

[a]American Occupational Therapy Association (2014).

increasing expectations over the course of the precepting period and with agency orientation content relevant to all clinical staff. Learning modules should each have a specific learning objective with associated goals and activities. The mentor might also consider building in expectations for the mentee to begin creating a sustainable support system within the local home health community and taking advantage of opportunities in state and national occupational therapy associations once the mentorship program has ended. Box 8.1 outlines a case example of a mentoring program developed and carried out by the first author and a recently graduated occupational therapy practitioner. Table 8.3 includes a list of suggested content topics, resources, and learning activities for a mentoring, precepting, or student fieldwork supervision program.

Box 8.1. Case Example of a Mentoring Program

Two home health occupational therapists engaged in a structured, 12-week, long-distance, formal mentoring program. The mentor had many years of home health experience in a nonprofit government home care system. The mentee was recently employed as the only occupational therapist for a hospital-based agency covering a rural four-county geographic area. Because these therapists were employed by competing agencies, meaning that the agencies both covered the same geographic area, the therapists first obtained the permission of their supervisors to participate.

They defined the program as consisting of the following components:

- Signed agreement between mentee and mentor
- Use of an activity log by mentee and mentor
- Outline of topics to be discussed
- Plan of action for each topic with goals and objectives
- Worksheet for each goal
- Pretest and posttest of the mentoring program content
- Evaluation.

Communication was weekly by telephone. The first part of each session was spent in a brief discussion of the mentee's current caseload, conducted similar to a case conference. The second part of the session covered the content topics, organized into learning modules, that had been assigned for the week. Each session lasted approximately 1.5 to 2 hours.

The two occupational therapists were aware that participation in a formal mentorship was recognized by the national professional credentialing entity and the state regulatory entity for recredentialing and licensure renewal. To maintain records required by those entities, the mentor and mentee kept an activity log documenting the date, time spent, and activity during the 12-week program.

Benefits of a Mentoring Program

Although developing and carrying out a mentoring program takes time and commitment for both mentor and mentee, it is an option worthy of consideration to enhance and expand the home health occupational therapy workforce. Establishing a precepting program based on this mentoring model not only enhances the home health occupational therapy workforce but may also strengthen the employer–employee relationship, promote retention, and support career development. Adapting this mentoring model to structure an occupational therapy fieldwork experience in home health would increase the number of new occupational therapy graduates interested in and prepared to join the home health workforce. As Robertson and Savio (2003) noted,

> Mentoring is a perpetually spiraling, evolutionary process. One mentoring experience leads to the next. Mentees become mentors, the cycle carries on, and each person's influence expands to have an impact on the lives of others. Mentors, too, become wiser guides with each mentoring experience. (p. 14)

Networking

Networking is another avenue to support professional development. Networking is informal and does not necessarily include an element of quality control. However, for home health practitioners, who spend most of their work day in isolation, networking is a way to build and feel part of a community of occupational therapy practitioners and, especially, of home health occupational therapy practitioners.

Table 8.3. Topics, Resources, and Learning Activities for an Occupational Therapy Mentoring, Precepting, or Student Fieldwork Supervision Program

Topic and Resources[a]	Suggested Learning Activities
General orientation to home health	
Chapter 4	Practice in the home vs. in a facility or clinic
Agency specific	Risk management: Clinician safety
Agency specific	Risk management: Equipment and supply management, universal precautions, and infection control
Agency specific	Scheduling
Agency specific	Intra-agency communication (including meetings)
Home health team	
Agency specific	Role of each discipline
Sections of Chapter 6 Agency specific	Case management
Sections of Chapter 8 State regulations	Occupational therapy assistant supervision
Sections of Chapter 6 Agency- and state-specific policies	Home health aide supervision
Medicare as payer and other key payer sources	
Appendix A	Medicare home health benefit
Agency specific	Definition of *homebound* Prospective payment system *Skilled therapy* definition Therapy reassessment requirements
Agency specific	Other major payers
Medicare as regulator	
Appendix B	Conditions of Participation
Appendix D	Comprehensive assessment and OASIS; medication regimen review
Chapters 4, 6, and 8 Agency specific	Integration with occupational therapy processes
Quality improvement: Outcomes and processes	
Appendix C	Agency-specific efforts related to medication management, fall prevention, pain management, hospitalization risk reduction
Sections of Chapters 4 and 5	Occupational therapy evaluation and intervention in relation to quality improvement efforts Self-management
Documentation	
Sections of Chapters 1, 4, and 5	Forms or technology
Agency specific	Time frames Support
Occupational therapy evaluation and intervention	
State-specific practice act and regulations	State regulation of occupational therapy services in home care
Chapter 4	Evaluation process in the home
Sections of Chapters 4 and 5	Identification of trajectories and projection of outcomes

(Continued)

Table 8.3. Topics, Resources, and Learning Activities for an Occupational Therapy Mentoring, Precepting, or Student Fieldwork Supervision Program *(cont.)*

Topic and Resources[a]	Suggested Learning Activities
Chapter 5 Agency specific	Intervention and care planning
Sections of Chapter 5	Use of the environment as an intervention strategy
Sections of Chapters 3, 4, and 5	Common diagnoses or health conditions and relation to self-management and outcomes
Agency and location specific	Community resources, home medical equipment vendors
Sections of Chapter 5	Use of the visit, phone monitoring, and client homework
Chapters 2 and 7	Work with caregivers
Sections of Chapters 2 and 5	Reassessment and revision of care plans as needed
Sections of Chapter 6 Agency specific	Team conferencing and collaboration
Chapters 2, 6, and 7	Discharge planning Community resources Caregiver supports
Referral sources; physicians and other external communications	
Agency specific	Criteria or screening for occupational therapy referrals
Sections of Chapters 1 and 8	Communications with acute and postacute (upstream) occupational therapists

Note. OASIS = Outcome and Assessment Information Set.
[a]References to chapters and appendixes refer to content in this text and Self-Paced Clinical Course. Agency-specific resources are developed by each agency to provide important information to the agency's employees.

AOTA offers opportunities to network electronically through OT Connections (http://otconnections.aota.org), a social media site for occupational therapy practitioners with groups and forums on a wide variety of topics, including home health practice. Participation allows a practitioner to pose questions or share ideas with practitioners from across the country. Topics may be related to specific clinical issues or to the pragmatics of home health practice.

Membership in AOTA offers the option of joining a Special Interest Section. The Home & Community Health Special Interest Section (HCHSIS) encompasses home health and similar practice areas. The HCHSIS provides the following benefits: It

- Contributes to a practice publication, *SIS Quarterly Practice Connections,* available in print or electronically;
- Sponsors a forum on OT Connections;
- Facilitates the publication of a continuing education article annually in *OT Practice;*
- Hosts an educational session and roundtables at the AOTA Annual Conference & Expo; and
- Seeks practitioners with relevant expertise to share that expertise in articles, as roundtable facilitators, and as presenters at the AOTA Annual Conference & Expo.

Membership in a state occupational therapy association offers opportunities for networking and continuing education at a more local level. Some state occupational therapy associations have a section focused on home health practice. State occupational therapy associations are also important resources for understanding and influencing occupational therapy practice acts or associated regulations relevant to home health practice.

Formal Continuing Professional Education

Participation in formal CPE is another means to develop and advance competencies. CPE participation may be face-to-face at conferences or workshops, mediated through electronic media such as webcasts or podcasts, or obtained through articles downloaded or distributed in professional publications. Occupational therapy practitioners working in home health need CPE specific both to occupational therapy practice and competencies and to home health practice, framed within the regulations and payment system that shape this practice setting. Resources for home health–specific content include the national home health trade associations (e.g., National Association for Home Care & Hospice; http://www.nahc.org) and similar state-level associations. It is important that HHAs extend opportunities for home health CPE to their occupational therapy practitioner staff. It is equally important that home health occupational therapy practitioners make their agencies aware of their interest in and need for such opportunities.

> It is important that HHAs extend opportunities for home health CPE to their occupational therapy practitioner staff. It is equally important that home health occupational therapy practitioners make their agencies aware of their interest in and need for such opportunities.

Home Health Community Perceptions of Occupational Therapy

As noted in the "Introduction" to this text and SPCC and in **Appendix A** (see the section "Skilled vs. Qualifying Service as a Continued Need for Occupational Therapy," pp. 181–188), occupational therapy is not an initial qualifying discipline for the Medicare Part A home health benefit, leading to a misperception by the home health industry that occupational therapy plays a limited role in home health. The misperception is fed by misunderstandings or inaccurate interpretations of the Medicare home health coverage criteria. It is important to put this issue in perspective by spelling out clearly how not being an initial qualifying discipline limits occupational therapy practice in home health and how it does not.

Medicare beneficiaries who are homebound, are under the care of a physician, and need only occupational therapy cannot qualify for the home health benefit. Under the current Medicare CoPs (CMS, 2011, § 484.55; see full regulation in **Appendix B,** pp. 202–204), occupational therapy cannot conduct the initial assessment visit or the start-of-care (SOC) comprehensive assessment for Medicare beneficiaries. This is where the limitation stops. Otherwise, occupational therapy carries out the same responsibilities as physical therapy or speech–language pathology.

The following statements correct common misperceptions:

- Occupational therapists may perform initial or SOC assessments for clients for whom occupational therapy establishes benefit eligibility.
- Occupational therapists may recertify a client for subsequent certifications (Medicare or not), and occupational therapists may perform OASIS assessments at any time point subsequent to the SOC, as noted in Chapter 4.

- Occupational therapists may supervise aides and aide care plans when nursing services are not provided and where permitted by state nursing regulations.
- Occupational therapy practitioners may serve as therapy or clinical managers or agency administrators.

The anomaly of occupational therapy's lack of status as an initial qualifying discipline under the Medicare home health benefit is a challenge, but it is a restriction only if occupational therapy practitioners and HHAs allow that status to limit the potential and benefits occupational therapy brings to home health clients and to HHAs.

Conclusion

Individual occupational therapy practitioners and the occupational therapy profession have a stake in a strong, well-equipped home health occupational therapy workforce. Shifts in demographics, in how health care is delivered, and in how health care consumers expect to receive care all point to continuing growth of the home health industry and an increasing demand for occupational therapy practitioners ready and invested in working in home health care. Home health is an ideal venue for occupation-based and contextually relevant occupational therapy intervention.

The days of working in home health occasionally or of agencies borrowing occupational therapy practitioners from an affiliated hospital or other facility are past. HHAs need occupational therapy practitioners competent in and committed to home health practice. Occupational therapy practitioners recognize that home health is a venue for establishing careers in client care, administration, and consulting. To achieve a viable professional status, occupational therapy practitioners and agencies must expect that occupational therapy is integrated into the provision of quality patient care through the home health team. Occupational therapy practitioners must expect, and agencies must provide, the support and structure to deliver occupational therapy services grounded in home health knowledge, skills, and competencies.

Occupational therapy educators have a role in addressing this need by increasing the presence of home health practice in educational curricula and supporting the establishment of home health fieldwork experiences. Occupational therapy scientists have a role in addressing this need by generating and translating evidence relevant to the occupational needs of the home health population and applicable to the home health service delivery model. Mentoring, precepting, and establishing home health student fieldwork opportunities offer means to meet the professional development needs of both occupational therapy practitioners and HHAs.

How occupational therapy is perceived by the home health industry should be dependent not on the status of occupational therapy under the Medicare home health benefit but on the day-to-day actions of the occupational therapy practitioners providing services on behalf of HHAs across the country. For agencies and practitioners who recognize the key role occupational therapy practitioners play in client outcomes and in agency success, there is no question that occupational therapy's current and future role in home health is strong and bright.

References

American Occupational Therapy Association. (2006). *Occupational therapy workforce and compensation report.* Bethesda, MD: Author.

American Occupational Therapy Association. (2010a). Guidelines for re-entry into the field of occupational therapy. *American Journal of Occupational Therapy, 64*(6, Suppl.), S27–S29. http://dx.doi.org/10.5014/ajot.2010.64S27

American Occupational Therapy Association. (2010b). *Occupational therapy compensation and workforce report.* Bethesda, MD: Author.

American Occupational Therapy Association. (2014). Occupational therapy practice framework: Domain and process (3rd ed.). *American Journal of Occupational Therapy, 68*(Suppl. 1), S1–48. http://dx.doi.org/10.5014/ajot.2014.682006

American Occupational Therapy Association. (2015a). Occupational therapy code of ethics (2015). *American Journal of Occupational Therapy, 69*(Suppl. 3), 6913410030. http://dx.doi.org/10.5014/ajot.2015.696S03

American Occupational Therapy Association. (2015b). Standards for continuing competence. *American Journal of Occupational Therapy, 69*(Suppl. 3), 6913410055. http://dx.doi.org/10.5014/ajot.2015.696S16

Cahill, L., & Blanchard, S. R. (2000). *Mentoring handbook.* Tempe: Arizona State University Graduate Women's Association.

Carnigan, S., Baker, L., Demers, K., & Samar, A. (2007). Home healthcare internship and preceptor programs: One organization's journey. *Home Healthcare Nurse, 25,* 439–447.

Centers for Medicare & Medicaid Services. (2010a). *Medicare and Medicaid statistical supplement, 2010 edition.* Retrieved from http://www.cms.gov/Research-Statistics-Data-and-Systems/Research/MedicareMedicaidStatSupp/2010.html

Centers for Medicare & Medicaid Services. (2010b). *Outcome-Based Quality Improvement (OBQI) manual.* Baltimore: Author. Retrieved from http://www.cms.gov/Medicare/Quality-Initiatives-Patient-Assessment-Instruments/HomeHealthQualityInits/Downloads/OBQI-Manual.pdf

Centers for Medicare & Medicaid Services. (2011). *Part 484: Home health services.* Washington, DC: Author. Retrieved from http://www.gpo.gov/fdsys/pkg/CFR-2011-title42-vol5/pdf/CFR-2011-title42-vol5-part484.pdf

Centers for Medicare & Medicaid Services. (2014a). *Home Health Compare: What is Home Health Compare?* Retrieved from http://www.medicare.gov/HomeHealthCompare/About/What-Is-HHC.html

Centers for Medicare & Medicaid Services. (2014b). *Medicare benefit policy manual: Chapter 7—Home health services.* Retrieved from https://www.cms.gov/Regulations-and-Guidance/Guidance/Manuals/downloads//bp102c07.pdf

Cisneros, A. (2008, October 5). *Therapy utilization.* Retrieved from http://www.homehealthstrategicmanagement.com/Articles/tabid/1520/articleType/ArticleView/articleId/285/Therapy-Utilization.aspx

Milner, T., & Bossers, A. (2004). Evaluation of the mentor–mentee relationship in an occupational therapy mentorship programme. *Occupational Therapy International, 11,* 96–111. http://dx.doi.org/10.1002/oti.200

National Association for Home Care & Hospice. (2010). *Basic statistics about home care.* Washington, DC: Author. Retrieved from http://www.nahc.org/assets/1/7/10HC_Stats.pdf

O'Neil, K. (2008). Preceptorship in home care. *Home Healthcare Nurse, 26,* 525–532. http://dx.doi.org/10.1097/01.NHH.0000338511.92946.ac

Robertson, S. C., & Savio, M. C. (2003, November 17). Mentoring as professional development. *OT Practice,* pp. 12–16.

Recommended Reading

Grindel-Waggoner, M. (1999). Home care: A history of caring, a future of challenges. *MedSurg Nursing, 8,* 118–120.

Metzler, C. A. (2003, November 17). Is OT performance in home health optimum? *OT Practice,* p. 7.

Strzelecki, M. V. (2006, April 17). The mentor connection: Boost your career. *OT Practice,* pp. 17–20.

Urish, C. (2004, February 9). Ongoing competence through mentoring. *OT Practice,* p. 10.

Wilding, C., Marais-Strydom, E., & Teo, N. (2003). MentorLink: Empowering occupational therapists through mentoring. *Australian Journal of Occupational Therapy, 50,* 259–261. http://dx.doi.org/10.1046/j.1440-1630.2003.00378.x

Appendixes

APPENDIX A

Medicare as Payer

Missi Zahoransky, MSHS, OTR/L, and
Karen Vance, BSOT

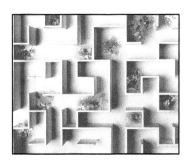

Contents

Overview of Medicare as Payer

Medicare is a federal program that, since the 1960s, has provided health insurance benefits to Americans ages 65 or older and to people with certain conditions and disabilities. Medicare specifies the services it will *cover*—that is, pay for—and the amounts it will pay for those services, and beneficiaries may pay a premium and are responsible for costs that Medicare does not cover. Medicare has multiple "Parts"— A through D—that cover different types of services.

This appendix first provides an overview of the coverage associated with Parts A through D of Medicare. It then introduces and reprints sections of the *Medicare Benefit Policy Manual,* Chapter 7—"Home Health Services" (Centers for Medicare & Medicaid Services [CMS], 2015), that are relevant to payment for home health occupational therapy services covered under the Part A Home Health Benefit. Next, Medicare program integrity contractors and the home health prospective payment system (PPS) are reviewed. Finally, payment for occupational therapy home health services under Part B Outpatient Therapy Services is discussed.

Part A

Medicare Part A is hospital insurance. Part A provides coverage for inpatient hospital care, limited skilled nursing facility care provided after a hospitalization (but not custodial or long-term care), home health agency (HHA) services, and hospice care. Specific criteria apply to coverage of care in each of these settings. Most beneficiaries pay no premium (i.e., monthly payment) for Part A because the beneficiary or a spouse paid Medicare taxes while working. To be eligible for Medicare Part A, a person must be

- Age 65 or older;
- Disabled (as defined in the Medicare Improvements for Patients and Providers Act of 2008, Pub. L. 110–275); or
- Diagnosed with end-stage renal disease (i.e., permanent kidney failure requiring dialysis or a kidney transplant; CMS, 2014a).

Part B

Medicare Part B is optional medical insurance that covers medically necessary services or supplies provided by a Medicare-certified provider. Part B covers

- *Medically necessary services:* Services or supplies that are needed to diagnose or treat [a] medical condition and that meet accepted standards of medical practice.
- *Preventive services:* Health care to prevent illness (like the flu) or detect it at an early stage, when treatment is most likely to work best. (Medicare.gov, 2014, para. 3)

Enrollment in Part B is voluntary. Beneficiaries pay a monthly premium for Part B that is adjusted annually (CMS, 2014b).

Part C

Medicare Part C is also known as "Medicare Advantage." A Medicare Advantage plan is offered by a private company that contracts with Medicare to provide all Part A and Part B benefits. Part C plans often have networks and require a beneficiary to use doctors, facilities, agencies, and providers within a particular network. Part C may have lower premiums and provide additional benefits that traditional Parts A and B may not include; Part C plans cannot offer benefits that are less than the traditional Part A and B benefits. Some Part C plans require beneficiaries to purchase Part D as a component of a total package of coverage.

Part D

Medicare Part D is a prescription drug coverage plan. Most beneficiaries pay a premium for Part D, and plans vary considerably in coverage. Each Medicare Part D plan has a list, or *formulary*, of the drugs covered by the plan.

Medicare Coverage Under the Part A Home Health Benefit

The following sections reprint text from the *Medicare Benefit Policy Manual* (CMS, 2015) pertinent to home health care occupational therapy. The sections of the manual are numbered for ease of location; in this appendix, these numbers are preceded by the section symbol (§), and sections omitted because they are not pertinent to home health occupational therapy are indicated by ellipses (spaced periods).

Conditions for Coverage

Parts of § 20 and § 30 of Chapter 7 of the *Medicare Benefit Policy Manual* (CMS, 2015) address the conditions HHAs must meet to be paid for their services.

§ 20—Conditions to Be Met for Coverage of Home Health Services

Medicare covers HHA services when the following criteria are met:

1. The person to whom the services are provided is an eligible Medicare beneficiary;
2. The HHA that is providing the services to the beneficiary has in effect a valid agreement to participate in the Medicare program;

3. The beneficiary qualifies for coverage of home health services as described in §30;

4. The services for which payment is claimed are covered as described in §§40 and 50;

5. Medicare is the appropriate payer; and

6. The services for which payment is claimed are not otherwise excluded from payment.

. . . .

§ 20.1.2—Determination of Coverage

The Medicare contractor's decision on whether care is reasonable and necessary is based on information reflected in the home health plan of care, the OASIS [Outcome and Assessment Information Set] as required by 42 CFR [*Code of Federal Regulations*] 484.55 or a medical record of the individual patient. Medicare does not deny coverage solely on the basis of the reviewer's general inferences about patients with similar diagnoses or on data related to utilization generally, but bases it upon objective clinical evidence regarding the patient's individual need for care. Coverage of skilled nursing care or therapy to perform a maintenance program does not turn on the presence or absence of a patient's potential for improvement from the nursing care or therapy, but rather on the patient's need for skilled care. Skilled care may be necessary to improve a patient's current condition, to maintain the patient's current condition, to prevent or slow further deterioration of the patient's condition.

This text was added to the *Medicare Benefit Policy Manual* after the *Jimmo v. Sebelius* settlement, which went into effect in January 2013. CMS issued a statement in response to the settlement that noted the following:

While an expectation of improvement would be a reasonable criterion to consider when evaluating, for example, a claim in which the goal of treatment is restoring a prior capability, Medicare policy has long recognized that there may also be specific instances where no improvement is expected but skilled care is, nevertheless, required in order to prevent or slow deterioration and maintain a beneficiary at the maximum practicable level of function. (CMS, 2013, p. 1)

§ 30—Conditions Patient Must Meet to Qualify for Coverage of Home Health Services

To qualify for the Medicare home health benefit, . . . a Medicare beneficiary must meet the following requirements:

- Be confined to the home;
- Under the care of a physician;
- Receiving services under a plan of care established and periodically reviewed by a physician;

- Be in need of skilled nursing care on an intermittent basis or physical therapy or speech–language pathology; or
- Have a continuing need for occupational therapy.

. . . .

§ 30.1.1—Patient Confined to the Home

For a patient to be eligible to receive covered home health services . . . , the law requires that a physician certify in all cases that the patient is confined to his/her home. For purposes of the statute, an individual shall be considered "confined to the home" (homebound) if the following two criteria are met:

1. Criteria-One:
   The patient must either:
   - Because of illness or injury, need the aid of supportive devices such as crutches, canes, wheelchairs, and walkers; the use of special transportation; or the assistance of another person in order to leave their place of residence
   OR
   - Have a condition such that leaving his or her home is medically contraindicated.

If the patient meets one of the Criteria-One conditions, then the patient must ALSO meet two additional requirements defined in Criteria-Two below.

2. Criteria-Two:
   - There must exist a normal inability to leave home;
   AND
   - Leaving home must require a considerable and taxing effort.

If the patient does in fact leave the home, the patient may nevertheless be considered homebound if the absences from the home are infrequent or for periods of relatively short duration, or are attributable to the need to receive health care treatment. Absences attributable to the need to receive health care treatment include, but are not limited to:

- Attendance at adult day centers to receive medical care;
- Ongoing receipt of outpatient kidney dialysis; or
- The receipt of outpatient chemotherapy or radiation therapy.

Any absence of an individual from the home attributable to the need to receive health care treatment, including regular absences for the purpose of participating in therapeutic, psychosocial, or medical treatment in an adult day-care program that is licensed or certified by a State, or accredited to furnish adult day-care services in a State, shall not disqualify an individual from being considered to be confined to his home. Any other absence of an individual from the home shall not so disqualify an individual if the absence is of an infrequent or of relatively short duration. For purposes of the preceding sentence, any absence for the purpose of attending a religious service shall be deemed to be an absence of infrequent or short duration. It is expected that in most instances, absences from the home that occur will be for the purpose of receiving health care treatment. However, occasional absences from the home for nonmedical purposes, e.g., an occasional trip to the barber, a walk around the block or a drive, attendance at a family reunion, funeral, graduation, or other infrequent or unique event would not necessitate a finding that the patient is not homebound if the absences are undertaken on an infrequent basis or are of relatively short duration and do not indicate that the patient has the capacity to obtain the health care provided outside rather than in the home.

Assessment Considerations for Homebound Status

Determining whether a patient is or continues to be homebound is based on a clinician's good assessment skills. Although assessing a patient's homebound status may be subjective, it is still based on assessment and observation, not on a patient's report or promise to be homebound. Certainly, interviewing patients may provide a picture of their abilities outside of a visit time frame, but relying on their report alone does not necessarily provide an accurate picture of their abilities, just their perception of their abilities.

As stated in the "Introduction" to this text and Self-Paced Clinical Course, the terms *evaluation* and *assessment* have meanings that are the reverse of those used in occupational therapy official documents. In the Medicare documents referred to in this appendix, *assessment* has the same meaning as *evaluation* as used in the occupational therapy official documents and refers to the overarching process of obtaining data with specific timelines about what data are to be collected and by whom.

An occupational therapist must investigate possible discrepancies in a patient's report, but HHA policies and procedures are varied regarding how the homebound status is verified. A common, but misguided, practice is to require a patient to declare homebound status to receive services, but the *Medicare Benefit Policy Manual* (CMS, 2015) does not require or imply that a patient should promise to be homebound. Rather, it is incumbent on the clinician to observe the patient's physical and cognitive status and document as objectively as possible the physical or behavioral attributes that indicate that a considerable and taxing effort is required for activities outside the home.

For example, assistive devices might reflect physical status, but the use of an assistive device in and of itself does not imply considerable and taxing effort without other accompanying descriptions, such as shortness of breath at short distances; elevated heart rate; frequent rest stops; or compromised balance, strength, or endurance. Describing potential risks in the documentation, such as wandering, supports the need for cognitive assistance for safety.

CMS (2015) does not specify how frequently such observations should occur in a clinician's documentation, but agency policy may dictate such requirements. Clinicians who include homebound status in documentation are expected to provide an adequate description of why the patient cannot receive health care services in another setting. The frequency of such documentation should match changes in the patient's progress to justify continuation of these services in the home.

Plan of Care

The HHA must establish a plan of care for (POC) each patient and have it signed by the certifying physician in a timely manner. The POC must be reviewed in consultation with other professionals at least every 60 days. The physician who signs the POC must be qualified to sign the physician certification as described in the Home Health Prospective Payment System (PPS) rule ("Home Health Prospective Payment System Rate Update," 2010). The POC must indicate in the orders section the types of services to be provided, including the discipline type, the nature of the services, and the frequency of provision (CMS, 2015). The following regulations in § 30 of Chapter 7 of the *Medicare Benefit Policy Manual* address the POC.

§ 30.2—Services Are Provided Under a Plan of Care Established and Approved by a Physician

§ 30.2.1—Content of the Plan of Care

The HHA must be acting upon a physician plan of care that meets the requirements of this section for HHA services to be covered.

The plan of care must contain all pertinent diagnoses, including:

- The patient's mental status;
- The types of services, supplies, and equipment required;
- The frequency of the visits to be made;
- Prognosis;
- Rehabilitation potential;
- Functional limitations;
- Activities permitted;
- Nutritional requirements;
- All medications and treatments;
- Safety measures to protect against injury;
- Instructions for timely discharge or referral; and
- Any additional items the HHA or physician chooses to include.

If the plan of care includes a course of treatment for therapy services:

- The course of therapy treatment must be established by the physician after any needed consultation with the qualified therapist;
- The plan must include measurable therapy treatment goals which pertain directly to the patient's illness or injury, and the patient's resultant impairments;
- The plan must include the expected duration of therapy services; and
- The plan must describe a course of treatment which is consistent with the qualified therapist's assessment of the patient's function.

. . . .

§ 30.3—Under the Care of a Physician

The patient must be under the care of a physician who is qualified to sign the physician certification and plan of care in accordance with 42 CFR 424.22.

A patient is expected to be under the care of the physician who signs the plan of care. It is expected that in most instances, the physician who certifies the patient's eligibility for Medicare home health services, in accordance with §30.5 below, will be the same physician who establishes and signs the plan of care.

. . . .

§ 30.5.1—Physician Certification

A certification (versus recertification) is considered to be anytime that a Start of Care OASIS is completed to initiate care. In such instances, a physician must certify (attest) that:

1. The home health services are or were needed because the patient is or was confined to the home as defined in §30.1;
2. The patient needs or needed skilled nursing services on an inter-mittent basis (other than solely venipuncture for the purposes of obtaining a blood sample), or physical therapy, or speech–language pathology services. Where a patient's sole skilled service need is for skilled oversight of unskilled services (management and evaluation of the care plan as defined in §40.1.2.2), the physician must include a brief narrative describing the clinical justification of this need as part of the certification; or as a signed addendum to the certification;
3. A plan of care has been established and is periodically reviewed by a physician;
4. The services are or were furnished while the patient is or was under the care of a physician;
5. For episodes with starts of care beginning January 1, 2011 and later, in accordance with §30.5.1.1 below, a face-to-face encounter oc-curred no more than 90 days prior to or within 30 days after the start of the home health care, was related to the primary reason the patient requires home health services, and was performed by an al-lowed provider type. The certifying physician must also document the date of the encounter.

   If the patient is starting home health directly after discharge from an acute/post-acute care setting where the physician, with privileges, that cared for the patient in that setting is certifying the patient's eligibility for the home health benefit, but will not be fol-lowing the patient after discharge, then the certifying physician must identify the community physician who will be following the patient after discharge. One of the criteria that must be met for a patient to be considered eligible for the home health benefit is that the patient must be under the care of a physician (number 4 listed above). Otherwise, the certification is not valid.

The certification must be complete prior to when an HHA bills Medicare for reimbursement; however, physicians should complete the certification when the plan of care is established, or as soon as possible thereafter. This is longstanding CMS policy as referenced in Pub 100-01, Medicare General Information, Eligibility, and Entitlement Manual, chapter 4, section 30.1. It is not acceptable for HHAs to wait until the end of a 60-day episode of care to obtain a completed certification/recertification.

Skilled vs. Qualifying Service as a Continued Need for Occupational Therapy

In addition to the patient being homebound and under the care of a physician, to qualify for the home health benefit, the services ordered on the physician's POC must include intermittent skilled nursing, physical therapy, speech–language pathology, or the continuing need for occupational therapy. For a continuing need for occupational therapy services to be covered under the Medicare home health benefit, a beneficiary's eligibility for home health services must first be established because the beneficiary requires the services of skilled nursing, speech–language pathology, or physical therapy at any time during the current or prior certification period. Occupational therapy alone does not establish initial Medicare home health eligibility, but it is considered a skilled service and, as such, can qualify the beneficiary for continued coverage of the home health benefit.

Medicare does not mandate which services or how many visits are required to establish eligibility but does recognize that once eligibility is established, occupational therapy, if a continued need, is a covered skilled service. The first ordered occupational therapy visit must occur after the qualifying service's first visit and before that qualifying service discharges. A beneficiary may then be discharged from skilled nursing, speech–language pathology, or physical therapy, and occupational therapy may remain as the only service on the POC. Medical social services and home health aide services are classified as dependent services and are covered under the home health benefit only if they are provided as dependent to a skilled service.

§ 30.4—Needs Skilled Nursing Care on an Intermittent Basis (Other Than Solely Venipuncture for the Purposes of Obtaining a Blood Sample), Physical Therapy, Speech–Language Pathology Services, or Has Continued Need for Occupational Therapy

The patient must need one of the following types of services:

1. Skilled nursing care that is

- Reasonable and necessary as defined in §40.1;
- Needed on an "intermittent" [basis] as defined in §40.1; and
- Not solely needed for venipuncture for the purposes of obtaining blood sample as defined in §40.1.2.13; or

2. Physical therapy as defined in §40.2.2; or
3. Speech–language pathology services as defined in §40.2.3; or
4. Have a continuing need for occupational therapy as defined in §§40.2.4.

The patient has a continued need for occupational therapy when:

1. The services which the patient requires meet the definition of "occupational therapy" services of §40.2, and
2. The patient's eligibility for home health services has been established by virtue of a prior need for skilled nursing care (other than solely venipuncture for the purposes of obtaining a blood sample), speech–language pathology services, or physical therapy in the current or prior certification period.

. . . .

§ 40—Covered Services Under a Qualifying Home Health Plan of Care

Section 1861(m) of the [Social Security] Act governs the Medicare home health services that may be provided to eligible beneficiaries by or under arrangements made by a participating home health agency (HHA). Section 1861(m) describes home health services as

- Part-time or intermittent skilled nursing care (other than solely venipuncture for the purposes of obtaining a blood sample);
- Part-time or intermittent home health aide services;
- Physical therapy;
- Speech–language pathology;
- Occupational therapy;
- Medical social services;
- Medical supplies (including catheters, catheter supplies, ostomy bags, supplies related to ostomy care, and a covered osteoporosis drug . . . , but excluding other drugs and biologicals);
- Durable medical equipment while under the plan of care established by a physician;
- Medical services provided by an intern or resident-in-training under an approved teaching program of the hospital in the case of an HHA which is affiliated or under common control with a hospital; and
- Services at hospitals, skilled nursing facilities, or rehabilitation centers when they involve equipment too cumbersome to bring to the home.

The term "part-time or intermittent" for purposes of coverage . . . means skilled nursing and home health aide services furnished any number of days per week as long as they are furnished (combined) less than 8 hours each day and 28 or fewer hours each week (or, subject to review on a case-by-case basis as to the need for care, less than 8 hours each day and 35 or fewer hours per week). . . .

For any home health services to be covered by Medicare, the patient must meet the qualifying criteria as specified in §30, including having a need for skilled nursing care on an intermittent basis, physical therapy, speech–language pathology services, or a continuing need for occupational therapy as defined in this section.

§ 40.1—Skilled Nursing Care

To be covered as skilled nursing services, the services must require the skills of a registered nurse, or a licensed practical (vocational) nurse under the supervision of a registered nurse, must be reasonable and necessary to the treatment of the patient's illness or injury as discussed in §40.1.1, below, and must be intermittent as discussed in §40.1.3. Coverage of skilled nursing care does not turn on the presence or absence of a patient's potential for improvement from the nursing care, but rather on the patient's need for skilled care.

. . . .

§ 40.2—Skilled Therapy Services

To be covered as skilled therapy, the services must require the skills of a qualified therapist and must be reasonable and necessary for the treatment of the patient's illness or injury as discussed below. Coverage does not turn on the presence or absence of an individual's potential for improvement, but rather on the beneficiary's need for skilled care.

§ 40.2.1—General Principles Governing Reasonable and Necessary Physical Therapy, Speech–Language Pathology Services, and Occupational Therapy

The service of a physical therapist, speech–language pathologist, or occupational therapist is a skilled therapy service if the inherent complexity of the service is such that it can be performed safely and/or effectively only by or under the general supervision of a skilled therapist. To be covered, assuming all other eligibility and coverage criteria have been met, the skilled services must also be reasonable and necessary to the treatment of the patient's illness or injury or to the restoration or maintenance of function affected by the patient's illness or injury. It is necessary to determine whether individual therapy services are skilled and whether, in view of the patient's overall condition, skilled management of the services provided is needed.

The development, implementation, management, and evaluation of a patient care plan based on the physician's orders constitute skilled therapy services when, because of the patient's clinical condition, those activities require the specialized skills, knowledge, and judgment of a qualified therapist to ensure the effectiveness of the treatment goals and ensure medical safety. Where the specialized skills, knowledge, and judgment of a therapist are needed to manage and periodically reevaluate the appropriateness of a maintenance program, such services would be covered, even if the skills of a therapist were not needed to carry out the activities performed as part of the maintenance program.

While a patient's particular medical condition is a valid factor in deciding if skilled therapy services are needed, a patient's diagnosis or prognosis should never be the sole factor in deciding that a service is or is not skilled. The key issue is whether the skills of a therapist are needed to treat the illness or injury, or whether the services can be carried out by unskilled personnel.

A service that is ordinarily considered unskilled could be considered a skilled therapy service in cases where there is clear documentation that, because of special medical complications, skilled rehabilitation personnel are required to perform the service. However, the importance of a particular service to a patient or the frequency with which it must be performed does not, by itself, make an unskilled service into a skilled service.

Assuming all other eligibility and coverage criteria have been met, the skilled therapy services must be reasonable and necessary to the treatment of the patient's illness or injury within the context of the patient's unique medical condition. To be considered reasonable and necessary for the treatment of the illness or injury:

a. The services must be consistent with the nature and severity of the illness or injury, the patient's particular medical needs, including the requirement that the amount, frequency, and duration of the services must be reasonable; and

b. The services must be considered, under accepted standards of medical practice, to be specific, safe, and effective treatment for the patient's condition, meeting the standards noted below. The home health record must specify the purpose of the skilled service provided.

1. Assessment, Measurement and Documentation of Therapy Effectiveness

To ensure therapy services are effective, at defined points during a course of treatment, for each therapy discipline for which services are provided, a qualified therapist (instead of an assistant) must perform the ordered therapy service. During this visit, the therapist must assess the patient using a method which allows for objective measurement of function and successive comparison of measurements. The therapist must document the measurement results in the clinical record. Specifically:

i. Initial Therapy Assessment

- For each therapy discipline for which services are provided, a qualified therapist (instead of an assistant) must assess the patient's function using a method which objectively measures activities of daily living such as, but not limited to, eating, swallowing, bathing, dressing, toileting, walking, climbing stairs, using assistive devices, and mental and cognitive factors. The measurement results must be documented in the clinical record.

- Where more than one discipline of therapy is being provided, a qualified therapist from each of the disciplines must functionally assess the patient. The therapist must document the measurement results which correspond to the therapist's discipline and care plan goals in the clinical record.

ii. Reassessment at least every 30 days (performed in conjunction with an ordered therapy service)

- At least once every 30 days, for each therapy discipline for which services are provided, a qualified therapist (instead of an assistant) must provide the ordered therapy service, functionally reassess the patient, and compare the resultant measurement to prior assessment measurements. The therapist must document in the clinical record the measurement results along with the therapist's determination of the effectiveness of therapy, or lack thereof.
- For multi-discipline therapy cases, a qualified therapist from each of the disciplines must functionally reassess the patient. The therapist must document the measurement results which correspond to the therapist's discipline and care plan goals in the clinical record.
- The 30-day clock begins with the first therapy service (of that discipline) and the clock resets with each therapist's visit/ assessment/measurement/documentation (of that discipline).

c. Services involving activities for the general welfare of any patient, e.g., general exercises to promote overall fitness or flexibility and activities to provide diversion or general motivation do not constitute skilled therapy. Unskilled individuals without the supervision of a therapist can perform those services.

d. Assuming all other eligibility and coverage requirements have been met, in order for therapy services to be covered, one of the following three conditions must be met:

1. The skills of a qualified therapist are needed to restore patient function:

- To meet this coverage condition, therapy services must be provided with the expectation, based on the assessment made by the physician of the patient's restorative potential that the condition of the patient will improve materially in a reasonable and generally predictable period of time. Improvement is evidenced by objective successive measurements.
- Therapy is not considered reasonable and necessary under this condition if the patient's expected restorative potential would be insignificant in relation to the extent and duration of therapy services required to reach such potential.

- Therapy is not required to effect improvement or restoration of function where a patient suffers a transient or easily reversible loss of function (such as temporary weakness following surgery) which could reasonably be expected to improve spontaneously as the patient gradually resumes normal activities. Therapy in such cases is not considered reasonable and necessary to treat the patient's illness or injury, under this condition. However, if the criteria for maintenance therapy described in (3) below is met, therapy could be covered under that condition.

2. The patient's clinical condition requires the specialized skills, knowledge, and judgment of a qualified therapist to establish or design a maintenance program, related to the patient's illness or injury, in order to ensure the safety of the patient and the effectiveness of the program, to the extent provided by regulation,

   - For patients receiving rehabilitative/restorative therapy services, if the specialized skills, knowledge, and judgment of a qualified therapist are required to develop a maintenance program, the expectation is that the development of that maintenance program would occur during the last visit(s) for rehabilitative/restorative treatment. The goals of a maintenance program would be to maintain the patient's current functional status or to prevent or slow further deterioration.
   - Necessary periodic reevaluations by a qualified therapist of the beneficiary and maintenance program are covered if the specialized skills, knowledge, and judgment of a qualified therapist are required.
   - Where a maintenance program is not established until after the rehabilitative/restorative therapy program has been completed, or where there was no rehabilitative/restorative therapy program, and the specialized skills, knowledge, and judgment of a qualified therapist are required to develop a maintenance program, such services would be considered reasonable and necessary for the treatment of the patient's condition in order to ensure the effectiveness of the treatment goals and ensure medical safety. When the development of a maintenance program could not be accomplished during the last visits(s) of rehabilitative/restorative treatment, the therapist must document why the maintenance program could not be developed during those last rehabilitative/restorative treatment visit(s).
   - When designing or establishing a maintenance program, the qualified therapist must teach the patient or the patient's family or [caregivers] necessary techniques, exercises or precautions

as necessary to treat the illness or injury. The instruction of the beneficiary or appropriate caregiver by a qualified therapist regarding a maintenance program is covered if the specialized skills, knowledge, and judgment of a qualified therapist are required. However, visits made by skilled therapists to a patient's home solely to train other HHA staff (e.g., home health aides) are not billable as visits since the HHA is responsible for ensuring that its staff is properly trained to perform any service it furnishes. The cost of a skilled therapist's visit for the purpose of training HHA staff is an administrative cost to the agency.

3. The skills of a qualified therapist (not an assistant) are needed to perform maintenance therapy:

- Coverage of therapy services to perform a maintenance program is not determined solely on the presence or absence of a beneficiary's potential for improvement from the therapy, but rather on the beneficiary's need for skilled care. Assuming all other eligibility and coverage requirements are met, skilled therapy services are covered when an individualized assessment of the patient's clinical condition demonstrates that the specialized judgment, knowledge, and skills of a qualified therapist ("skilled care") are necessary for the performance of a safe and effective maintenance program. Such a maintenance program to maintain the patient's current condition or to prevent or slow further deterioration is covered so long as the beneficiary requires skilled care for the safe and effective performance of the program. When, however, the individualized assessment does not demonstrate such a necessity for skilled care, including when the performance of a maintenance program does not require the skills of a therapist because it could safely and effectively be accomplished by the patient or with the assistance of non-therapists, including unskilled caregivers, such maintenance services will not be covered.
- Further, under the standard set forth in the previous paragraph, skilled care is necessary for the performance of a safe and effective maintenance program only when (a) the particular patient's special medical complications require the skills of a qualified therapist to perform a therapy service that would otherwise be considered non-skilled; or (b) the needed therapy procedures are of such complexity that the skills of a qualified therapist are required to perform the procedure.

e. The amount, frequency, and duration of the services must be reasonable.

As is outlined in home health regulations, as part of the home health agency (HHA) Conditions of Participation (CoPs), the clinical record of the patient must contain progress and clinical notes. Additionally, in Pub. 100-04, Medicare Claims Processing Manual, Chapter 10, "Home Health Agency Billing" [CMS, 2014c], instructions specify that for each claim, HHAs are required to report all services provided to the beneficiary during each episode[;] this includes reporting each visit in line-item detail. As such, it is expected that the home health records for every visit will reflect the need for the skilled medical care provided. These clinical notes are also expected to provide important communication among all members of the home care team regarding the development, course and outcomes of the skilled observations, assessments, treatment and training performed. Taken as a whole then, the clinical notes are expected to tell the story of the patient's achievement towards his/her goals as outlined in the Plan of Care. In this way, the notes will serve to demonstrate why a skilled service is needed.

Therefore the home health clinical notes must document as appropriate:

- the history and physical exam pertinent to the day's visit . . . (including the response or changes in behavior to previously administered skilled services)[,] and
- the skilled services applied on the current visit, and
- the patient/caregiver's immediate response to the skilled services provided, and
- the plan for the next visit based on the rationale of prior results.

Clinical notes should be written such that they adequately describe the reaction of a patient to his/her skilled care. Clinical notes should also provide a clear picture of the treatment, as well as "next steps" to be taken. Vague or subjective descriptions of the patient's care should not be used. For example terminology such as the following would not adequately describe the need for skilled care:

- Patient tolerated treatment well
- Caregiver instructed in medication management
- Continue with POC

Objective measurements of physical outcomes of treatment should be provided and/or a clear description of the changed behaviors due to education programs should be recorded in order that all concerned can follow the results of the applied services.

When the skilled service is being provided to either maintain the patient's condition or prevent or slow further deterioration, the clinical notes must also describe:

- A detailed rationale that explains the need for the skilled service in light of the patient's overall medical condition and experiences,
- the complexity of the service to be performed, and
- any other pertinent characteristics of the beneficiary or home.

Medicare Program Integrity Contractors

Decisions about whether provided services are reasonable and necessary ultimately reside with the agency's Medicare contractor who pays the claims. CMS has several types of contractors that focus on ensuring accurate payment for provided services. These contractors conduct reviews of an agency's documentation to ensure that all provided services are reasonable and necessary and fall within coverage guidelines on the basis of information from the beneficiary's POC and the medical record. These reviews are generally retroactive, so the accuracy and completeness of documentation from the beginning of care influence whether a review is "clean" (i.e., has no problems) or results in financial or other compliance penalties. Although each Medicare contractor may have specific review criteria,

> Medicare does not deny coverage solely on the basis of the reviewer's general inferences about patients with similar diagnoses or on data related to utilization generally, but bases it upon objective clinical evidence regarding the patient's individual need for care. (CMS, 2015, § 20.1.2)

Therefore, coverage is determined in large part by the thoroughness and accuracy of the occupational therapist's documentation of the individual patient's progress toward his or her goals.

Home Health Prospective Payment System

The home health PPS, implemented on October 1, 2000, is the methodology Medicare uses to pay an HHA. Reimbursement to an HHA is determined prospectively, or at the beginning of a 60-day episode of home health care. The amount of the payment is based on characteristics of the patient and expected service utilization. The prospective payment covers all costs associated with home health care provision, including routine and nonroutine medical supplies, but excludes all durable medical equipment, which is covered by a separate fee schedule. Six disciplines are covered under the home health PPS:

1. Skilled nursing services
2. Home health aide services
3. Physical therapy services
4. Speech–language pathology services
5. Occupational therapy services
6. Medical social services.

Medicare beneficiaries are eligible to receive coverage for home health services for a 60-day episode of care. A beneficiary who continues to meet the coverage criteria remains eligible for subsequent episodes. There is no limit on how many episodes a beneficiary may have; coverage is based on eligibility as determined by the criteria set forth for coverage by Medicare in the *Medicare Benefit Policy Manual,* Chapter 7, § 20 (CMS, 2015).

Payment Rate

The PPS base payment rate is a national rate established annually. The base rate is adjusted on the basis of the beneficiary's geographic area (i.e., labor adjustment) and the beneficiary's care needs and health condition (i.e., case-mix adjustment). Medicare determined that a beneficiary's location was a determining factor in the cost of providing home health services, so the labor adjustment reflects the agency's wage index on the basis of the location of service provision (i.e., core-based statistical area) as defined by Medicare.

The case-mix adjustment to the base payment rate reflects the beneficiary's individual clinical characteristics and specific service needs indicated by data collected through OASIS. The case-mix data are organized into three dimensions—(1) clinical, (2) functional, and (3) service utilization—and each dimension is assigned a score value. The scores for each of these dimensions are tabulated to determine the beneficiary's case-mix adjustment score, and the payment amount is adjusted accordingly.

Consolidated Billing

Consolidated billing of all home health services is required while a beneficiary is under a home health POC. *Consolidated billing* means that HHAs are fiscally responsible for the cost of all services and supplies provided to beneficiaries covered under a POC. Medicare provides payment for all covered services only to the HHA overseeing the beneficiary's POC, and these anticipated costs are included in the PPS payment rate. The payment is made to the HHA regardless of whether the service or item was furnished directly by the agency or under arrangement with others (CMS, 2014c, § 10.11). Services subject to the home health consolidated billing provision are

- Skilled nursing care;
- Home health aide services;
- Physical therapy;
- Speech–language pathology;
- Occupational therapy;
- Medical social services;
- Routine and nonroutine medical supplies; and
- Home health services to homebound patients provided under arrangement with hospitals, skilled nursing facilities, or rehabilitation centers when they involve equipment too cumbersome to bring to the home or are furnished while the patient is at the facility to receive such services.

The last bullet would apply when a patient under a home health POC (Part A) needs a whirlpool treatment for a wound, for example, that would be too cumbersome to perform in the home. In this case, the HHA might have a contract with a hospital therapy clinic to perform the whirlpool treatment at the facility. The caregiver would transport the patient to and from the facility, the facility would bill the HHA for payment, and the HHA would be reimbursed under consolidated billing. (Two exceptions to consolidated billing include therapy services performed by a physician and durable medical equipment.)

Therapy services on a home health POC (Part A) must be provided directly by or under arrangement with the HHA and cannot be billed to an outpatient facility under Part B while a beneficiary is under the active care of an HHA. If a secondary physician orders outpatient therapy (Part B) while the patient is under a home health POC (Part A), the outpatient provider will not be reimbursed because the treatment rendered by the outpatient provider was not under arrangement with the HHA as part of the home health POC. It is the responsibility of the outpatient therapy provider or supplier (Part B) to investigate whether a beneficiary is under the care of an HHA (Part A) before beginning outpatient services.

Home Health Resource Groups

Home health resource groups (HHRGs) are a way of classifying patients by personal characteristics and health status. HHRGs represent the dimensions from the case-mix weight as well as other factors, such as a regional wage index scoring. The home health PPS uses HHRGs, reflected on the claim as Health Insurance Prospective Payment System (HIPPS) codes, to calculate payment. OASIS data are used to automatically create a distinct alphanumeric home health HIPPS code that provides a snapshot of each beneficiary. This process occurs automatically once the patient's OASIS data have been electronically transmitted, and the HIPPS code registers in the HHA's billing system. The accuracy of the OASIS data thus drives the accuracy of the episode payment.

HHRG payment groupings are determined on the basis of several factors to provide the beneficiary snapshot:

- *Dimensions:* The HHRG has three dimensions: (1) clinical, (2) functional, and (3) service utilization. Each has severity categories within them corresponding to one portion of the HHRG code.
- *Severity points:* The severity points are derived from OASIS data collected by the HHA, which assigns a level of severity to each data item.
- *Early or later episodes:* An *early episode* is defined as the "1st or 2nd episode in a sequence of adjacent covered episodes" and a *later episode* as the "3rd episode and beyond in a sequence of adjacent covered episodes" (CMS, 2014c, § 10.1.19.2). An episode is considered adjacent if separated by fewer than 60 days. The adjacent episodes may not necessarily be provided by the same HHA. It is the responsibility of the HHA to record accurately whether an episode is early or later in the OASIS documentation because it affects the PPS payment.
- *Therapy utilization:* Early research for the home health prospective payment model revealed that therapy services in the POC had a significant impact on the utilization costs for an episode of care. Therefore, the home health PPS model has accounted for therapy costs in the episode payment formula on the basis of total combined therapy utilization. As evidence of the impact of therapy on home health evolved, the representation of therapy utilization in the HHRG has been adjusted.

Data provided for each of these factors are coded and grouped to determine what the payment will be.

Billing Procedures

PPS billing is a two-part process. At the beginning of the episode, the HHA submits a *request for anticipated payment* (RAP), which is the request to the Medicare contractor for the initial split payment percentage for that 60-day episode (CMS, 2014c,

§ 10.1.12). The HHA submits a RAP and receives a split payment estimate. The *Medicare Claims Processing Manual* mandates that an HHA can submit a RAP when all four of the following conditions are met:

1. The OASIS assessment has been transmitted to the state according to OASIS regulations.
2. A physician's verbal order to initiate home care has been received and documented by the HHA.
3. A POC has been established and sent to the physician for signature.
4. The first billable service visit has occurred (CMS, 2014c, § 10.1.10.3).

The HHA submits the final claim at the end of the episode to receive the remaining portion of the split payment (CMS, 2014c). The final payment is adjusted for any changes that occurred during the episode that affected the anticipated claim amount (e.g., therapy visits changed from the anticipated number established at start of care [SOC]). The HHA submits a final claim

- At the end of the 60-day period, or after the patient is discharged, whichever is earlier;
- Once all services are provided for the episode; and
- After the physician has signed the POC and any subsequent verbal orders (CMS, 2014c, § 10.1.10.4).

Circumstances that will cause the final payment to be adjusted include a partial episode payment (PEP), low utilization payment adjustments (LUPAs), death, and outliers.

Partial Episode Payment

A PEP occurs when a patient transfers to a different agency or is discharged (but not for admission to an inpatient facility) and readmitted to the same agency within a 60-day period. This scenario creates two separate episodes, and a PEP results in a payment adjustment for the first episode. The first episode receives only a partial prorated payment according to the number of days before transfer or discharge. The second episode receives a full episodic payment for the entirely new episode, regardless of whether it is the same or a different HHA or whether the reason for home health care is the same or different.

For example, a patient receiving home health services for an exacerbation of diabetes is discharged with all goals met on Day 30 of an episode. On Day 40, a new home health referral is received after hospitalization for a fractured hip. The HHA receives a prorated 30-day payment for the first segment, and the same (or different) agency then begins a new 60-day episode with the new referral (CMS, 2014c, § 10.1.15).

Low Utilization Payment Adjustment

A LUPA occurs when a beneficiary receives four or fewer visits by the HHA in a given 60-day episode. In this instance, the HHA is reimbursed for the visits with a predetermined, standardized, per-discipline rate annually established by CMS. If a LUPA is unplanned (e.g., if the patient goes to the hospital and does not return during the

60-day episode) and the RAP resulted in a payment to the agency, the difference between the RAP payment and the LUPA payment is recouped on a future payment (CMS, 2014c, § 10.1.17).

Death

Death of a beneficiary during an episode results in full payment for the episode or a LUPA payment if fewer than five total visits were made (CMS, 2014c, § 10.1.16).

Outliers

Outliers occur when beneficiaries require an unusually high level of care in the 60-day episode. For these beneficiaries, Medicare has established outlier payments in addition to the case-mix–adjusted episode payment. These additional service needs can be met by any of the six covered disciplines. Outliers are calculated automatically by the system on final claim submission. The formula is designed to help the HHA with excessive costs but does not reimburse the total amount, thus encouraging the HHA to be as cost efficient as possible (CMS, 2014c, § 10.1.21).

Part B Outpatient Therapy Services Provided by a Home Health Agency

Delivering Part B outpatient therapy in the context of their own home to patients who do not meet the criteria for *homebound* can increase the sustainability of outcomes. Part B therapy allows an HHA to provide the patient with the option of completing the POC with a familiar occupational therapist, which can be a powerful transition tool to community living.

An HHA may bill for Part B outpatient therapy if no Medicare Part A home health services are billed under a home health POC at the same time (e.g., the patient is not homebound) and there is a valid therapy POC. If a Medicare beneficiary is receiving any Part A home health services, he or she is ineligible to receive therapy under the Part B benefit (see the "Consolidated Billing" section in this appendix). An HHA must discharge a patient from Part A services before Part B outpatient rehabilitation can be initiated. Box A.1 provides a case example of a patient who transitioned from Part A to Part B therapy services delivered by an HHA.

Box A.1. Transition From Part A to Part B Outpatient Therapy Provided by a Home Health Agency

A primary care physician ordered home health skilled nursing, physical therapy, and occupational therapy for **Mrs. M** after cardiac surgery. The skilled nursing services in the home health plan of care (POC) were completed and discontinued before completion of therapy. Therapy continued on Mrs. M's home health POC, but she was nearing nonhomebound status.

Mrs. M visited her cardiac physician, who ordered outpatient physical and occupational therapy. The home health agency (HHA) discharged Mrs. M from Part A home health services and then commenced outpatient therapy under Part B coverage.

Although the cardiac physician made the referral for Part B outpatient services, Mrs. M was still under the POC of the Part A primary care physician. The HHA was responsible for communicating with both the primary care physician and the cardiac physician to coordinate care. All communication among the HHA, physicians, and outpatient therapists was clearly documented in Mrs. M's clinical record.

A physician-signed POC and specific documentation different from home health documentation are required for reimbursement of Part B outpatient services provided by an HHA. The POC for outpatient therapy provided by an HHA must be reviewed at least every 30 days by the therapist and certifying physician. The HHA bills the outpatient services on a different claim than Medicare Part A home health; outpatient billing uses the Healthcare Common Procedure Coding System, which is different from the HIPPS code for home health.

For reimbursement of outpatient therapy services, the Medicare Physician Fee Schedule (CMS, 2014d) is the method of payment and specifies any existing caps or other limitations that apply to the benefit. The beneficiary would need to meet his or her Part B deductible and pay a coinsurance (CMS, 2014b, § 10.2).

References

Centers for Medicare & Medicaid Services. (2013). Jimmo v. Sebelius *settlement agreement fact sheet*. Retrieved from http://www.cms.gov/Medicare/Medicare-Fee-for-Service-Payment/ SNFPPS/Downloads/Jimmo-FactSheet.pdf

Centers for Medicare & Medicaid Services. (2014a). *Medicare claims processing manual: Chapter 3—Inpatient hospital billing*. Retrieved from http://www.cms.gov/manuals/ downloads/clm104c03.pdf

Centers for Medicare & Medicaid Services. (2014b). *Medicare claims processing manual: Chapter 5—Part B outpatient rehabilitation and CORF/OPT services*. Retrieved from https://www.cms. gov/manuals/downloads/clm104c05.pdf

Centers for Medicare & Medicaid Services. (2014c). *Medicare claims processing manual: Chapter 10—Home health agency billing*. Retrieved from www.cms.gov/manuals/downloads/ clm104c10.pdf

Centers for Medicare & Medicaid Services. (2014d). *Physician fee schedule*. Retrieved from http://www.cms.gov/Medicare/Medicare-Fee-for-Service-Payment/PhysicianFeeSched

Centers for Medicare & Medicaid Services. (2015). *Medicare benefit policy manual: Chapter 7— Home health services*. Retrieved from https://www.cms.gov/Regulations-and-Guidance/ Guidance/Manuals/downloads//bp102c07.pdf

Home Health Prospective Payment System Rate Update for Calendar Year 2011; Changes in Certification Requirements for Home Health Agencies and Hospices, 42 CFR § 424.22. (2010).

Medicare.gov. (2014). *What Part B covers*. Retrieved from http://www.medicare.gov/what-medicare-covers/part-b/what-medicare-part-b-covers.html

APPENDIX B

Medicare as Regulator

*Missi Zahoransky, MSHS, OTR/L, and
Karen Vance, BSOT*

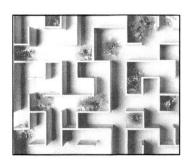

Contents

Overview of Medicare as Regulator

Medicare provides regulatory oversight for home health care providers and suppliers to ensure the quality and effectiveness of the services they provide. *Medicare providers* are "patient care institutions such as hospitals, critical access hospitals, hospices, nursing homes, and home health agencies" (Centers for Medicare & Medicaid Services [CMS], 2012, para. 2). *Medicare suppliers* are "agencies for diagnosis and therapy rather than sustained patient care, such as laboratories, clinics, and ambulatory surgery centers" (CMS, 2012, para. 2). The providers and suppliers must be participating in the Medicare program and must maintain quality standards to remain in it.

The *Conditions of Participation* (CoPs) are the minimum health and safety regulations that home health agencies (HHAs) must continually meet to remain in the Medicare and Medicaid programs. The CoPs can be found in the *Code of Federal*

Regulations (CFR), which has many sections and parts. Title 42 of the CFR, Part 484, cited as *42 CFR Part 484,* deals specifically with home health (CMS, 2011). The sections of the CFR are numbered for ease of location; in this appendix, these numbers are preceded by the section symbol (§), and sections omitted because they are not pertinent to home health occupational therapy are indicated by ellipses (spaced periods). Other regulations governing the organization and delivery of service by HHAs come from federal or state entities.

Regulations apply to all services provided by the agency, facility, and individual clinician. An agency may provide services to patients with various insurances and must be aware of the coverage criteria for each individual insurance. However, the regulations, unlike coverage criteria, apply to the treatment of all of a provider's patients, regardless of payer source, and HHAs must comply with all of the regulations to be a Medicare-certified provider of home health services. This appendix first defines Medicare-certified HHAs and then reprints the sections of the CoPs that are relevant to home health occupational therapy.

Medicare-Certified Home Health Agencies

The term *home health services* typically refers to Medicare-certified home health services. Although other organizations use the terms *home health* or *home care* when describing their services, they may be providing private-duty care or nonmedical services such as companion care, housekeeping, or chore services. The services provided by non–Medicare-certified organizations are paid for out of pocket or may be covered under a state Medicaid program or other insurance program.

A Medicare-certified HHA may be public (operated by state or local government), nonprofit (private, exempt from federal income taxation, and often supported by private contributions or foundations), or proprietary (private, profit making, and not exempt from taxation). Some HHAs choose to provide additional services outside the scope of the home health services listed in § 1861(m) of the Medicare Improvements for Patients and Providers Act of 2008 (Pub. L. 110–275); agencies are responsible for billing patients or other insurances for all noncovered services or supplies rendered. A Medicare-certified HHA

- Is primarily engaged in providing skilled nursing services and other therapeutic services;
- Has policies established by a group of professionals (associated with the agency or organization), including one or more physicians and one or more registered professional nurses, to govern the services which it provides;
- Provides for supervision of above-mentioned services by a physician or registered professional nurse;
- Maintains clinical records on all patients;
- Is licensed pursuant to State or local law, or has approval as meeting the standards established for licensing by the State or locality;
- Has in effect an overall plan and budget for institutional planning;
- Meets the federal requirements in the interest of the health and safety of individuals who are furnished services by the HHA; and
- Meets additional requirements as the Secretary finds necessary for the effective and efficient operation of the program. (CMS, 2013, para. 2)

The HHA must meet these requirements to be certified as a home health provider by Medicare, regardless of what insurances it bills or what types of patient the HHA provides services to.

Medicare Conditions of Participation

An HHA must comply with the CoPs to continue as a Medicare-certified agency, and the agency is dependent on its clinicians to maintain that compliance. Again, the HHA must adhere to these conditions for all patients served, regardless of payer source.

Locating and Identifying the Conditions of Participation

The intent of the CoPs is to ensure quality care provision for and protect the safety of Medicare beneficiaries. The sections in 42 CFR Part 484 pertaining to HHAs are as follows:

- Subpart A—General Provisions
  - 484.1   Basis and scope
  - 484.2   Definitions
  - 484.4   Personnel qualifications
- Subpart B—Administration
  - 484.10 Patient rights
  - 484.11 Release of patient identifiable Outcome and Assessment Information Set (OASIS) information
  - 484.12 Compliance with federal, state, and local laws, disclosure and ownership information, and accepted professional standards and principles
  - 484.14 Organization, services, and administration
  - 484.16 Group of professional personnel
  - 484.18 Acceptance of patients, plan of care, and medical supervision
  - 484.20 Reporting OASIS information
- Subpart C—Furnishing of Services
  - 484.30 Skilled nursing services
  - 484.32 Therapy services
  - 484.34 Medical social services
  - 484.36 Home health aide services
  - 484.38 Qualifying to furnish outpatient physical therapy or speech pathology services
  - 484.48 Clinical records
  - 484.52 Evaluation of the agency's program
  - 484.55 Comprehensive assessment of patients.

Two terms are used to describe the CoPs: (1) *conditions* and (2) *standards*. For example, Section § 484.55 addresses the condition *comprehensive assessment of patients* but includes many standards that are separately surveyed and assessed, such as the timing of the updates to the comprehensive assessment. As stated in the "Introduction" to this text and Self-Paced Clinical Course, the terms *evaluation* and *assessment* have meanings that are the reverse of those used in occupational therapy official documents. In the Medicare documents referred to in this appendix, *assessment* has the same meaning as *evaluation* as used in the occupational therapy official documents and refers to the overarching process of obtaining data with specific timelines about what data are to be collected and by whom.

Excerpts of the Conditions of Participation

The following CoPs are excerpted in this appendix for readers to reference:

- 484.4　　　　Personnel qualifications
- 484.14(g)　Standard: Coordination of patient services
- 484.18　　　Acceptance of patients, plan of care, and medical supervision
- 484.32　　　Therapy services
- 484.55　　　Comprehensive assessment of patients

42 CFR § 484.4　Personnel qualifications.

. . . .

Occupational therapist. A person who—

(a) (1) Is licensed or otherwise regulated, if applicable, as an occupational therapist by the State in which practicing, unless licensure does not apply;

(2) Graduated after successful completion of an occupational therapist education program accredited by the Accreditation Council for Occupational Therapy Education (ACOTE) of the American Occupational Therapy Association, Inc. (AOTA), or successor organizations of ACOTE; and

(3) Is eligible to take, or has successfully completed the entry-level certification examination for occupational therapists developed and administered by the National Board for Certification in Occupational Therapy, Inc. (NBCOT).

(b) On or before December 31, 2009—

(1) Is licensed or otherwise regulated, if applicable, as an occupational therapist by the State in which practicing; or

(2) When licensure or other regulation does not apply—

(i) Graduated after successful completion of an occupational therapist education program accredited by the Accreditation Council for Occupational Therapy Education (ACOTE) of the American Occupational Therapy Association, Inc. (AOTA) or successor organizations of ACOTE; and

(ii) Is eligible to take, or has successfully completed the entry-level certification examination for occupational therapists developed and administered by the National Board for Certification in Occupational Therapy, Inc., (NBCOT).

(c) On or before January 1, 2008—

(1) Graduated after successful completion of an occupational therapy program accredited jointly by the committee on Allied Health Education and Accreditation of the American Medical Association and the American Occupational Therapy Association; or

(2) Is eligible for the National Registration Examination of the American Occupational Therapy Association or the National Board for Certification in Occupational Therapy.

(d) On or before December 31, 1977—

(1) Had 2 years of appropriate experience as an occupational therapist; and

(2) Had achieved a satisfactory grade on an occupational therapist proficiency examination conducted, approved, or sponsored by the U.S. Public Health Service.

(e) If educated outside the United States, must meet all of the following:

(1) Graduated after successful completion of an occupational therapist education program accredited as substantially equivalent to occupational therapist entry level education in the United States by one of the following:

   (i) The Accreditation Council for Occupational Therapy Education (ACOTE).

   (ii) Successor organizations of ACOTE.

   (iii) The World Federation of Occupational Therapists.

   (iv) A credentialing body approved by the American Occupational Therapy Association.

(2) Successfully completed the entry-level certification examination for occupational therapists developed and administered by the National Board for Certification in Occupational Therapy, Inc. (NBCOT).

(3) On or before December 31, 2009, is licensed or otherwise regulated, if applicable, as an occupational therapist by the State in which practicing.

Occupational therapy assistant. A person who—

(a) Meets all of the following:

(1) Is licensed, unless licensure does not apply, or otherwise regulated, if applicable, as an occupational therapy assistant by the State in which practicing.

(2) Graduated after successful completion of an occupational therapy assistant education program accredited by the Accreditation Council for Occupational Therapy Education, (ACOTE) of the American Occupational Therapy Association, Inc. (AOTA) or its successor organizations.

(3) Is eligible to take or successfully completed the entry-level certification examination for occupational therapy assistants developed and administered by the National Board for Certification in Occupational Therapy, Inc. (NBCOT).

(b) On or before December 31, 2009—

(1) Is licensed or otherwise regulated as an occupational therapy assistant, if applicable, by the State in which practicing; or any qualifications defined by the State in which practicing, unless licensure does not apply; or

(2) Must meet both of the following:
  (i) Completed certification requirements to practice as an occupational therapy assistant established by a credentialing organization approved by the American Occupational Therapy Association.
  (ii) After January 1, 2010, meets the requirements in paragraph (a) of this section.

(c) After December 31, 1977 and on or before December 31, 2007—
  (1) Completed certification requirements to practice as an occupational therapy assistant established by a credentialing organization approved by the American Occupational Therapy Association; or
  (2) Completed the requirements to practice as an occupational therapy assistant applicable in the State in which practicing.

(d) On or before December 31, 1977—
  (1) Had 2 years of appropriate experience as an occupational therapy assistant; and
  (2) Had achieved a satisfactory grade on an occupational therapy assistant proficiency examination conducted, approved, or sponsored by the U.S. Public Health Service.

(e) If educated outside the United States, on or after January 1, 2008—
  (1) Graduated after successful completion of an occupational therapy assistant education program that is accredited as substantially equivalent to occupational therapist assistant entry level education in the United States by—
    (i)   The Accreditation Council for Occupational Therapy Education (ACOTE).
    (ii) Its successor organizations.
    (iii) The World Federation of Occupational Therapists.
    (iv) By a credentialing body approved by the American Occupational Therapy Association; and
  (2) Successfully completed the entry-level certification examination for occupational therapy assistants developed and administered by the National Board for Certification in Occupational Therapy, Inc. (NBCOT).

· · · ·

42 CFR § 484.14(g)   Standard: Coordination of patient services.

All personnel furnishing services maintain liaison to ensure that their efforts are coordinated effectively and support the objectives outlined in the plan of care. The clinical record or minutes of case conferences establish that effective interchange, reporting, and coordination of patient care does occur. A written summary report for each patient is sent to the attending physician at least every 60 days.

. . . .

42 CFR § 484.18   Condition of participation: Acceptance of patients, plan of care, and medical supervision.

Patients are accepted for treatment on the basis of a reasonable expectation that the patient's medical, nursing, and social needs can be met adequately by the agency in the patient's place of residence. Care follows a written plan of care established and periodically reviewed by a doctor of medicine, osteopathy, or podiatric medicine.

(a) *Standard: Plan of care.* The plan of care developed in consultation with the agency staff covers all pertinent diagnoses, including mental status, types of services and equipment required, frequency of visits, prognosis, rehabilitation potential, functional limitations, activities permitted, nutritional requirements, medications and treatments, any safety measures to protect against injury, instructions for timely discharge or referral, and any other appropriate items. If a physician refers a patient under a plan of care that cannot be completed until after an evaluation visit, the physician is consulted to approve additions or modifications to the original plan. Orders for therapy services include the specific procedures and modalities to be used and the amount, frequency, and duration. The therapist and other agency personnel participate in developing the plan of care.

(b) *Standard: Periodic review of plan of care.* The total plan of care is reviewed by the attending physician and HHA personnel as often as the severity of the patient's condition requires, but at least once every 60 days or more frequently when there is a beneficiary elected transfer; a significant change in condition resulting in a change in the case-mix assignment; or a discharge and return to the same HHA during the 60-day episode. Agency professional staff promptly alert the physician to any changes that suggest a need to alter the plan of care.

(c) *Standard: Conformance with physician orders.* Drugs and treatments are administered by agency staff only as ordered by the physician with the exception of influenza and pneumococcal polysaccharide vaccines, which may be administered per agency policy developed in consultation with a physician, and after an assessment for contraindications. Verbal orders are put in writing and signed and dated with the date of receipt by the registered nurse or qualified therapist (as defined in § 484.4 of this chapter) responsible for furnishing or supervising the ordered services. Verbal orders are only accepted by personnel authorized to do so by applicable State and Federal laws and regulations as well as by the HHA's internal policies.

. . . .

42 CFR § 484.32   Condition of participation: Therapy services.

Any therapy services offered by the HHA directly or under arrangement are given by a qualified therapist or by a qualified therapy assistant under the supervision of a qualified therapist and in accordance with the plan of care. The qualified therapist assists the physician in evaluating level of function, helps develop the plan of care (revising it as necessary), prepares clinical and progress notes, advises and consults with the family and other agency personnel, and participates in in-service programs.

(a) *Standard: Supervision of physical therapy assistant and occupational therapy assistant.* Services furnished by a qualified physical therapy assistant or qualified occupational therapy assistant may be furnished under the supervision of a qualified physical or occupational therapist. A physical therapy assistant or occupational therapy assistant performs services planned, delegated, and supervised by the therapist, assists in preparing clinical notes and progress reports, and participates in educating the patient and family, and in in-service programs.

. . . .

42 CFR § 484.55   Condition of participation: Comprehensive assessment of patients.

Each patient must receive, and an HHA must provide, a patient-specific, comprehensive assessment that accurately reflects the patient's current health status and includes information that may be used to demonstrate the patient's progress toward achievement of desired outcomes. The comprehensive assessment must identify the patient's continuing need for home care and meet the patient's medical, nursing, rehabilitative, social, and discharge planning needs. For Medicare beneficiaries, the HHA must verify the patient's eligibility for the Medicare home health benefit including homebound status, both at the time of the initial assessment visit and at the time of the comprehensive assessment. The comprehensive assessment must also incorporate the use of the current version of the Outcome and Assessment Information Set (OASIS) items, using the language and groupings of the OASIS items, as specified by the Secretary.

(a) *Standard: Initial assessment visit.*
   (1) A registered nurse must conduct an initial assessment visit to determine the immediate care and support needs of the patient; and, for Medicare patients, to determine eligibility for the Medicare home health benefit, including homebound status. The initial assessment visit must be held either within 48 hours of referral, or within 48 hours of the patient's return home, or on the physician-ordered start of care date.

(2) When rehabilitation therapy service (speech language pathology, physical therapy, or occupational therapy) is the only service ordered by the physician, and if the need for that service establishes program eligibility, the initial assessment visit may be made by the appropriate rehabilitation skilled professional.

(b) *Standard: Completion of the comprehensive assessment.*

(1) The comprehensive assessment must be completed in a timely manner, consistent with the patient's immediate needs, but no later than 5 calendar days after the start of care.

(2) Except as provided in paragraph (b)(3) of this section, a registered nurse must complete the comprehensive assessment and for Medicare patients, determine eligibility for the Medicare home health benefit, including homebound status.

(3) When physical therapy, speech–language pathology, or occupational therapy is the only service ordered by the physician, a physical therapist, speech–language pathologist or occupational therapist may complete the comprehensive assessment, and for Medicare patients, determine eligibility for the Medicare home health benefit, including homebound status. The occupational therapist may complete the comprehensive assessment if the need for occupational therapy establishes program eligibility.

(c) *Standard: Drug regimen review.* The comprehensive assessment must include a review of all medications the patient is currently using in order to identify any potential adverse effects and drug reactions, including ineffective drug therapy, significant side effects, significant drug interactions, duplicate drug therapy, and noncompliance with drug therapy.

(d) *Standard: Update of the comprehensive assessment.* The comprehensive assessment must be updated and revised (including the administration of the OASIS) as frequently as the patient's condition warrants due to a major decline or improvement in the patient's health status, but not less frequently than—

(1) The last five days of every 60 days beginning with the start-of-care date, unless there is a—

(i)   Beneficiary elected transfer;

(ii) Significant change in condition; or

(iii) Discharge and return to the same HHA during the 60-day episode.

(2) Within 48 hours of the patient's return to the home from a hospital admission of 24 hours or more for any reason other than diagnostic tests;

(3) At discharge.

(e) *Standard: Incorporation of OASIS data items.* The OASIS data items determined by the Secretary must be incorporated into the HHA's own assessment and must include: clinical record items, demographics and patient history, living arrangements, supportive assistance, sensory status, integumentary status, respiratory status, elimination status, neuro/emotional/behavioral status, activities of daily living, medications, equipment management, emergent care, and data items collected at inpatient facility admission or discharge only.

References

Centers for Medicare & Medicaid Services. (2011). *Part 484: Home health services.* Washington, DC: Author. Retrieved from http://www.gpo.gov/fdsys/pkg/CFR-2011-title42-vol5/pdf/CFR-2011-title42-vol5-part484.pdf

Centers for Medicare & Medicaid Services. (2012). *Survey and certification: Certification and compliance.* Retrieved from http://cms.gov/Medicare/Provider-Enrollment-and-Certification/CertificationandComplianc/index.html?redirect=/CertificationandComplianc

Centers for Medicare & Medicaid Services. (2013). *Home health providers.* Retrieved from https://www.cms.gov/Medicare/Provider-Enrollment-and-Certification/CertificationandComplianc/HHAs.html

Medicare Improvements for Patients and Providers Act of 2008, Pub. L. 110–275, 122 Stat. 2494.

APPENDIX C

Medicare as Quality Monitor

Karen Vance, BSOT

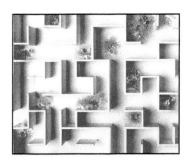

Contents

Overview of Medicare as Quality Monitor

Medicare has always had a role in monitoring the quality of service delivery by home health agencies (HHAs). Although Medicare's role in monitoring quality has not changed, the methods and measures by which quality is monitored have changed with advances in evidence and technology. Quality standards and measures are influenced by evidence from health care–related studies, analysis from the

Institute of Medicine (IOM), and electronically gathered evidence from the Outcome and Assessment Information Set (OASIS).

The IOM, a nonprofit nongovernmental organization that provides unbiased and authoritative advice to decision makers and the public to promote informed health care–related decisions, informed the Centers for Medicare & Medicaid Services' (CMS's) designs for quality measurement and control in home health (IOM, 2014). In a 2001 report titled *Crossing the Quality Chasm: A New Health System for the 21st Century,* the IOM called on all health care constituencies to support six aims for improvement based on the need for health care to be

1. *Safe:* avoiding injuries to patients from the care that is intended to help them.
2. *Effective:* providing services based on scientific knowledge to all who could benefit, and refraining from providing services to those not likely to benefit.
3. *Patient-centered:* providing care that is respectful of and responsive to individual patient preferences, needs, and values, and ensuring that patient values guide all clinical decisions.
4. *Timely:* reducing waits and sometimes harmful delays for both those who receive and those who give care.
5. *Efficient:* avoiding waste, including waste of equipment, supplies, ideas, and energy.
6. *Equitable:* providing care that does not vary in quality because of personal characteristics such as gender, ethnicity, geographic location, and socioeconomic status. (p. 3)

The IOM created this list of performance characteristics as a specific agenda for improvement across all sectors, forms of payment, types of organization, and clinical disciplines.

In 2001, the U.S. Department of Health and Human Services and CMS announced the Quality Initiative, launched nationally for several sectors of health care, and the Home Health Quality Initiative (HHQI) began in 2003 (CMS, 2014). The process of the HHQI begins with data collection to measure Outcome-Based Quality Improvement (OBQI). Medicare mandates and provides the technology for HHA-level quality improvement efforts for OBQI. OBQI is an ongoing process of outcome data collection, data analysis, and report generation to help agencies target outcomes needing improvement and develop action plans to improve the targeted outcomes. OBQI is essential to agencies' performance improvement activities and a key to unlocking many opportunities for occupational therapy practitioners to help their agencies improve outcomes. This appendix introduces the HHQI and discusses the OBQI process in detail.

As stated in the "Introduction" to this text and Self-Paced Clinical Course, the terms *evaluation* and *assessment* have meanings that are the reverse of those used in occupational therapy official documents. In the Medicare documents referred to in this appendix, *assessment* has the same meaning as *evaluation* as used in the occupational therapy official documents and refers to the overarching process of obtaining data with specific timelines about what data are to be collected and by whom.

Home Health Quality Initiative

The HHQI was designed with two purposes: (1) to enable consumers to make better-informed decisions about their health care by making available information about quality of care and (2) to stimulate and support providers and clinicians in improving the quality of health care. The sections that follow describe how these two purposes are promoted in home health care.

Empowerment of Consumers Through Public Disclosure

As discussed in Section I of this text, there are many stakeholders in the quality of home health care. For patients (i.e., consumers) and their caregivers, effectiveness of care registers as an individual human metric. For other stakeholders, including payers, regulators, researchers, and policymakers, effectiveness of care is measured on a broader scale that weighs it against the value gained as shown by the metrics of a population. To measure effectiveness at the population level, the metrics used must be well defined, consistent, comparable, and quantifiable. The *OBQI Manual* (CMS, 2010a) lists three perspectives on quality measures:

1. *Structural measures of quality* "assess the adequacy of the 'inputs' to care such as the care setting, the qualifications of care providers, and the equipment and technical devices used" and include "measures . . . such as percentage of [registered nurses] with bachelor's degrees at a given home health agency" (CMS, 2010a, p. 2-1).
2. *Process measures of quality* are the "'throughputs' to care such as specific interventions, comprehensiveness of assessment, and adequacy of care planning" and include measures "such as whether a depression assessment is conducted at admission" (CMS, 2010a, p. 2-1).
3. *Outcome measures of quality* are the "outputs" of care—that is, "what happens to the health status of patients as a result of care"—and include measures "such as whether a surgical wound healed during the care interval" (CMS, 2010a, p. 2-1).

Public disclosure of quality information is done through the CMS website Home Health Compare (HHC; Medicare.gov, n.d.), where consumers can compare the performance of different HHAs to make more-informed choices among them. Box C.1 shows a sample list of home health measures that have been publicly disclosed on HHC. These measures evolve as updates occur to OASIS and as evidence unfolds from the data.

Additional quality reporting requirements began in the third quarter of calendar year 2010. The Home Health Consumer Assessment of Healthcare Providers and Systems (HHCAHPS) Home Health Care Survey measures the experiences of people receiving home health care from Medicare-certified HHAs. The survey has three goals:

1. To produce comparable data on the patient's perspective that allows objective and meaningful comparisons between home health agencies on domains that are important to consumers.
2. Public reporting of survey results will create incentives for agencies to improve their quality of care.
3. Public reporting will enhance public accountability in health care by increasing the transparency of the quality of care provided in return for public investment. (Home Health Care CAHPS Survey, 2014, para. 1)

Box C.1. List of Home Health Compare Measures Publicly Reported

Measures of home health agencies' performance are publicly disclosed on the Centers for Medicare & Medicaid Services website Home Health Compare (http://www.medicare.gov/HomeHealthCompare) to enable consumers to make more informed choices. Agencies' performance is reported on measures such as the following:

- How often patients got better at walking or moving around
- How often patients got better at getting in and out of bed
- How often patients got better at bathing
- How often the home health team checked patients for pain
- How often the home health team treated patients' pain
- How often patients had less pain when moving around
- How often the home health team treated heart failure patients' symptoms
- How often patients' breathing improved
- How often patients' wounds improved or healed after an operation
- How often the home health team checked patients for the risk of developing pressure sores
- How often the home health team included treatments to prevent pressure sores in the plan of care
- How often the home health team took doctor-ordered action to prevent pressure sores
- How often patients had more pressure sores when home health care ended
- How often the home health team began patients' care in a timely manner
- How often the home health team taught patients (or their family caregivers) about their drugs
- How often patients got better at taking their drugs correctly by mouth
- How often the home health team checked patients' risk of falling
- How often the home health team checked patients for depression
- How often the home health team determined whether patients received a flu shot for the current flu season
- How often the home health team determined whether their patients received a pneumococcal vaccine (pneumonia shot)
- For patients with diabetes, how often the home health team got doctor's orders, gave foot care, and taught patients about foot care
- How often patients receiving home health care needed urgent, unplanned care in the hospital emergency room without being admitted to the hospital
- How often home health patients had to be admitted to the hospital.

Source. Medicare.gov (2014). In the public domain.

CMS began publicly reporting home health results from the HHCAHPS survey on HHC in April 2012.

Support for Providers' Quality Improvement Efforts

Support from CMS to enable providers and clinicians to improve the quality of the care they provide can be found in a set of manuals that provide tools to measure, monitor, and manage their performance. The manuals are available online and are briefly described below and reviewed in greater detail later in this appendix:

- The *OASIS–C1/ICD–10 Version Guidance Manual* (CMS, 2015) describes the use of OASIS to collect uniform health status data on patients receiving home health care.
- The *OBQI Manual* (CMS, 2010a) describes the OBQI Outcome Report in detail and helps HHAs use the data in this report and implement the steps in OBQI.
- The *Outcome-Based Quality Monitoring (OBQM) Manual* (CMS, 2010b) helps HHAs understand and use the information in the Agency Patient-Related

Characteristics Report and the Potentially Avoidable Event Report (discussed later in this appendix).
- The *Process-Based Quality Improvement (PBQI) Manual* (CMS, 2010c) describes the Process Quality Measure Report (discussed later in this appendix) and its use for quality improvement purposes.

OASIS data collection, the first step in the OBQI process, is detailed in **Appendix D.** The remainder of this appendix provides an overview of the OBQI framework and introduces the tools necessary to participate in the pursuit of quality at HHAs.

Outcome-Based Quality Improvement

OBQI focuses on ongoing data collection and analysis and the generation of reports to help agencies identify outcomes needing improvement. Monitoring the quality of home health service delivery is complex. As Shaughnessy, Crisler, Hittle, and Schlenker (2002) put it,

> In all, the nature, environment, and interpersonal circumstances of home care delivery are unique. It is extremely difficult and challenging to monitor the quality and effectiveness of care provided in the home. For this reason, monitoring patient outcomes is particularly useful in home care. Because the interval over which home care is provided should be characterized by improvement, stabilization, or a minimal rate of decline in functioning, health and functional status should be measured at a minimum of two time points: start of care and discharge. This is necessary to monitor change in health status over the care interval and evaluate the effectiveness of care. Changes in health status or patient outcomes can then be measured across large groups of patients cared for by a particular agency in order to judge whether its home care is effective relative to other agencies. (p. 3)

Outcome Definition

CMS (2010a) uses multiple definitions of *outcomes:*

- Outcomes are health status changes between two or more time points, where the term "health status" encompasses physiologic, functional, cognitive, emotional, and behavioral health.
- Outcomes are changes that are intrinsic to the patient.
- Outcomes are positive, negative, or neutral changes in health status.
- Outcomes are changes that result from care provided, from natural pro- gression of disease and disability, or from both. (p. 2-2)

The change between two time points can be "positive, negative, or neutral" (p. 2-2), so change in patient health status can be improvement, decline, or maintenance (i.e., no change). Maintenance is important to home health patients with chronic conditions whose desired outcome is to stabilize in order to remain safely in their own homes.

Measurement Time Points

To begin operationalizing the OBQI framework, occupational therapy practitioners need to know the time points implied in CMS's definitions of outcomes and under- stand when health status is to be measured to enable tracking of change. These time points are (1) start of care (SOC), (2) resumption of care (ROC), and (3) discharge. *Start of care* is the time of admission to an HHA, when OASIS assessment and data collection occur to establish the patient's baseline health status against which change will be measured. If the patient's home health episode is interrupted by an inpatient facility stay, the baseline is reset at the ROC OASIS assessment. The discharge OASIS data collection is the end point at which the patient's health status is measured. Outcome measurement begins at SOC or resets at ROC data collection and ends at discharge from the HHA, no matter how many times a patient is recertified for a new payment episode.

A payment episode is always 60 days, so if a patient is recertified and continues receiving services for a second payment episode, the span between the beginning and ending time points of the quality episode is 120 days. Even when a clinician other than an occupational therapist collects data at SOC, occupational therapy may be the only discipline remaining on the plan of care (POC) at the end of the episode to perform the discharge OASIS data collection. The data collected at discharge indicate whether the patient improved, stabilized, or declined in each of the outcome measures and are included in the HHA's publicly reported outcomes on HHC. Accurate data collection is critical to ensuring that the measures accurately reflect the patient's progress during a home health stay.

Two-Stage Framework: Outcome Analysis and Outcome Enhancement

OBQI has two stages: (1) *outcome analysis,* or analysis of the data collected by the HHA, and (2) *outcome enhancement,* or the steps the HHA takes to improve the outcomes the analysis identifies as in need of improvement (see Figure C.1).

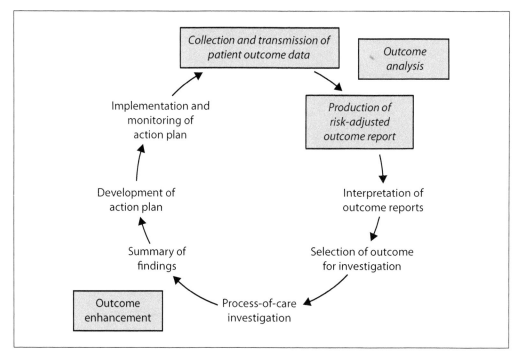

Figure C.1. Two-Stage Outcome-Based Quality Improvement (OBQI) framework.

Source. From *Outcome-Based Quality Improvement (OBQI) Manual* (p. 2-3), by Centers for Medicare & Medicaid Services, 2010, Baltimore: Author. Retrieved from http://www.cms.gov/HomeHealthQualityInits/Downloads/ HHQIOBQIManual.pdf. In the public domain.

Outcome Analysis

Outcome analysis is the first stage in OBQI. It is critical to be able to distinguish changes in a patient's health status that are attributable to the care provided from those attributable to the natural progression of the patient's condition. This distinction is accomplished through *risk adjustment,* which is the statistical process of compensating or controlling for the potential influence of non–care-related variables that can affect outcomes. Risk adjustment enables HHC to report changes that resulted from the care that an HHA provided and allows consumers to compare those outcomes among HHAs. The data are risk adjusted for the reports that describe outcome measures (discussed later in this section) but not for those that describe the process measures.

Risk adjustment prevents home health clinicians from being able to explain away poor performance outcomes by claiming that their patients are older or sicker or by citing some other risk factor that is outside their control. These factors are adjusted for in the data, so reported outcomes do not reflect the effect of factors HHAs cannot influence. Excusing a lower score on a particular outcome on the basis of patient age or presence of a chronic disease prevents the HHA from targeting that outcome for improvement; risk adjustment forces an objective, open-minded look at opportunities for performance improvement.

The data transmitted by the HHA are analyzed to produce aggregate reports that show the HHA's present performance in terms of total agency patient outcomes for a defined date range. The risk-adjusted outcome data allow comparison of the HHA's present performance with two references: (1) a national sample of home care patients and (2) the preceding time period for the HHA. The HHA's analyzed data are returned to the agency in the form of four different reports:

1. Outcome Report (addressed in detail in the *OBQI Manual* [CMS, 2010a])
2. Potentially Avoidable Event Report (addressed in detail in the *OBQM Manual* [CMS, 2010b])
3. Agency Patient-Related Characteristics Report (addressed in detail in the *OBQM Manual* [CMS, 2010b])
4. Process Quality Measure Report (addressed in detail in the *PBQI Manual* [CMS, 2010c]).

The date ranges reflected in these reports are chosen by the HHA when pulling the reports for review, and the current and prior reference periods are labeled with the selected dates. The number of eligible cases shows only the number of patients whose data are eligible to appear for each outcome measure. For example, when a patient scores the highest possible response for lower-body dressing, he or she cannot improve and therefore is not eligible to be counted in the pool of data for that measure.

When selecting outcomes for investigation, agencies consider the level of significance for each measure comparison. If the significance is greater than .10, the probability is high that any difference is attributable to some factor (e.g., a statistical artifact) other than the care provided. A significance level of .10 or less means that the difference between the HHA's current performance and its prior performance or national reference data is likely the result of the care provided. If the agency's current performance is significantly lower than the national reference data, the agency should target this outcome for improvement. The manuals corresponding to each report provide ample instructions and frequently asked questions explaining how to read and interpret the reports and how to use them to select outcomes for investigation.

Outcome Report

The Outcome Report displays clinical outcomes that meet the following criteria:

- They display sufficient variation within the home care patient population (i.e., they are neither extremely rare nor universally common).
- They can be affected by the care provided by a home care agency.
- They are amenable to risk adjustment (i.e., risk factors are readily measured and empirically demonstrate a statistical relationship with the outcome).
- They reflect meaningful aspects of health status or quality of life for home care patients. (CMS, 2010a, p. 2-5)

Table C.1 provides a complete list of end-result and utilization outcomes included in the Outcome Report. For each occupational therapy POC, practitioners should identify the outcome measures that target a performance area within the domain of occupational therapy and focus intervention on those measures to improve not only the patient's outcomes but also the HHA's overall outcomes.

Exhibit C.1 is an excerpt from an Outcome Report showing two end-result outcomes of interest to occupational therapy practitioners: (1) improvement in lower-body dressing and (2) improvement in bathing. In both of these reported outcomes, the HHA's current performance is lower than the national reference, indicating that these outcomes could be targeted for improvement. The improvement in lower-body dressing compared with the HHA's performance in the previous reference period may indicate that this measure had already been targeted and an action plan was currently in place; the improvement is significant at the .05 level, indicating that patient improvements likely occurred in response to the provided care.

Potentially Avoidable Event Report

The Potentially Avoidable Event Report is used to identify negative events (e.g., injury from a fall, decline in three or more activities of daily living, development of a pressure ulcer) experienced by an HHA's patients that could have been avoided. Attached to the report is a list of the patients who experienced each negative event reflected in the report; HHAs can use this list to investigate the patients' clinical records to ascertain whether the event might have been avoided with more appropriate care, thus contributing to improved quality of care. Exhibit C.2 shows a sample excerpt from this report.

Agency Patient-Related Characteristics Report

The Agency Patient-Related Characteristics Report is a summary of the characteristics, circumstances, disabilities, and diseases of the patients that an HHA serves. HHAs can compare data on patients admitted over a specific period with a national sample of patients and with the HHA's patients from a prior time period. These data help identify differences in a specific HHA's patient population and those of other HHAs, and trends and patterns seen in this report can inform agency decisions

Table C.1. OASIS-Based Outcome Measures

Outcome Category[a]	Measure
End-result outcomes	
Clinical status improvement	Improvement in anxiety level
	Improvement in behavior problem frequency
	Improvement in bowel incontinence
	Improvement in confusion frequency
	Improvement in dyspnea[b]
	Improvement in pain interfering with activity[b]
	Improvement in speech and language
	Improvement in status of surgical wounds[b]
	Improvement in urinary incontinence
	Improvement in urinary tract infection
Clinical status stabilization	Stabilization in anxiety level
	Stabilization in cognitive functioning
	Stabilization in speech and language
Functional status improvement	Improvement in ambulation/locomotion[b]
	Improvement in bathing[b]
	Improvement in bed transferring[b]
	Improvement in dressing—lower body
	Improvement in dressing—upper body
	Improvement in eating
	Improvement in grooming
	Improvement in management of oral medications[b]
	Improvement in light meal preparation
	Improvement in phone use
	Improvement in toileting hygiene
	Improvement in toilet transferring
Functional status stabilization	Stabilization in bathing
	Stabilization in bed transferring
	Stabilization in grooming
	Stabilization in light meal preparation
	Stabilization in management of oral medications
	Stabilization in phone use
	Stabilization in toileting hygiene
	Stabilization in toilet transferring
Utilization outcomes	
	Acute care hospitalization[b]
	Discharged to community
	Emergency department use without hospitalization[b]
	Emergency department use with hospitalization

Source. Adapted from *Outcome-Based Quality Improvement (OBQI) Manual* (p. 2-6), by Centers for Medicare & Medicaid Services, 2010, Baltimore: Author. Retrieved from http://www.cms.gov/HomeHealthQualityInits/Downloads/HHQIOBQIManual.pdf. In the public domain.
Note. OASIS = Outcome and Assessment Information Set.
[a]*End-result outcomes* are health status outcomes. *Utilization outcomes* suggest but do not unequivocally reflect health status changes (and, as a result, can be regarded as proxy or surrogate outcomes).
[b]These measures are publicly reported for each agency on Home Health Compare (Medicare.gov, n.d.).

about program development. Exhibit C.3 shows an example of an Agency Patient-Related Characteristics Report.

Process Quality Measure Report
The Process Quality Measure Report provides the rates of use of specific best practices for home health care. OASIS process measures address timeliness of care, care coordination, population health and prevention, effectiveness of care, and safety. Process quality measures are not risk adjusted like the outcome measures. Exhibit C.4 provides an excerpt from a Process Quality Measure Report. More detail on this report can be found in the *PBQI Manual* (CMS, 2010c).

Exhibit C.1. Excerpt From an Outcome Report

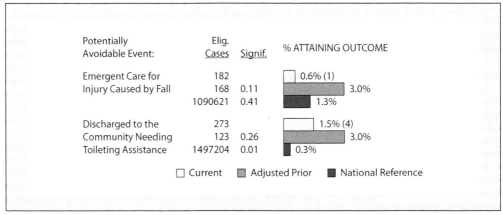

End Result Outcomes:	Elig. Cases	Signif.	% ATTAINING OUTCOME
Improvement in	203		59.5% (121)
Lower Body Dressing	183	0.05++	49.1%
	1473483	0.14	64.6%
Improvement in	262		59.5% (156)
Bathing	253	0.38	55.2%
	1994597	0.21	63.3%

☐ Current   ▨ Adjusted Prior   ■ National Reference

++ The probability is 5% or less that this difference is due to chance, and 95% or more that the difference is real.

Source. From *Outcome-Based Quality Improvement (OBQI) Manual* (p. 4-9), by Centers for Medicare & Medicaid Services, 2010, Baltimore: Author. Retrieved from http://www.cms.gov/HomeHealthQualityInits/Downloads/HHQIOBQIManual.pdf. In the public domain.

Outcome Enhancement

The second stage of the OBQI framework is *outcome enhancement,* or use of collected, analyzed, and reported data to improve an HHA's performance and enhance the outcomes reported. Many HHAs have OBQI committees to review reports and suggest ways to enhance outcomes. Sitting on the OBQI committee provides occupational therapy practitioners with opportunities to demonstrate the appropriate use of their services and identify ways occupational therapy can contribute to outcome improvement.

The four steps in outcome enhancement are

- Selecting specific outcomes from the risk-adjusted or descriptive Outcome Reports;
- Evaluating the care that produced these outcomes in your agency;
- Developing a plan of action to improve care (or to reinforce care where outcomes are superior to the reference); and
- Implementing and monitoring the plan of action in the agency. (CMS, 2010a, p. 4-1)

Exhibit C.2. Excerpt From a Potentially Avoidable Event Report

Potentially Avoidable Event:	Elig. Cases	Signif.	% ATTAINING OUTCOME
Emergent Care for	182		0.6% (1)
Injury Caused by Fall	168	0.11	3.0%
	1090621	0.41	1.3%
Discharged to the	273		1.5% (4)
Community Needing	123	0.26	3.0%
Toileting Assistance	1497204	0.01	0.3%

☐ Current   ▨ Adjusted Prior   ■ National Reference

Source. From *Outcome-Based Quality Monitoring (OBQM) Manual: Agency Patient-Related Characteristics Reports and Potentially Avoidable Event Reports* (p. 3-3), by Centers for Medicare & Medicaid Services, 2010, Baltimore: Author. Retrieved from http://www.cms.gov/HomeHealthQualityInits/Downloads/HHQIOBQMManual.pdf. In the public domain.

Exhibit C.3. Excerpt From an Agency Patient-Related Characteristics Report

	Current Mean	Prior Mean	Ref. Mean		Current Mean	Prior Mean	Ref. Mean
PATIENT HISTORY				**LIVING ARRANGEMENT / ASSISTANCE**			
Demographics				**Current Situation**			
Age (years)	70.75	70.96	72.78*	Lives alone (%)	33.3%	32.8%	32.4%
Gender: Female (%)	69.4%	66.6%	62.9%**	Lives with others (%)	34.7%	32.4%+	34.9%
Race: Black (%)	1.7%	1.6%	10.7%**	Lives in congregate situation (%)	32.0%	34.8%	32.7%
Race: White (%)	97.5%	97.8%	85.5%**	**Availability**			
Race: Other (%)	0.8%	0.7%	3.8%**	Around the clock (%)	39.0%	40.2%	38.2%
Payment Source				Regular daytime (%)	0.9%	0.7%	3.9%
Any Medicare (%)	80.4%	81.5%	82.6%	Regular nighttime (%)	0.5%	0.3%	2.0%
Any Medicaid (%)	12.9%	14.4%	14.3%	Occasional (%)	22.0%	21.6%	21.3%
Any HMO (%)	3.0%	2.9%	5.8%**	None (%)	37.7%	37.2%	34.5%**
Medicare HMO (%)	1.3%	1.2%	2.2%				
Other (%)	19.9%	23.5%+	21.9%	**CARE MANAGEMENT**			
Episode Start				**ADLs**			
Episode timing: Early (%)	74.7%	73.1%	78.7%*	None needed (%)	63.4%	60.3%	71.9%**
Episode timing: Later (%)	20.5%	21.1%	14.1%**	Caregiver currently provides (%)	21.9%	23.8%	16.9%
Episode timing: Unknown (%)	4.8%	5.8%	7.2%	Caregiver training needed (%)	10.0%	10.8%	7.4%
Inpatient Discharge /				Uncertain/Unlikely to be provided (%)	3.7%	4.0%	2.0%
Medical Regimen Change				Needed, but not available (%)	1.0%	1.1%	1.8%
Long-term nursing facility (%)	1.3%	1.2%	2.2%	**IADLs**			
Skilled nursing facility (%)	2.1%	1.9%	2.1%	None needed (%)	77.1%	80.9%	67.5%**
Short-stay acute hospital (%)	27.3%	30.0%	27.2%	Caregiver currently provides (%)	13.1%	10.8%	18.9%*
Long-term care hospital (%)	64.6%	60.9%	62.2%	Caregiver training needed (%)	6.6%	5.4%	9.4%
Inpatient rehab hospital/unit (%)	2.3%	2.0%	3.3%	Uncertain/Unlikely to be provided (%)	2.2%	1.8%	3.1%
Psychiatric hospital/unit (%)	1.3%	1.3%	1.6%	Needed, but not available (%)	1.0%	1.1%	1.1%
Medical regimen change (%)	99.2%	98.5%	86.5%*	Frequency of ADL/IADL (1–5)	2.89	2.68	2.68

Source. From *Outcome-Based Quality Monitoring (OBQM) Manual: Agency Patient-Related Characteristics Reports and Potentially Avoidable Event Reports* (p. 2-2, Table 2.1), by Centers for Medicare & Medicaid Services, 2010, Baltimore: Author. Retrieved from http://www.cms.gov/HomeHealthQualityInits/Downloads/ HHQIOBQMManual.pdf. In the public domain.

Note. ADLs = activities of daily living; HMO = health maintenance organization; IADLs = instrumental activities of daily living. A single asterisk [*] corresponds to the 0.01 level of significance (i.e., a 1% probability that the observed difference is due to chance or a 99% probability that the difference is real). A double asterisk [**] corresponds to the 0.001 level of significance (0.1% probability).

Exhibit C.4. Excerpt From a Process Quality Measure Report

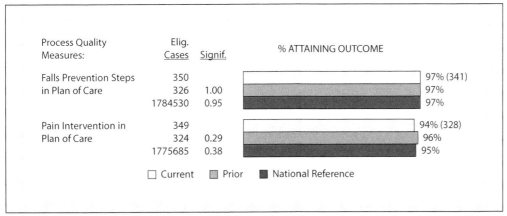

Source. From *Process-Based Quality Improvement (PBQI) Manual* (p. 2-11), by Centers for Medicare & Medicaid Services, 2010, Baltimore: Author. Retrieved from http://www.cms.gov/HomeHealthQualityInits/Downloads/HHQIOASIS-PBQI.pdf. In the public domain.

The sections that follow discuss each of these steps in turn.

Selection of Outcomes for Investigation

The *OBQI Manual* lists six criteria, in the order to be considered, for HHAs to use in selecting outcomes to investigate for enhancement (CMS, 2010b, p. 4-2–4-4):

1. *Statistically significant outcome differences.* Outcomes selected should be those in which the agency's performance is significantly lower than either the agency's previous performance or the national reference data.
2. *Larger magnitude of outcome differences.* Because the level of statistical significance varies according to sample size, comparing the magnitude of differences in outcomes (e.g., percentage of patients achieving the outcomes) between the groups is also a consideration in selecting an outcome for investigation.
3. *Adequate number of cases.* At least 30 eligible cases should be represented in the outcome data when evaluating potential target outcomes. A smaller sample size can result in an outcome percentage that may inaccurately reflect the real level of the problem.
4. *Significance levels of outcome differences.* When the Outcome Reports show no statistically significant differences at the .10 level, the HHA can target the outcome measures with significance levels closest to .10 (but no greater than .25).
5. *Importance or relevance to the agency's goals.* The HHA may select outcome measures for investigation that have importance for its strategic planning goals or specific objectives in a quality initiative program.
6. *Clinical significance.* An HHA may select an outcome measure for investigation when either outcome differences indicate potentially serious clinical problems or an HHA wants to focus on specific outcomes important for special programs or patient or payer types.

Using these criteria, an HHA can focus time and energy on the outcomes that are most relevant and critical to improving its delivery of quality home health services.

Evaluation of Care Processes

Once the HHA has selected outcomes to target for improvement, the momentum toward improved patient care continues with the *process-of-care investigation,* in which the HHA systematically investigates the clinical actions contributing to targeted outcomes and identifies the aspects of care provision it must change or reinforce to improve those outcomes (see Figure C.2). The process-of-care investigation includes

- Identifying pertinent important clinical actions that are anticipated to occur when providing care,
- Determining the specific aspects of a problem (or strength) in care delivery that contribute to the outcome results after investigating the care that was provided, and
- Specifying best practices to be implemented (CMS, 2010a).

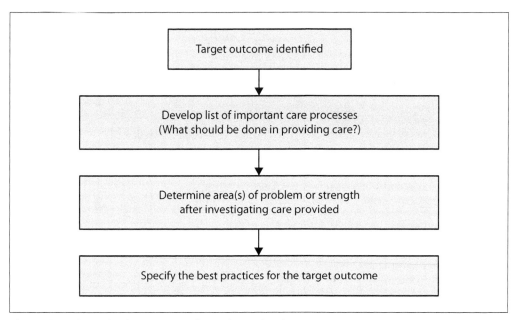

Figure C.2. Steps in the process-of-care investigation.

Source. From *Outcome-Based Quality Improvement (OBQI) Manual* (p. 5-5), by Centers for Medicare & Medicaid Services, 2010, Baltimore: Author. Retrieved from http://www.cms.gov/HomeHealthQualityInits/Downloads/HHQIOBQIManual.pdf. In the public domain.

Unlike OBQI, which targets outcomes, PBQI starts with rates of compliance with best practices that have already been identified by the process measures in the OASIS. The process of investigation then identifies the reasons for low rates of compliance with the best care practices chosen by the agency for implementation. Table C.2 compares the steps in the two processes.

HHAs may take PBQI one step further and investigate process quality measures in conjunction with relevant outcomes. For example, the measure *improvement in pain interfering with activity* might have an associated process quality measure such as

- Pain assessment conducted,
- Pain interventions in POC, or
- Pain interventions implemented during all episodes of care.

Table C.2. Comparison of Outcome- and Process-Based Quality Improvement Actions

Outcome-Based Quality Improvement Actions	Process-Based Quality Improvement Actions
Selection of specific outcomes from the Outcome Reports	Selection of specific care processes from the Process Quality Measure Report
Evaluation of the care that produced these outcomes in the agency	Assessment of reasons for low rates of compliance with the best-practice care processes
Development of a plan of action to improve care (or to reinforce care when outcomes are superior to national reference data), focusing on best-care practices	Development of a plan of action to improve rates of compliance with best-practice care processes
Implementation and monitoring of the plan of action	Implementation of a plan of action and monitoring for improvement in rates of compliance with best-practice care processes

Source. Adapted from *Process-Based Quality Improvement (PBQI) Manual* (p. 3-1), by Centers for Medicare & Medicaid Services, 2010, Baltimore: Author. Retrieved from http://www.cms.gov/HomeHealthQualityInits/Downloads/HHQIOASIS-PBQI.pdf. In the public domain.

The *PBQI Manual* (CMS, 2010c, p. 3-2) provides several more examples.

If the HHA is investigating a lower-than-desired rate of improvement in pain interfering with activity (outcome), as part of the OBQI investigation it can identify specific process quality measure findings that may be related to the low rate. If the HHA has low rates of compliance with the process quality measure *pain interventions* implemented during all episodes of care, then during the process-of-care investigation, the HHA could determine whether patients for whom the best practices were not implemented were also those patients whose pain interfering with activity did not improve. If the investigation finds that the low rates of compliance with the process quality measures have affected the target outcome of pain interfering with activity, the HHA can develop and implement a plan of action to improve the use of the best care practices with the specific goal of decreasing pain interfering with activity.

Not every outcome measure has specific process quality measures associated with it, but best practices measured in the Process Quality Measure Report may affect several of the OBQI outcome measures and potentially avoidable event (adverse event or OBQM) outcomes. The *OBQI Manual* provides guidance for accessing the reports, selecting charts for the process-of-care investigation, selecting tools to use for chart review, and drawing conclusions to take the process-of-care investigation to the next step—development of a plan of action.

Development of a Plan of Action

A plan of action is written for each targeted outcome to guide the agency's outcome enhancement activities. A standard format for plans of action is first to summarize the findings of the process-of-care investigation and then to delineate the clinical practices the HHA desires to put into place (examples can be found in the *OBQI Manual;* CMS, 2010a, p. 7-4). A plan of action includes

- Designation as an OBQI or PBQI activity
- Type of activity targeted
- Target outcome
- Statement of the identified problem
- Development of best practices
- Action strategies and monitoring approaches
- Evaluation (CMS, 2010a).

The plan of action first provides a problem statement identifying the type of activity targeted for action and its outcome. It then identifies best practices to address the problem, which lead to guidelines for implementing the plan that identify the exact clinical actions clinicians should take and when and how to do so.

Occupational therapy practitioners' identification of best practices to be added to the plan of action is critical to improve the HHA's performance relative to target outcomes and to strengthen the position of occupational therapy in the home health setting. For example, a common diagnosis in home health is chronic obstructive pulmonary disease. Implementing energy conservation strategies is a best-practice intervention for occupational therapy practitioners working with a patient who has limited energy for daily routines. Suggesting this best practice as a clinical action for this diagnosis on a regular basis could improve both functional outcome and dyspnea outcome measures for the HHA.

Implementation and Monitoring of the Plan of Action

The plan of action specifies *action strategies*, or activities that facilitate the specified best practices identified in the plan. Action strategies must be related to the best practices, practical and achievable, adequate to change care, and scheduled to begin immediately. To implement the plan of action, all appropriate clinicians perform the specific action strategies the team has identified as necessary to enhance the target outcome.

Changing care processes is complex, and the *OBQI Manual* encourages HHAs to move beyond traditional in-service approaches when designing the interventions to spread designated best practices across the HHA. Standardizing best practices among clinicians in an HHA will facilitate changes in care behaviors and result in improved patient outcomes.

Approaches to monitoring the plan of action and obtaining information about staff use of best practices include

- Quarterly record review,
- Peer review,
- Supervisory visits for periodic evaluations,
- Staff meetings, and
- Case conferences.

These approaches are easily incorporated into the HHA's normal operations, which helps ensure that the monitoring steps actually occur.

References

Centers for Medicare & Medicaid Services. (2010a). *Outcome-Based Quality Improvement (OBQI) manual*. Baltimore: Author. Retrieved from http://www.cms.gov/HomeHealthQualityInits/Downloads/HHQIOBQIManual.pdf

Centers for Medicare & Medicaid Services. (2010b). *Outcome-Based Quality Monitoring (OBQM) manual: Agency patient-related characteristics reports and potentially avoidable event reports*. Baltimore: Author. Retrieved from http://www.cms.gov/HomeHealthQualityInits/Downloads/HHQIOBQMManual.pdf

Centers for Medicare & Medicaid Services. (2010c). *Process-Based Quality Improvement (PBQI) manual*. Baltimore: Author. Retrieved from http://www.cms.gov/HomeHealthQualityInits/Downloads/HHQIOASIS-PBQI.pdf

Centers for Medicare & Medicaid Services. (2014). *Home Health Quality Initiative*. Retrieved from http://www.cms.gov/Medicare/Quality-Initiatives-Patient-Assessment-Instruments/HomeHealthQualityInits/index.html?redirect=/HomeHealthQualityInits

Centers for Medicare & Medicaid Services. (2015). *OASIS–C1/ICD–10 version guidance manual*. Retrieved from http://www.cms.gov/Medicare/Quality-Initiatives-Patient-Assessment-Instruments/HomeHealthQualityInits/HHQIOASISUserManual.html

Home Health Care CAHPS Survey. (2014). *Overview*. Retrieved from https://homehealthcahps.org/GeneralInformation/AboutHomeHealthCareCAHPSSurvey.aspx

Institute of Medicine. (2001). *Crossing the quality chasm: A new health system for the 21st century*. Washington, DC: National Academy Press.

Institute of Medicine. (2014). *About the IOM*. Retrieved from http://www.iom.edu/About-IOM.aspx

Medicare.gov. (n.d.). *Home Health Compare: Process of care and outcome of care quality measures*. Retrieved from http://www.medicare.gov/homehealthcompare/Data/Quality-Measures-List.html

Shaughnessy, P., Crisler, K., Hittle, D., & Schlenker, R. (2002). *Summary of the report on OASIS and Outcome-Based Quality Improvement in home health care: Research and demonstration findings, policy implications, and considerations for future change*. Denver: University of Colorado Health Sciences Center, Center for Health Services Research.

APPENDIX D

Outcome and Assessment Information Set (OASIS)

Karen Vance, BSOT

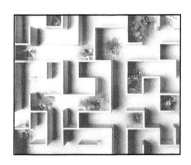

Contents

Overview of OASIS

The Outcome and Assessment Information Set (OASIS) is a data collection set that captures a picture of the home health population and measures the success of the services provided in home health settings. As described on the website of the Centers for Medicare & Medicaid Services (CMS; 2012),

> OASIS is a group of data items . . . designed for the purpose of enabling the rigorous and systematic measurement of patient home health care outcomes, with appropriate adjustment for patient risk factors affecting those outcomes. Outcomes have been defined in many ways, but those derived from OASIS items have a very specific definition: they measure changes in a patient's health status between two or more time points. . . . OASIS data items address sociodemographic, environmental, support system, health status, functional status, and health service utilization characteristics of the patient. The data are collected at start of care, 60-day follow-ups, and discharge (and surrounding an inpatient facility stay). (paras. 1–2)

OASIS is the first step, measurement (data collection), in Outcome-Based Quality Improvement (OBQI; CMS, 2010a), discussed in **Appendix C.** The OASIS data set was developed by the Center for Health Services Research at the University of Colorado Health Sciences Center through a research and demonstration program funded primarily by CMS, with additional funding from the Robert Wood Johnson Foundation and the New York State Department of Health.

Together with agency- and discipline-specific content, OASIS is part of the home health comprehensive assessment. The measure of success in home health is the *outcome*, defined as a change in a patient's health status between a beginning and an ending time point. OASIS contains a group of standard items designed to enable systematic measurement, documentation, reporting, and analysis of home health patient outcomes, with adjustment for patient characteristics affecting those outcomes (CMS, 2015).

In addition to outcomes, OASIS includes measures of processes of care that reflect best practices. Process measures were identified through a literature review and by industry experts for the *OBQI Manual* (CMS, 2010a). In particular, the process data elements reflect the recommendations of the Institute of Medicine (IOM; 2000) and of the Medicare Payment Advisory Commission (2015), a congressional agency that provides analysis and policy advice on Medicare, to focus on high-risk, high-volume, problem-prone conditions in home health. OASIS process measures capture such domains as

- Timeliness of care,
- Care coordination,
- Population health and prevention,
- Effectiveness of care, and
- Safety.

Certain OASIS items can be used to predict the amount of resources a home health agency (HHA) will need to serve a patient for a 60-day episode of care, given the clinical, functional, and service need characteristics of that patient. Therefore, OASIS data are also a part of the prospective payment system (PPS) formula that helps determine the amount of predetermined Medicare payments for home health services. Payment for every 60-day episode in every agency across the nation begins with the same dollar amount (the PPS base payment). This dollar amount is multiplied by a regional wage index that reflects labor costs in the specific geographic region. The resulting amount is then multiplied by the case-mix weight, which individualizes the payment to the characteristics and conditions of the particular patient. The case-mix weight is derived from specific OASIS items that create a clinical and functional picture of the patient, referred to as *case-mix items*. HHA personnel often refer to case-mix items as *payment items*. Many OASIS forms or electronic databases highlight case-mix items in some way to ensure that clinicians pay extra attention to completing them accurately.

Thus, occupational therapy practitioners use OASIS to create a picture of the patient through accurate documentation, which translates to the bottom line: a PPS payment. Occupational therapists need to understand how to collect OASIS data accurately to practice effectively within the regulatory and payment requirements of the home health setting. Accurate data collection reflects Standard I, Professional Standing and Responsibility, in the *Standards of Practice for Occupational Therapy* (American Occupational Therapy Association [AOTA], 2015), which states, "An occupational therapy practitioner is knowledgeable about and delivers occupational therapy services in accordance with AOTA standards, policies, and guidelines and state, federal, and other regulatory and payer requirements relevant to practice and service delivery" (p. 3). This appendix describes the accurate and effective use of OASIS in home health occupational therapy.

As stated in the "Introduction" to this text and Self-Paced Clinical Course (SPCC), the terms *evaluation* and *assessment* have meanings that are the reverse of those used in occupational therapy official documents. In the Medicare documents referred to in this appendix, *assessment* has the same meaning as *evaluation* as used in the occupational therapy official documents and refers to the overarching process of obtaining data with specific timelines about what data are to be collected and by whom.

OASIS Guidance Manual

The first resource and last word on OASIS data collection is the *OASIS Guidance Manual,* available for free on CMS's website (CMS, 2015). The *OASIS Guidance Manual,* one of four manuals, addresses data collection as the first step in outcome measurement; the other three manuals focus on the subsequent steps in OBQI:

- The *OBQI Manual* (CMS, 2010a) describes how agencies can use OASIS to improve outcomes.
- The *Outcome-Based Quality Monitoring (OBQM) Manual: Agency Patient-Related Characteristics Reports and Potentially Avoidable Event Reports* (CMS, 2010b) describes the use of two OASIS-based reports in the agency's quality monitoring program.
- The *Process-Based Quality Improvement (PBQI) Manual* (CMS, 2010c) describes the use of process-of-care best practices in home health care delivery.

Although OASIS data are also used as part of the PPS payment formula, this set of manuals emphasizes the original intent of OASIS: to provide a measurement tool to aid in the pursuit of quality home health service delivery.

OASIS has gone through several versions since its original development and will continue to evolve. This text references the most current version of the *OASIS Guidance Manual* at the time of this writing (CMS, 2015) to enable readers to locate greater detail on the topics under discussion.

How to Retrieve the *OASIS Guidance Manual*

The CMS website provides the current version of the *OASIS Guidance Manual* (see CMS, 2015). HHAs commonly provide clinicians with versions of the *OASIS Guidance Manual,* but clinicians should ensure that the printed versions match those on the CMS website, which is the only reliable source of the most current version.

How to Navigate the *OASIS Guidance Manual*

Downloading the manual opens a compressed folder containing pdf files for each part of the *OASIS Guidance Manual.* Among the files are the following:

- "Manual Cover and TOC" provides a preface and a detailed table of contents for the entire *OASIS Guidance Manual.*
- "Chapter1" provides an overview of the manual, an explanation of the revisions reflected in the current version, a summary of facts, and instructions for collecting and transmitting accurate data.
- "Chapter2_Intro" introduces the separate files for OASIS items required at specific time points. "Chapter2_OASIS-C1 ICD-10_ALL" provides a tracking sheet with an overview of items required at all time points.
- "Chapter3_Intro" introduces the OASIS item-specific guidance, provided in separate files labeled with a section letter and item category. The item-specific guidance discussed later in this appendix is from the Chapter 3 files.
- "Chapter4" contains sample clinical record forms incorporating OASIS items that agencies can use as guidance in developing their own forms.
- "Chapter5" contains citations and links to resources that support agencies' use of OASIS.
- Appendix files address comprehensive assessment, accuracy of OASIS data, guidance on which items to report at each time point, regulations on data reporting, background on OASIS and OBQI, and changes made in recent versions of OASIS.

Hereinafter in this appendix, the term *OASIS Guidance Manual* refers to the item-specific guidance found in Chapter 3 of the manual, including the separate section files, which readers should download before continuing to read this appendix. OASIS items have numbers consisting of the letter M and four numerals corresponding to the section topics (see Table D.1). Because new items may be added in future updates, the numbers within each section are not necessarily continuous.

Regulations Governing OASIS Data Collection

OASIS data collection and transmission are required for all nonmaternity patients age 18 years or older who are receiving skilled services covered by Medicare or Medicaid (CMS, 2015, p. 1-2). OASIS data must be integrated into an HHA's comprehensive assessment. Although OASIS data collection is not required for non-Medicare and non-Medicaid beneficiaries, Medicare-certified agencies are required to perform the comprehensive assessment, including OASIS data collection, for all patients receiving their services as a Condition of Participation (CoP; CMS, 2011). Thus, all patients receiving skilled care from an HHA are expected to receive the

Table D.1. OASIS–C1 Numbering System

Section	Item Numbers
A. Patient tracking	M0010–M0069; M0140–M0150
B. Clinical record	M0080–M0110
C. Patient history and diagnoses	M1000–M1056
D. Living arrangements	M1100
E. Sensory status	M1200–M1242
F. Integumentary status	M1300–M1350
G. Respiratory status	M1400–M1410
H. Cardiac status	M1500–M1510
I. Elimination status	M1600–M1630
J. Neuro/emotional/behavioral status	M1700–M1750
K. ADLs/IADLs	M1800–M1910
L. Medications	M2000–M2040
M. Care management	M2102–M2110
N. Therapy need and plan of care	M2200–M2250
O. Emergent care	M2300–M2310
P. Discharge (also data collected at transfer or death)	M0903, M0906, M2400–M2430

Source. From Centers for Medicare & Medicaid Services, *OASIS–C1/ICD–10 Guidance Manual,* 2015, Baltimore: Author. Retrieved from http://www.cms.gov/Medicare/Quality-Initiatives-Patient-Assessment-Instruments/ HomeHealthQualityInits/HHQIOASISUserManual.html. In the public domain.
Note. ADLs = activities of daily living; IADLs = instrumental activities of daily living; OASIS = Outcome and Assessment Information Set.

comprehensive assessment, regardless of diagnosis or services ordered. Needs for referral to additional services are also identified through the comprehensive assessment.

Incorporating OASIS Data Into the Comprehensive Assessment

Regulations mandate that Medicare-certified agencies incorporate OASIS items into the comprehensive assessment and that in doing so they maintain the exact item number, wording, and skip pattern. The HHA, however, may arrange the sequence of the numbered items and the format of the comprehensive assessment according to agency preferences. The electronic software an HHA uses often dictates the sequence and formatting of a clinician's documentation. HHAs are required to incorporate the OASIS data set when developing the content of the comprehensive assessment, but they may choose the sequencing of items. The original *OASIS Implementation Manual* (Health Care Financing Administration, 1999) recommended that agencies begin with the required OASIS items and then add the assessment items the agency deems necessary to meet clinical, regulatory, or accreditation requirements (e.g., status, vital signs at rest and after activity, cultural or educational barriers that might affect progress toward goals).

The required OASIS items and agency-specific assessment items comprise a discipline-neutral core assessment that all qualifying disciplines are (or can become) competent in performing. To this core comprehensive assessment, the agency then adds discipline-specific assessment items that supplement, not duplicate, the core assessment items. For example, the discipline-specific items for occupational therapy might include assessment items necessary to develop the occupational therapy treatment plan, such as cognitive or vision assessments. The discipline-specific assessment items together with the OASIS items and the agency-specific assessment items constitute a full comprehensive assessment for a given discipline.

Many HHAs develop individual comprehensive assessments for each discipline that may complete such an assessment. An occupational therapist completing a comprehensive assessment for the purposes of recertifying a patient, for example, would use the comprehensive assessment specific to occupational therapy, not the assessment previously completed by a registered nurse (RN). An occupational therapist can and should provide input on development of the occupational therapy–specific portion of a comprehensive assessment, including content, format, and flow of items, for paper or electronic documentation. As stated earlier, the sequence of the OASIS items may follow the logic of the individual HHA's comprehensive assessment, rather than be inserted in numeric order. However, the *M* label of each OASIS item must remain unaltered.

Who May Complete OASIS Data Collection

OASIS items were designed to be discipline neutral and were tested and validated with clinicians from all disciplines. The comprehensive assessment and OASIS data collection may be completed by an RN, physical therapist, speech–language pathologist, or occupational therapist. A licensed practical nurse or licensed vocational nurse, physical therapy assistant, occupational therapy assistant, social worker, or aide may not complete the assessments (CMS, 2015, p. 1-3).

According to the CoP standard for comprehensive assessment (§ 484.55; CMS, 2011), if nursing is on the referring order, an RN must complete the start-of-care (SOC) assessment and data collection, regardless of frequency or required start date (e.g., "RN to remove staples on Day 10 of episode"). Subsequent assessments may be completed by any qualified discipline active on the plan of care (POC). If nursing is not on the referring order, the appropriate therapist who establishes program eligibility completes the SOC comprehensive assessment and collects OASIS data.

Occupational therapy by itself cannot establish initial Medicare program eligibility. However, once program eligibility is established, occupational therapists may complete assessments at subsequent time points, regardless of what disciplines are active. Most important, occupational therapists can assess patients to recertify for another episode, but most frequently they complete the discharge assessment.

OASIS assessments and data are collected only once by the agency at each specified time point, although individual disciplines and HHAs may require additional documentation at those and other time points. Employees must follow HHA policy dictating practices other than those specified in the regulations as a condition of employment. When agency policy differs significantly from the regulations, however, occupational therapists can advocate for changes in agency policy to promote more appropriate occupational therapy utilization. For example, an HHA may have a policy that occupational therapists may not complete comprehensive assessments for any patients; this policy is more restrictive than the regulation (§ 484.55), which allows any skilled discipline to complete the comprehensive assessment after benefit eligibility has been established, and occupational therapists can advocate to change this agency policy. For example, occupational therapy establishes eligibility for many payers other than Medicare and could complete the comprehensive assessment under the regulation, whereas the agency policy in this scenario restricts such practice.

Data Collection Time Points

Data collection is required at the following time points for Medicare and Medicaid beneficiaries and must be completed within a specified time frame:

- *SOC:* within 5 days of SOC date
- *Transfer to inpatient facility:* within 48 hours of becoming aware of the transfer
- *Resumption of care (ROC) after an inpatient stay:* within 48 hours of discharge from an inpatient facility
- *Recertification:* within the last 5 days of each 60-day certification period
- *Other follow-up:* within 48 hours of becoming aware of a significant change in condition
- *Discharge from home care:* within 48 hours of becoming aware of discharge
- *Death at home:* within 48 hours of becoming aware of death (CMS, 2011, § 484.55).

The assessments and corresponding data collection completed at these time points should occur during a visit because they require an in-person encounter with the patient. For two exceptions—transfer to inpatient facility and death at home—the data items are limited and can be obtained through a phone call.

Compliance with the required timing of each of the assessments is captured by the following OASIS items:

- *M0030 (A. Patient Tracking):* SOC date—date of the first reimbursable visit delivered; must be within 48 hours of the referral date or discharge from inpatient facility or on a physician-ordered date
- *M0032 (A. Patient Tracking):* ROC date—date of the first visit after an inpatient stay; must be within 48 hours of inpatient facility discharge
- *M0090 (B. Clinical Record):* Date assessment is completed—date the final data are collected from the patient and through care coordination with the physician and other disciplines on the POC (not the date of documenting or entering data from the assessment)
- *M0102 (B. Clinical Record):* Date of physician-ordered SOC (or ROC)—date specified by the physician that ordered services are to begin, regardless of which service
- *M0104 (B. Clinical Record):* Date of referral—most recent date (if updated) the verbal, written, or electronic referral to begin home care was received by the HHA.

Noncompliance with required timing of the assessments is reported back to the HHA in the form of an error report when data are submitted.

On occasion, a visit becomes the discharge visit, but this is not known until after the fact. For example, a physician visit might result in orders to continue therapy on an outpatient basis, and the patient must be discharged from home health care before an outpatient therapy visit to the home can be made. On these occasions, the information gathered during the last visit made to the patient is used to complete the discharge OASIS data. In such a scenario, the clinician should take care to correctly enter dates in the following items on the discharge OASIS:

- *M0090 (B. Clinical Record):* In the case of an unplanned discharge, this is the date the assessment is completed and recorded, based on documentation from the last or most recent home visit.

- *M0903 (P. Discharge):* Date of the last or most recent visit to the patient.
- *M0906 (P. Discharge):* Date of discharge (e.g., phone discharge from the physician), transfer, or death, determined by agency policy or physician order.

Release of Patient-Identifiable OASIS Information

The Health Insurance Portability and Accountability Act of 1996 (HIPAA; Pub. L. 104–191) affects the ways HHAs handle patient confidentiality. The HHA and any agent acting on behalf of the HHA must ensure that all protected (i.e., patient-identifiable) health information in the clinical record, including OASIS data, remains confidential and is not released to the public. The data, whether in hard-copy or electronic format, must be secured and controlled. All HHAs are required to adhere to the provisions of HIPAA to ensure patient confidentiality and the security of patient information.

Data Transmission Requirements

There are four standards in the CoPs for data transmission (CMS, 2011, § 484.20):

(a) *Standard: Encoding and transmitting OASIS data.* An HHA must encode and electronically transmit each completed OASIS assessment to the State agency or the CMS OASIS contractor, regarding each beneficiary with respect to which such information is required to be transmitted (as determined by the Secretary), within 30 days of completing the assessment of the beneficiary.

(b) *Standard: Accuracy of encoded OASIS data.* The encoded OASIS data must accurately reflect the patient's status at the time of assessment.

(c) *Standard: Transmittal of OASIS data.* An HHA must—
   (1) For all completed assessments, transmit OASIS data in a format that meets the requirements of paragraph (d) of this section.
   (2) Successfully transmit test data to the State agency or CMS OASIS contractor.
   (3) Transmit data using electronics communications software that provides a direct telephone connection from the HHA to the State agency or CMS OASIS contractor.
   (4) Transmit data that includes the CMS-assigned branch identification number, as applicable.

(d) *Standard: Data format.* The HHA must encode and transmit data using the software available from CMS or software that conforms to CMS standard electronic record layout, edit specifications, and data dictionary, and that includes the required OASIS data set.

Role of Occupational Therapy in OASIS Data Collection

OASIS data accuracy drives not only accurate payment but also accurate reporting of outcomes in the agency's OBQI reports and to the public on Home Health Compare (CMS, 2010a). Occupational therapists play a role in data accuracy on three levels:

1. By collecting data during one of the assessment time points
2. By contributing an accurate clinical picture of a patient in documentation and communication with team members who are collecting data

3. By offering formal or informal training to agency team members regarding strategies for accurate data collection in domains of greater occupational therapy expertise (e.g., activities of daily living [ADLs], instrumental activities of daily living [IADLs]).

Collecting Data During Assessments

To collect accurate data during an assessment, occupational therapists must be familiar with each OASIS item covered in Chapter 3 of the *OASIS Guidance Manual*. Each OASIS item-specific guidance page follows a specific format that includes

- OASIS item,
- Item intent,
- Time points at which the item or items were completed,
- Response-specific instructions, and
- Data sources and resources.

Familiarity with Chapter 3 of the *OASIS Guidance Manual* is particularly helpful when discrepancies occur in how clinicians describe a patient using OASIS data. The OASIS as a data collection set was validated with a high degree of interrater reliability, but data are reliable only when the data collector strictly adheres to the item description. The item language is very specific, and knowledge of each item guidance provided in Chapter 3 assists occupational therapists in providing an accurate clinical picture of the patient.

Contributing to an Accurate Clinical Picture

Occupational therapy documentation in home health, as in other settings, is guided by the *Occupational Therapy Practice Framework: Domain and Process* (3rd ed.; AOTA, 2014) and by the HHA's requirements for occupational therapy documentation. Even when an occupational therapist is not collecting data directly at an assessment time point, the occupational therapy evaluation is important in painting a clear picture of the patient. For example, OASIS items assessing how a patient dresses the upper or lower body include obtaining the clothes (i.e., retrieving them from where they are stored), not just donning and doffing the clothing items. An assessing clinician may score the patient as needing assistance on OASIS. If, however, an occupational therapist documents that patient as independent in dressing but does not include information about how the patient obtains the clothes, the occupational therapy documentation may appear to be contradictory to the OASIS response selected by the other clinician.

Additionally, occupational therapists can contribute to an accurate clinical picture by educating other clinicians in the nuances of the patient's performance to improve the accuracy of their data collection. For example, in case conferences, occupational therapists can show how an occupational therapy description of a patient's ADL and IADL performance can help another clinician select the correct OASIS response items. During such opportunities, occupational therapists can provide insights or strategies to other clinicians to ensure accurate data collection for the ADL and IADL items under a tight time frame. In another example, an occupational therapist can explain how other clinicians can use their observations of a patient's balance, strength, and mobility and the presence of equipment to extrapolate about the patient's ability to get in and out of the tub. During conferences, occupational therapists may share their own previous observations of the patient's performance and conditions present at the time and other variables that could provide a larger, more rounded picture of the patient during the assessment time frame.

Offering Agency Training

OASIS training varies widely among HHAs, and many clinicians get little support in developing good data collection skills. When teachable moments such as formal conferences on a patient are not a convenient option, occupational therapists can offer an in-service to HHA staff to provide insights and strategies for accurate and time-efficient assessment data collection. Occupational therapists can also help other clinicians assess the following patient factors and performance skills to determine whether a patient is safe bathing in a shower or tub:

- Impaired balance with no presence of adaptive equipment or handrails for stepping in and out or for leaning forward to adjust water temperature
- Need for cognitive cuing to remember how to use adaptive equipment
- Presence of pulmonary disease limiting the amount of time the patient may safely stand in a warm, moist, slippery environment
- Joint limitations that prevent reaching hard-to-wash areas.

Providing such training is not handing the profession's domain over to other disciplines; it is using the knowledge and experience of one's own profession to assist colleagues in collecting accurate data for an assessment designed for discipline neutrality.

Conventions in OASIS Data Collection

Consistency is critical to the validity and reliability of analysis and comparison of data from the collective national database. *OASIS conventions* are a set of general rules for consistently completing OASIS data collection; the entire list of conventions is reprinted in Box D.1. Clinicians must measure the same defined activity across patients for the measured outcomes to be comparable. The conventions ensure that rather than simply assessing a patient, clinicians collect data in a consistent manner to ensure valid and reliable reporting of outcomes and to enable comparisons across patients. The *OASIS Guidance Manual* conventions (see Item 10 in Box D.1) include following the item-specific guidance in the manual, so reading the item and response descriptions alone (e.g., on an agency form) is inadequate for data accuracy.

OASIS Outcome Measure Item Guidance

This section provides a detailed overview of the OASIS data items that are most salient in occupational therapy practice. Although an occupational therapist must be knowledgeable and familiar with the entire data set, it is beyond the scope of this text and SPCC to review the entire OASIS. Reviewing the highlighted items is intended to increase readers' familiarity with the specific items most relevant to occupational therapy for improved data accuracy and provide guidance on how to use the *OASIS Guidance Manual* to encourage readers to undertake further independent review of the entire data set.

Box D.1. Conventions for Completing OASIS Items

General OASIS Item Conventions

1. Understand the time period under consideration for each item. Report what is true on the day of assessment unless a different time period has been indicated in the item or related guidance. Day of assessment is defined as the 24 hours immediately preceding the home visit and the time spent by the clinician in the home.

2. For OASIS purposes, a care episode (also referred to as a quality episode) must have a beginning (that is, an SOC or ROC assessment) and a conclusion (that is, a Transfer or Discharge assessment) to be considered a complete care episode.

3. If the patient's ability or status varies on the day of the assessment, report the patient's "usual status" or what is true greater than 50% of the assessment time frame, unless the item specifies differently (for example, for M2020 Management of Oral Medications, M2030 Management of Injectable Medications, and M2100e Management of Equipment, instead of "usual status" or "greater than 50% of the time," consider the medication or equipment for which the most assistance is needed).

4. Minimize the use of NA and Unknown responses.

5. Responses to items documenting a patient's current status should be based on independent observation of the patient's condition and ability at the time of the assessment without referring back to prior assessments. Several process items require documentation of prior care, at the time of or since the time of the most recent SOC, ROC, or FU OASIS assessment. These instructions are included in item guidance for the relevant OASIS questions.

6. Combine observation, interview, and other relevant strategies to complete OASIS data items as needed (for example, it is acceptable to review the hospital discharge summary to identify inpatient procedures and diagnoses at Start of Care, or to examine the care notes to determine if a physician-ordered intervention was implemented at Transfer or Discharge). However, when assessing physiologic or functional health status, direct observation is the preferred strategy.

7. When an OASIS item refers to assistance, this means assistance from another person unless otherwise specified within the item. Assistance is not limited to physical contact and includes both verbal cues and supervision.

8. Complete OASIS items accurately and comprehensively, and adhere to skip patterns.

9. Understand the definitions of words as used in the OASIS.

10. Follow rules included in the Item Specific Guidance (Chapter 3 of this manual).

11. Stay current with evolving CMS OASIS guidance updates. CMS may post updates up to twice per year, in June and December.

12. Only one clinician may take responsibility for accurately completing a comprehensive assessment. However, for selected items, collaboration is appropriate (for example, Medication items M2000–M2004). These exceptions are noted in the Item Specific Guidance.

13. When the OASIS item includes language specifying "one calendar day" (for example, M2002 Medication Follow-up), this means until the end of the next calendar day. When the language specifies "same day" (for example, M1510 Heart Failure Follow-up), this means by the end of today.

14. The use of "that is" or "specifically," means scoring of the item should be limited to only the circumstances listed. The use of "for example," means the clinician may consider other relevant circumstances or attributes when scoring the item.

Conventions Specific to ADL/IADL Items

1. Report the patient's ability, not actual performance or willingness, to perform a task. While the presence or absence of a caregiver may impact actual performance of activities, it does not impact the patient's ability to perform a task.

2. The level of ability refers to the patient's ability to safely complete specified activities.

3. Understand what tasks are included and excluded in each item and select the OASIS response based only on included tasks.

4. If the patient's ability varies between the different tasks included in a multi-task item, report what is true in a majority of the included tasks, giving more weight to tasks that are more frequently performed.

5. Consider medical restrictions when determining ability. For example, if the physician has ordered activity restrictions, consider this when selecting the best response to functional items related to ambulation, transferring, etc.

Source. Reprinted from Table 2 (pp. 1-6–1-7), in Centers for Medicare & Medicaid Services, *OASIS–C1/ICD–10 Guidance Manual,* 2015, Baltimore: Author. Retrieved from http://www.cms.gov/Medicare/Quality-Initiatives-Patient-Assessment-Instruments/HomeHealthQualityInits/HHQIOASISUserManual.html. In the public domain.
Note. ADL = activity of daily living; CMS = Centers for Medicare & Medicaid Services; FU = follow-up; IADL = instrumental activity of daily living; NA = not applicable; OASIS = Outcome and Assessment Information Set; ROC = resumption of care; SOC = start of care.

Although ADLs and IADLs are the most obvious and significant sections relevant to occupational therapy, other OASIS items can benefit from occupational therapists' insights to increase accuracy of data collection. The items reviewed here were also selected because

- Occupational therapists can provide relevant input needed for accurate responses to the items;
- Occupational therapists may be less familiar with the items;
- The items reflect publicly reported outcomes;
- The items may affect the PPS episode payment; and
- Clinicians often answer these items incorrectly.

Certain items are typically maintained by clinical or nonclinical personnel in the HHA office. For example, the patient's demographic information may be entered by nonclinical office personnel setting up an electronic clinical record, and *International Statistical Classification of Diseases and Related Health Problems,* 10th Revision (*ICD–10;* World Health Organization, 2010), coding is often handled by specialized personnel who review patient assessment data and referral documents and code the diagnoses, conditions, and procedures appropriately. If personnel other than the assessing clinician make coding recommendations or corrections, they must follow agency policy to ensure that the changes have been discussed with and approved by the original assessing clinician.

A. Patient Tracking, B. Clinical Record

Many of the items included in Section A, "Patient Tracking," and Section B, "Clinical Record," of the *OASIS Guidance Manual* involve demographics and record-keeping information captured by an HHA from the beginning of the referral and intake process. Many of the items, such as patient identification number or date of birth, do not change during or across episodes.

C. Patient History and Diagnoses

Section C, "Patient History and Diagnoses," elicits information about the patient's condition just before the admission to home health care and identifies the diagnoses or conditions warranting the home health episode. Items M1011–M1018 involve inpatient diagnoses and diagnoses requiring a recent change in treatment regimen and are intended to help clinicians develop an appropriate POC.

Assessing clinicians are required to list the diagnoses or procedures and their *ICD–10* codes in accordance with the coding conventions in the *ICD–10–CM Official Guidelines for Coding and Reporting* (CMS & National Center for Health Statistics [NCHS], 2014). Instructions for *ICD–10* coding are beyond the scope of this text; moreover, ascribing the actual *ICD–10* code to the diagnosis list is not typically a function of an occupational therapist. However, occupational therapists can and should help inform what diagnoses should be included on the list and lend information to help sequence them in accordance with relevance to the POC.

(M1011) List each **Inpatient Diagnosis** and ICD–10–CM code at the level of highest specificity for only those conditions treated during an inpatient stay within the last 14 days (no V, W, X, Y or Z codes or surgical codes).

(M1017) Diagnoses Requiring Medical or Treatment Regimen Change Within Past 14 Days: List the patient's Medical Diagnoses and ICD–10–CM codes at the level of highest specificity for those conditions requiring changed medical or treatment regimen within the past 14 days (no V, W, X, Y, or Z codes or surgical codes).

(M1018) Conditions Prior to Medical or Treatment Regimen Change or Inpatient Stay Within Past 14 Days: If this patient experienced an inpatient facility discharge or change in medical or treatment regimen within the past 14 days, indicate any conditions that existed prior to the inpatient stay or change in medical or treatment regimen.

The specific instructions for these items explain that the day of the home health admission is considered Day 0, the day immediately before that is Day 1, and so on to Day 14 preceding admission. For consistent data collection, a clinician must know how to consider which conditions to include in the list.

An occupational therapist may be aware of diagnoses, conditions, or procedures gleaned from a thorough assessment of a patient who required treatment within 14 days before the home health admission but that the clinician performing the SOC assessment might not have noted. For example, the occupational therapist might detect a low vision diagnosis that the assessing clinician missed. The occupational therapist should communicate any missed information to the assessing clinician or to agency personnel.

M1017 provides an opportunity to list recent conditions (within the past 14 days) requiring a change in medical or treatment regimen without a corresponding inpatient stay. In many cases, the lists in M1011 and M1017 are the same, but if the patient did not have an inpatient stay (M1011), M1017 provides the opportunity to capture this recent medical and treatment history.

(M1021/1023/1025) Diagnoses, Symptom Control, and Optional Diagnoses: List each diagnosis for which the patient is receiving home care in Column 1, and enter its ICD–10–CM code at the level of highest specificity in Column 2 (diagnosis codes only—no surgical or procedure codes allowed). Diagnoses are listed in the order that best reflects the seriousness of each condition and supports the disciplines and services provided. Rate the degree of symptom control for each condition in Column 2. ICD–10–CM sequencing requirements must be followed if multiple coding is indicated for any diagnoses. If a Z-code is reported in Column 2 in place of a diagnosis that is no longer active (a resolved condition), then optional item M1025 (Optional Diagnoses—Columns 3 and 4) may be completed. Diagnoses reported in M1025 will not impact payment.

Code each row according to the following directions for each column:

Column 1:   Enter the description of the diagnosis. Sequencing of diagnoses should reflect the seriousness of each condition and support the disciplines and services provided.

Column 2:   Enter the ICD–10–CM code for the condition described in Column 1—no surgical or procedure codes allowed. Codes must be entered at the level of highest specificity and ICD–10–CM coding rules and sequencing requirements must be followed. Note that external cause codes (ICD–10–CM codes beginning with V, W, X, or Y) may not be reported in M1021 (Primary Diagnosis) but may be reported in M1023 (Secondary Diagnoses). Also note that when a Z-code is reported in Column 2, the code for the underlying condition can often be entered in Column 2, as long as it is an active on-going condition impacting home health care.

Rate the degree of symptom control for the condition listed in Column 1. Do not assign a symptom control rating if the diagnosis code is a V, W, X, Y or Z-code. Choose one value that represents the degree of symptom control appropriate for each diagnosis using the following scale:

0—Asymptomatic, no treatment needed at this time
1—Symptoms well controlled with current therapy
2—Symptoms controlled with difficulty, affecting daily functioning; patient needs ongoing monitoring
3—Symptoms poorly controlled; patient needs frequent adjustment in treatment and dose monitoring
4—Symptoms poorly controlled; history of re-hospitalizations

Note that the rating for symptom control in Column 2 should not be used to determine the sequencing of the diagnoses listed in Column 1. These are separate items and sequencing may not coincide.

Column 3:   (OPTIONAL) There is no requirement that HHAs enter a diagnosis code in M1025 (Columns 3 and 4). Diagnoses reported in M1025 will not impact payment.

Agencies may choose to report an underlying condition in M1025 (Columns 3 and 4) when:

• a Z-code is reported in Column 2 AND
• the underlying condition for the Z-code in Column 2 is a resolved condition. An example of a resolved condition is uterine cancer that is no longer being treated following a hysterectomy.

Column 4:   (OPTIONAL) If a Z-code is reported in M1021/M1023 (Column 2) and the agency chooses to report a resolved underlying condition that requires multiple diagnosis codes under ICD–10–CM coding guidelines, enter the diagnosis descriptions and the ICD–10–CM codes in the same row in Columns 3 and 4. For example, if the resolved condition is a manifestation code, record the diagnosis description and ICD–10–CM code for the underlying condition in Column 3 of that row and the diagnosis description and ICD–10–CM code for the manifestation in Column 4 of that row. Otherwise, leave Column 4 blank in that row.

The intent of M1021, M1023, and M1025 is to accurately code each diagnosis in compliance with Medicare's regulations for coverage and payment. M1021 is the primary diagnosis, the one most acute and related to the patient's current POC and, therefore, the chief reason for providing home care. The guidance for these items states, "The assessing clinician is expected to complete the patient's comprehensive assessment and understand the patient's overall medical condition and care needs before selecting and assigning diagnoses" (CMS, 2015, p. C-9). In other words, simply listing the diagnoses responsible for an inpatient stay or mentioned on a home health referral is not the intent of this OASIS item.

Two points are made clear in the primary diagnosis selection criteria. First, although information regarding the reason for a recent inpatient stay immediately precedes M1021, "the primary diagnosis may or may not relate to the patient's most recent hospital stay, but must relate to the skilled services (skilled nursing, physical therapy, occupational therapy, and speech language pathology) rendered by the HHA" (CMS, 2015, p. C-9). Second, if more than one diagnosis is concurrently treated, "the patient's primary home health diagnosis is defined as the chief reason the patient is receiving home care and the diagnosis most related to the current home health Plan of Care" (p. C-9).

Secondary diagnoses listed in M1023 "are comorbid conditions that exist at the time of the assessment, that are actively addressed in the patient's Plan of Care, or that have the potential to affect the patient's responsiveness to treatment and rehabilitative prognosis" (CMS, 2015, p. C-8). The HHA must ensure that the secondary diagnoses are listed in the order that best reflects "the degree [to which] they impact the patient's health and need for home health care, rather than the degree of symptom control" (CMS, 2015, p. C-10).

The home health occupational therapist performing the comprehensive assessment is responsible for the selection, sequencing, and coding of diagnoses on the basis of an assessment, but he or she includes a review of referral information and the history and physical examination to ensure that the selection is supported by medical record documentation. The physician is responsible for diagnosing the patient, but the occupational therapist selects, sequences, rates the severity of, and codes the diagnoses provided by the physician. When sufficient documentation from the medical record is not consistent with the home health POC, it is incumbent on the HHA to either pursue clarification from the physician regarding a condition or reconsider the appropriateness of the home health POC.

The sequence of diagnoses listed in OASIS is governed by three types of logic: (1) coverage regulations, (2) *ICD–10–CM* coding conventions, and (3) payment requirements. Coverage regulations are discussed in **Appendix A** of this text. For a Medicare beneficiary to receive covered services under the home health benefit, the services must be reasonable and necessary for the condition being treated. The conditions or diagnoses are listed and sequenced to reflect the intensity of services needed for the home health episode of care.

The second type of logic is found in the *ICD–10–CM* coding manual conventions (CMS & NCHS, 2014). As noted in the *OASIS Guidance Manual,* HIPAA requires adherence to the rules governing diagnosis sequencing and coding by all health care settings (CMS, 2015, p. C-9). For health information to be electronically portable across settings, data coding conventions must be accurately and consistently applied by all clinicians across all health care settings.

The third type of logic governing the sequence of diagnoses is payment consideration. The primary diagnosis (M1021) and the secondary diagnoses (M1023) are important in creating a picture of the patient that helps establish an accurate, individualized payment for that 60-day home health episode of care. Years of statistical analysis by CMS have indicated that certain diagnoses cost more to provide care for than others. These diagnoses add money to the case-mix weight and are therefore called *case-mix diagnoses.* Examples include patients with a primary diagnosis of diabetes or with certain neurological diagnoses.

Changes to M1021, M1023, and M1025 are frequently recommended on the basis of review by an expert coder or deliberation about the individual disciplines' plans of care. It is incumbent on occupational therapists to be aware of and adhere to the HHA OASIS correction policy.

E. Sensory Status

Because a patient's impaired vision or significant pain will affect his or her POC, occupational therapy practitioners must understand two items: M1200, vision, and M1242, frequency of pain interfering with the patient's activity or movement. In addition, these items add to the case-mix weight, and therefore the PPS payment calculation, depending on the responses selected.

(**M1200**) **Vision** (with corrective lenses if the patient usually wears them):

- ☐ 0 - Normal vision: sees adequately in most situations; can see medication labels, newsprint.
- ☐ 1 - Partially impaired: cannot see medication labels or newsprint, but <u>can</u> see obstacles in path, and the surrounding layout; can count fingers at arm's length.
- ☐ 2 - Severely impaired: cannot locate objects without hearing or touching them or patient nonresponsive.

The *OASIS Guidance Manual* provides specific guidance regarding what are considered corrective lenses, and each response provides examples or illustrations suggesting how to assess whether the patient has normal, partially impaired, or severely impaired vision. The key to accurately recording this item is to assess actual vision, not a compensatory strategy the patient has developed to cope with vision loss.

Occupational therapists have a vast cadre of methods to ascertain a patient's level of functional vision, but during the home health admission process, it is important to be able to use these methods swiftly and accurately. For example, clinicians are required to collect medicine bottles and copy down the information from the label during the admission, so they can ask the patient to read the information on the labels to assess vision while completing the medication component. Normal functional vision may be indicated if the patient provides the correct information, but the clinician must consider that the patient may have memorized the type of medication, prescription number, or physician phone number, as opposed to actually reading the label. Vision is a critical safety element for any person desiring to remain in his or her own home, so the clinician may need to use other evaluative strategies to gain an accurate assessment of a patient's vision and its influence on the safety of remaining at home.

Occupational therapists have many opportunities to observe how a patient's vision impedes safety or any type of performance. Such observations and the effectiveness of existing compensatory strategies are important to communicate to the rest of the home health team. However, clinicians must remember that this OASIS item assesses vision, not compensatory strategies.

(M1242) Frequency of Pain Interfering with patient's activity or movement

    ☐ 0 - Patient has no pain
    ☐ 1 - Patient has pain that does not interfere with activity or movement
    ☐ 2 - Less often than daily
    ☐ 3 - Daily, but not constantly
    ☐ 4 - All of the time

The key to selecting the most appropriate response to M1242 is to recognize the distinction between M1242 and the data item immediately preceding it, M1240, which asks whether the patient has had a pain assessment using a standardized tool. Every HHA should have a standardized pain assessment included in its policies, and every clinician should have training in proper administration of the standardized scale. Many standardized scales instruct the clinician to ask the patient to rate his or her pain according to the scale provided. In other words, the patient self-reports his or her perception of the pain experience.

M1242 involves not a standardized pain scale, but rather an assessment by the clinician based on observation and interview to determine the frequency with which a patient's pain interferes with activity or movement. For example, a patient who has a high pain tolerance and perceives little pain may subconsciously make changes in his or her daily life to deal with pain he or she does not acknowledge. The clinician, however, can identify these changes as interference with activity or movement even though the patient does not report a significant level of pain.

The *OASIS Guidance Manual* indicates that *interference* "results in the activity being performed less often than otherwise desired, requires the patient to have additional assistance in performing the activity, or causes the activity to take longer to complete" (CMS, 2015, p. E-6). Moreover, occupational therapists must consider all activities, not just ADLs. Two types of activity often not considered are (1) sleep and (2) recreational activities. Although little movement is involved in sleep, pain often interrupts this activity. Guidance for M1242 clarifies that if pain is well controlled with pharmacological or nonpharmacological treatments, this control should be considered when evaluating for interference with activity. So if a nighttime pain medication helps the patient successfully sleep through the night, then the pain does not interfere with the activity of sleep.

Thorough assessment of a patient's occupational profile for typically performed activities (leisure or otherwise) and assessment of his or her current occupational performance helps the clinician know how to begin observing for interference from pain. Observing patients during assessment of ADL and IADL routines provides a more accurate picture of pain interference than simply asking them whether pain keeps them from doing things they want to do.

G. Respiratory Status

(M1400) When is the patient dyspneic or noticeably **Short of Breath**?

☐ 0 - Patient is not short of breath
☐ 1 - When walking more than 20 feet, climbing stairs
☐ 2 - With moderate exertion (for example, while dressing, using commode or bedpan, walking distances less than 20 feet)
☐ 3 - With minimal exertion (for example, while eating, talking, or performing other ADLs) or with agitation
☐ 4 - At rest (during day or night)

Identifying whether a patient has dyspnea or is noticeably short of breath is difficult unless the occupational therapist observes the patient in various situations. Despite the complexity and length of a comprehensive assessment, it may not allow the clinician an opportunity to observe the patient in many situations. The value of an occupational therapy assessment is that the patient is observed in situations that are integral to his or her context.

Several specific instructions in the *OASIS Guidance Manual* are worth pointing out. First, the clinician is to note whether the patient is on continuous oxygen; if so, then shortness of breath must be assessed while the patient uses the oxygen. However, if there are physician orders for continuous oxygen, the clinician should also observe whether the patient actually continuously uses the oxygen; if the patient uses it only intermittently, then the shortness of breath should be assessed when he or she is not on the oxygen. Second, when assessing patients who are bedfast or chairfast, the clinician may need to pay attention to subtle changes in respiration or request that the patient perform such activities as transferring, repositioning, or getting on and off a bedpan to fully assess possible dyspnea.

In the author's experience, a good rule for OASIS data collection is to begin at the bottom response and work up to select the first response that most appropriately applies to a patient. As in item M1400, the bottom response represents the poorest performance in most OASIS items, and the assessing clinician may not consider it if he or she begins with the top response and stops short of reading all the available responses. For example, a clinician observing a patient climbing stairs might scan the responses and select 1 for M1400, failing to consider that much less exertion than climbing stairs might cause the patient to become dyspneic. In such a case, the clinician would not report the true picture of the patient (e.g., 2 or 3) at the beginning of the episode, meaning that potential progress would not be captured at the end of the episode when data are collected again.

I. Elimination Status

Elimination items are reflected in the case-mix weight but are often hastily assessed. Many clinicians have their own method of assessing for incontinence in a respectful and discreet manner, but some skim past the issue and therefore collect incorrect data. HHAs whose reports indicate a lack of improvement in elimination outcomes should investigate whether clinicians are inadequately assessing and incorrectly scoring the status at baseline.

Assessing for possible incontinence requires tact as well as clinical reasoning and perceptive multisensory observation. The accuracy of OASIS items related to incontinence suffers when clinicians use the common but misguided technique of administering the data set as a questionnaire. Patients may not be honest in answering questions about incontinence because of embarrassment or shame, denial, or fear (real or perceived) that incontinence might precipitate admission to a nursing home. Clinicians may start the assessment with a tactful inquiry about this clinical factor, but clinical reasoning must prevail. For example, an 85-year-old patient may insist she has no problem with leaking, but the clinician should also check the bathroom, possibly while performing other ADL assessments, and be alert to the presence of pads in the closet or trash, the smell of urine, and other signs of a problem.

> **(M1610)** Urinary Incontinence or **Urinary Catheter Presence:**
>
> ☐ 0 - No incontinence or catheter (includes anuria or ostomy for urinary drainage) *[Go to M1620]*
> ☐ 1 - Patient is incontinent
> ☐ 2 - Patient requires a urinary catheter (specifically: external, indwelling, intermittent, or suprapubic) *[Go to M1620]*
>
> **(M1615) When** does **Urinary Incontinence** occur?
>
> ☐ 0 - Timed-voiding defers incontinence
> ☐ 1 - Occasional stress incontinence
> ☐ 2 - During the night only
> ☐ 3 - During the day only
> ☐ 4 - During the day and night

The instructions for M1610 state that patients with any incontinence at all, including stress incontinence, are to be scored as incontinent (1), so the clinician needs to both ask the patient directly and be alert to evidence to identify the correct response. If no incontinence (0) is erroneously selected in M1610, the skip pattern (i.e., "[Go to M1620]") would prevent the assessing clinician from finding that indeed the patient has stress incontinence in M1615. Instructions for M1615 note that timed voiding is more than simply making it to the toilet on time; it is a compensatory strategy used to manage incontinence through a planned, scheduled voiding pattern.

> **(M1620) Bowel Incontinence Frequency:**
>
> ☐ 0 - Very rarely or never has bowel incontinence
> ☐ 1 - Less than once weekly

☐ 2 - One to three times weekly
☐ 3 - Four to six times weekly
☐ 4 - On a daily basis
☐ 5 - More often than once daily
☐ NA - Patient has ostomy for bowel elimination
☐ UK - Unknown *[Omit "UK" option on (follow-up), (discharge)]*

M1620 does not address treatment of incontinence, such as a bowel program. Because M1620 identifies the frequency of bowel incontinence, not just the presence, accurate data collection is reliant on patient or caregiver report.

K. Activities of Daily Living and Instrumental Activities of Daily Living

OASIS items do not capture, describe, or measure ADLs in the same way most occupational therapists do. Assessing a patient's ADLs and IADLs and documenting objective, measurable progress are skills required of occupational therapists in all health care settings. However, to accurately collect data regarding ADLs and IADLs in OASIS, occupational therapists must be familiar with each OASIS item and understand the nuances of every incremental response level.

Conventions Specific to ADL and IADL Items

Several OASIS conventions are specific to the ADL and IADL items (see Box D.1). One convention requires that the clinician assess the patient's actual ability to do the activity, not willingness or preference for long-standing routines. For example, although a patient may prefer to sponge bathe at the sink and has done so for years, the OASIS bathing item (M1830) requires that he or she be assessed for the ability to bathe in the shower or tub.

Another convention specific to the ADL and IADL items clarifies that occupational therapists assess the patient's ability to safely perform the activity. This convention is relevant, for example, when a therapist is greeted at the door by a fully dressed patient who lives alone and uses no assistive ambulation device. The therapist cannot report that the patient is independent in dressing and ambulation until the assessment shows that he or she is safe doing so. If the patient demonstrates poor balance and has difficulty reaching without losing his or her balance, it may not be safe for him or her to reach into the closet for clothing without some type of assistance. The most appropriate response item would describe the level at which the patient can safely perform the activity—for example, after someone has laid the clothing out. Another ADL and IADL convention states that if the patient's ability varies among the different tasks included in a multitask item, the assessor should report what is true in a majority of the included tasks, giving more weight to tasks that are more frequently performed, such as particular types of transfers or types of equipment.

Implications of ADL and IADL Data for Allocating Resources

ADL and IADL data for OASIS help identify the resources a family may need to maintain a patient safely in his or her own home. These resources may be financial or human. A family might need to pay for or provide assistance requiring the physical presence of another person on a daily basis, or intermittent phone supervision for reminders may be the only assistance needed.

Caregiver burden is part of what is measured in the ADL and IADL items. For example, the first response option (0) in the dressing items (M1810 and M1820) indicates that no assistance of any type is necessary for the entire dressing activity, including obtaining the clothes from where they are stored, so no caregiver resource of any type is required. The next response option (1) indicates that occasional caregiver assistance is needed to lay out clothing for the patient but not to don and doff the clothes. The next response (2) indicates that someone must be present to provide either physical or supervisory assistance for the patient to safely complete the dressing task. The last response (3) indicates that the caregiver must entirely complete the task.

An occupational therapist might describe many increments of improvement in his or her documentation within any one of these response options. Although the occupational therapist would document smaller increments of measurable, objective progress elsewhere in the medical record, he or she needs to be mindful of how much progress is needed before a change occurs in the level of resources required to maintain the patient at home. For example, a therapist assessing a patient who has improved from requiring moderate physical assistance with dressing to needing only verbal cuing for safety might not be able to reflect this change using the response OASIS items, but the lack of change in response would accurately reflect the caregiver's perspective, which is that the resource of a human being's presence in the same room is still required every time the patient dresses. Understanding what an OASIS data item actually measures and recognizing its difference from conventional occupational therapy documentation increases the occupational therapist's accuracy in collecting data.

(M1800) Grooming: Current ability to tend safely to personal hygiene needs (specifically: washing face and hands, hair care, shaving or make up, teeth or denture care, or fingernail care).

☐ 0 - Able to groom self unaided, with or without the use of assistive devices or adapted methods.
☐ 1 - Grooming utensils must be placed within reach before able to complete grooming activities.
☐ 2 - Someone must assist the patient to groom self.
☐ 3 - Patient depends entirely upon someone else for grooming needs.

(M1810) Current **Ability to Dress Upper Body** safely (with or without dressing aids) including undergarments, pullovers, front-opening shirts and blouses, managing zippers, buttons, and snaps:

☐ 0 - Able to get clothes out of closets and drawers, put them on and remove them from the upper body without assistance.
☐ 1 - Able to dress upper body without assistance if clothing is laid out or handed to the patient.
☐ 2 - Someone must help the patient put on upper body clothing.
☐ 3 - Patient depends entirely upon another person to dress the upper body.

(M1820) Current **Ability to Dress <u>Lower</u> Body** safely (with or without dressing aids) including undergarments, slacks, socks or nylons, shoes:

- ☐ 0 - Able to obtain, put on, and remove clothing and shoes without assistance.
- ☐ 1 - Able to dress lower body without assistance if clothing and shoes are laid out or handed to the patient.
- ☐ 2 - Someone must help the patient put on undergarments, slacks, socks or nylons, and shoes.
- ☐ 3 - Patient depends entirely upon another person to dress lower body.

The OASIS items assessing a patient's ability to dress the upper and lower body specify that both articles of clothing and their closures are to be included in the assessment. Each item description also specifies that the performance is to be assessed with or without dressing aids; conventional occupational therapy documentation and occupational therapists often consider the use of adaptive equipment to be modified independent.

Items M1810 and M1820 exemplify the importance of knowing the details of each response option. The first response option indicates that the patient can perform the described activity without assistance from another person. However, the first response option for dressing also implies independence in getting clothing items out of closets and drawers. Conventional occupational therapy documentation typically separates the task of retrieving articles of clothing from storage from the task of donning and doffing the clothing when assigning a measurable level of assistance to the activity of dressing, but the OASIS includes both aspects of dressing in the measure. Awareness of this detail is essential to accurate data collection.

Item-specific guidance for both of the dressing items instructs clinicians to assess the patient's ability to dress in what would be considered routine articles of clothing. *Routine clothing* is defined as what the patient usually wears or will wear if a change in clothing is part of a new routine. If a patient has modified what he or she wears to accommodate a recent physical limitation and the limitation is expected to be temporary (e.g., a fracture), then the modified clothing would not be considered routine clothing; therefore, assessing ability to dress would involve use of the clothing he or she wore before the physical limitation. If, however, the physical limitation is expected to be permanent or to worsen (e.g., severe rheumatoid arthritis), then any modification to clothing will most likely be part of a new routine, and the assessment of dressing would measure use of the recently modified clothing. The item-specific guidance also specifies that dressing assessment includes use of any prosthetic, orthotic, or support devices for the lower body (e.g., foot orthoses, compression stockings), which could influence what response the occupational therapist selects.

(M1830) Bathing: Current ability to wash entire body safely. <u>**Excludes**</u> **grooming (washing face, washing hands, and shampooing hair).**

- ☐ 0 - Able to bathe self in <u>shower or tub</u> independently, including getting in and out of tub/shower.

    ☐ 1 - With the use of devices, is able to bathe self in shower or tub independently, including getting in and out of the tub/shower.

    ☐ 2 - Able to bathe in shower or tub with the intermittent assistance of another person:

       (a) for intermittent supervision or encouragement or reminders, <u>OR</u>

       (b) to get in and out of the shower or tub, <u>OR</u>

       (c) for washing difficult to reach areas.

    ☐ 3 - Able to participate in bathing self in shower or tub, <u>but</u> requires presence of another person throughout the bath for assistance or supervision.

    ☐ 4 - Unable to use the shower or tub, but able to bathe self independently with or without the use of devices at the sink, in chair, or on commode.

    ☐ 5 - Unable to use the shower or tub, but able to participate in bathing self in bed, at the sink, in bedside chair, or on commode, with the assistance or supervision of another person.

    ☐ 6 - Unable to participate effectively in bathing and is bathed totally by another person.

The intent of M1830 is to assess the patient's ability to perform the activity described in the OASIS item, not the patient's preferred bathing routine. M1830 assesses the patient's ability to safely wash his or her entire body, excluding washing face, hands, and hair. Each of the response options explains that the patient's ability to bathe is to be assessed using the shower or tub, even though that may not be where the patient typically bathes. For example, selecting the response option indicating that the patient can participate in bathing at the sink (4) is appropriate only if he or she is unable to use the shower or tub.

If the patient's ability to bathe varies over time, the clinician should select the response that represents the patient's ability more than 50% of the time period under consideration. Patients' routines vary greatly (e.g., some bathe early in the morning and others just before going to bed), and the demands and working hours of a home health clinician's schedule rarely coincide with a patient's bathing routine, which often results in an inability to observe the patient's performance in its natural temporal context. For some patients, such as those with chronic obstructive pulmonary disease or congestive heart failure, endurance and time of day are critical to performance; in these cases, assessing the patient in his or her natural temporal context may give the clinician a better picture of how the patient more naturally performs.

Unlike the dressing items (M1810 and M1820), which include the qualifier *with or without dressing aids* in the item description, M1830 specifies the use of devices within the response options; therefore, whether devices are used must be considered with each individual response. Again, considering each response option beginning with the bottom response and working up is more likely to result in the most appropriate response for each patient. The item-specific guidance for this item is extensive, and clinicians should closely review the instructions for each specific response.

(M1840) Toilet Transferring: Current ability to get to and from the toilet or bedside commode safely <u>and</u> transfer on and off toilet/commode.

☐ 0 - Able to get to and from the toilet and transfer independently with or without a device.
☐ 1 - When reminded, assisted, or supervised by another person, able to get to and from the toilet and transfer.
☐ 2 - <u>Unable</u> to get to and from the toilet but is able to use a bedside commode (with or without assistance).
☐ 3 - <u>Unable</u> to get to and from the toilet or bedside commode but is able to use a bedpan/urinal independently.
☐ 4 - Is totally dependent in toileting.

The toilet transferring item measures ability using different types of equipment, so familiarity with each response option is key. The item includes getting to and transferring on and off both the toilet and the bedside commode. (The patient's toileting hygiene ability is measured in a separate OASIS item, M1845).

A common mistake in data collection for M1840 occurs when the occupational therapist misses the fact that the first two responses refer only to the toilet and that use of the bedside commode is not reflected until the third response option. Use of the bedside commode is not measured unless the patient cannot get to and transfer on and off the toilet. The item-specific guidance notes that if the patient can get to the toilet during the day but uses the bedside commode at night for convenience, ability to get to the toilet is considered in selecting the most appropriate response. The response selected should represent the patient's ability more than 50% of the time.

(M1845) Toileting Hygiene: Current ability to maintain perineal hygiene safely, adjust clothes and/or incontinence pads before and after using toilet, commode, bedpan, urinal. If managing ostomy, includes cleaning area around stoma, but not managing equipment.

☐ 0 - Able to manage toileting hygiene and clothing management without assistance.
☐ 1 - Able to manage toileting hygiene and clothing management without assistance if supplies/implements are laid out for the patient.
☐ 2 - Someone must help the patient to maintain toileting hygiene and/or adjust clothing.
☐ 3 - Patient depends entirely upon another person to maintain toileting hygiene.

(M1850) Transferring: Current ability to move safely from bed to chair, or ability to turn and position self in bed if patient is bedfast.

☐ 0 - Able to independently transfer.
☐ 1 - Able to transfer with minimal human assistance or with use of an assistive device.

☐ 2 - Able to bear weight and pivot during the transfer process but unable to transfer self.

☐ 3 - Unable to transfer self and is unable to bear weight or pivot when transferred by another person.

☐ 4 - Bedfast, unable to transfer but is able to turn and position self in bed.

☐ 5 - Bedfast, unable to transfer and is unable to turn and position self.

M1850 measures transferring from bed to chair or repositioning if the patient is bedfast. The item-specific guidance clarifies that *bedfast* refers to being confined to the bed because of either a physician restriction or the patient's inability to tolerate being out of the bed. A patient is not bedfast simply because he or she spends most of his or her time in bed or requires a hydraulic lift and two people to get in and out of bed.

Use of equipment or devices does not appear until the second response option (1) in M1850, so indicating that the patient can independently transfer means that he or she can do so without an assistive device. When a patient uses the arms of a chair to push up and augment the transfer to stand or pivot, doing so does not necessarily constitute use of an assistive device according to item-specific guidance.

Extensive specific instructions are included for M1850, and the occupational therapist may find opportunities to assist team members in understanding the nuances of the guidance. For example, *assistance* includes any combination of verbal cuing, environmental setup, and hands-on assistance. *Minimal assistance* indicates that the person assisting the patient is contributing less than 25% of the total effort required to perform the transfer. An occupational therapist can provide examples for team members of what less than 25% assistance might look like in the context of a shared patient.

(M1860) Ambulation/Locomotion: Current ability to walk safely, once in a standing position, or use a wheelchair, once in a seated position, on a variety of surfaces.

☐ 0 - Able to independently walk on even and uneven surfaces and negotiate stairs with or without railings (specifically: needs no human assistance or assistive device).

☐ 1 - With the use of a one-handed device (for example, cane, single crutch, hemi-walker), able to independently walk on even and uneven surfaces and negotiate stairs with or without railings.

☐ 2 - Requires use of a two-handed device (for example, walker or crutches) to walk alone on a level surface and/or requires human supervision or assistance to negotiate stairs or steps or uneven surfaces.

☐ 3 - Able to walk only with the supervision or assistance of another person at all times.

☐ 4 - Chairfast, <u>unable</u> to ambulate but is able to wheel self independently.

☐ 5 - Chairfast, unable to ambulate and is <u>unable</u> to wheel self.

☐ 6 - Bedfast, unable to ambulate or be up in a chair.

Item M1860 measures mobility once the patient is in position to ambulate or use a wheelchair, separating the transfer from the activity. The response options are different for when assistive devices are used and when they are not. Assistive devices are not mentioned until the second (1) and third (2) response options, and the responses distinguish between one-handed and two-handed devices. Clinicians must carefully read the responses, though, because more than just the type of device differentiates the second and third responses. The second response indicates that the patient uses a one-handed device but can independently walk on even or uneven surfaces and negotiate stairs with or without railings. However, the third response describes the use of a two-handed device to walk alone only on a level surface and requires supervision or assistance for uneven surfaces or negotiating stairs. Unless the occupational therapist carefully reads these responses and considers all of the detailed variables, he or she risks answering M1860 incorrectly.

L. Medications

Occupational therapists must understand the distinctions between the items in the medications section both to collect accurate data and to capture improvement in these outcomes. Quality improvement efforts have emphasized medication management and its impact on the outcomes and cost of health care delivery since the IOM released its 2000 report *To Err Is Human*. In response to this report's account of medication errors, all health care settings established processes focused on medication reconciliation, drug regimen review, and education to promote patients' ability to manage their medications. The first OASIS item in the medications section, M2000, is one of the few OASIS items that reflect a CoP required for the home health care setting (§ 484.55[c]).

(M2000) Drug Regimen Review: Does a complete drug regimen review indicate potential clinically significant medication issues (for example, adverse drug reactions, ineffective drug therapy, significant side effects, drug interactions, duplicate therapy, omissions, dosage errors, or noncompliance [nonadherence])?

- ☐ 0 - Not assessed/reviewed *[Go to M2010]*
- ☐ 1 - No problems found during review *[Go to M2010]*
- ☐ 2 - Problems found during review
- ☐ NA - Patient is not taking any medications *[Go to M2040]*

As noted in the *Framework* (AOTA, 2014, p. S19), developing, managing, and maintaining medication routines is an IADL within the domain of occupational therapy. As Siebert (2010) observed,

> In order to complete the drug regimen review accurately, an occupational therapist must analyze the patient's performance (e.g., does the patient report symptoms or exhibit signs that medication is ineffective or producing side effects?), collaborate with other clinicians, or use pharmaceutical software to address the required elements of the review. (p. 31)

Most HHAs have policies in place addressing completion of the drug regimen review by an occupational therapist rather than a nurse and specifying the vehicle for communicating the necessary information for compliance with this CoP.

(M2020) Management of Oral Medications: Patient's current ability to prepare and take all oral medications reliably and safely, including administration of the correct dosage at the appropriate times/intervals. **Excludes injectable and IV medications. (NOTE: This refers to ability, not compliance or willingness.)**

☐ 0 - Able to independently take the correct oral medication(s) and proper dosage(s) at the correct times.

☐ 1 - Able to take medication(s) at the correct times if:
(a) individual dosages are prepared in advance by another person; OR
(b) another person develops a drug diary or chart.

☐ 2 - Able to take medication(s) at the correct times if given reminders by another person at the appropriate times

☐ 3 - Unable to take medication unless administered by another person.

☐ NA - No oral medications prescribed.

The medication-related item in which occupational therapists can have the most influence in improving outcomes is M2020. Siebert (2010) noted,

> In order to accurately assess the patient's ability to manage medication routines, the occupational therapist must identify the patient's existing routines, analyze the activity demands associated with administering and managing medications, and assess the patient's skills in relation to the activity demands. From this evaluation process, the therapist then selects appropriate intervention approaches (e.g., remediation, establishment, compensation, adaptation) to best support the patient's performance of medication routines. In many cases, this intervention is coordinated with nursing intervention focused on medication teaching. (p. 31)

OASIS Process Measure Item Guidance

OASIS process items addressing vaccines, pressure ulcers, heart failure symptoms, POC and intervention synopses, medication intervention, and patient or caregiver drug education intervention require the occupational therapist to look back in the medical record to select the correct response. Occupational therapists often collect OASIS data at the end of the episode, when many of these look-back process measures are being collected. The occupational therapist should identify the HHA's look-back tools or strategies. For example, an HHA may keep a record of patients to whom a vaccine has been delivered, or the documentation software may link visits documenting heart failure symptoms. Therefore, it is beneficial to be familiar with which OASIS items require a look back and to have strategies to improve the efficiency of collecting the correct response item. The following sections address the process measure items.

Vaccines

OASIS items M1041 through M1056 in Section C of Chapter 3 address population health and prevention and are harmonized with similar measures in other health care settings and collected at transfer and discharge time points. The instructions for these items contain information integral to answering them correctly. Each year, the Centers for Disease Control and Prevention (CDC) identifies the year's influenza season, declares when there is a shortage of influenza vaccines, provides age and condition guidelines for the influenza and pneumococcal vaccines, and compiles a list of medical contraindications for each vaccine. The HHA should make the necessary CDC information available to clinicians, and occupational therapists should identify where in the medical record the HHA typically documents whether either of the vaccines were delivered to the patient during the defined episode.

(M1041) Influenza Vaccine Data Collection Period: Does this episode of care (SOC/ROC to Transfer/Discharge) include any dates on or between October 1 and March 31?

☐ 0 - No *[Go to M1051]*
☐ 1 - Yes

(M1046) Influenza Vaccine Received: Did the patient receive the influenza vaccine for this year's flu season?

☐ 1 - Yes; received from your agency during this episode of care (SOC/ROC to Transfer/Discharge)
☐ 2 - Yes; received from your agency during a prior episode of care (SOC/ROC to Transfer/Discharge)
☐ 3 - Yes; received from another health care provider (for example: physician, pharmacist)
☐ 4 - No; patient offered and declined
☐ 5 - No; patient assessed and determined to have medical contraindication(s)
☐ 6 - No; not indicated - patient does not meet age/condition guidelines for influenza vaccine
☐ 7 - No; inability to obtain vaccine due to declared shortage
☐ 8 - No; patient did not receive the vaccine due to reasons other than those listed in Responses 4–7.

(M1051) Pneumococcal Vaccine: Has the patient ever received the pneumococcal vaccination (for example, pneumovax)?

☐ 0 - No
☐ 1 - Yes *[Go to M1500 at (transfer); Go to M1230 at (discharge)]*

(M1056) Reason Pneumococcal Vaccine not received: If patient has never received the pneumococcal vaccination (for example, pneumovax), state reason:

☐ 1 - Offered and declined
☐ 2 - Assessed and determined to have medical contraindication(s)

☐ 3 - Not indicated; patient does not meet age/condition guidelines for pneumococcal vaccination

☐ 4 - None of the above

Pressure Ulcers

CMS (2010a), informed by the National Pressure Ulcer Advisory Panel, has encouraged pressure ulcer risk assessments to reduce the overall incidence of pressure ulcers. The measures in M1307 through M1309 in Section F of Chapter 3 require the clinician to look back in the medical record to identify the presence or development of pressure ulcers during a home health episode and to estimate the length of time the pressure ulcer remained unhealed. Nursing orders on the home health POC to address pressure ulcers may have been discharged before establishing the ongoing need for occupational therapy, so knowing where to look back for this information is necessary.

(M1307) The **Oldest Stage II Pressure Ulcer** that is present at discharge: (Excludes healed Stage II Pressure Ulcers)

☐ 1 - Was present at the most recent SOC/ROC assessment

☐ 2 - Developed since the most recent SOC/ROC assessment. Record date pressure ulcer first identified: __/__/__ (month / day / year)

☐ NA - No Stage II pressure ulcers are present at discharge

(M1308) Current Number of Unhealed Pressure Ulcers at Each Stage or Unstageable:

(Enter "0" if none; Excludes Stage I pressure ulcers and healed Stage II pressure ulcers)

Stage Descriptions – unhealed pressure ulcers	Number Currently Present
a. **Stage II:** Partial thickness loss of dermis presenting as a shallow open ulcer with red pink wound bed, without slough. May also present as an intact or open/ruptured serum-filled blister.	
b. **Stage III:** Full thickness tissue loss. Subcutaneous fat may be visible but bone, tendon, or muscles are not exposed. Slough may be present but does not obscure the depth of tissue loss. May include undermining and tunneling.	
c. **Stage IV:** Full thickness tissue loss with visible bone, tendon, or muscle. Slough or eschar may be present on some parts of the wound bed. Often includes undermining and tunneling.	
d.1 Unstageable: Known or likely but Unstageable due to non-removable dressing or device.	
d.2 Unstageable: Known or likely but Unstageable due to coverage of wound bed by slough and/or eschar.	
d.3 Unstageable: Suspected deep tissue injury in evolution.	

(M1309) Worsening in Pressure Ulcer Status since SOC/ROC:

Instructions for a–c: For Stage II, III and IV pressure ulcers, report the number that are new or have increased in numerical stage since the most recent SOC/ROC	
	Enter Number (Enter "0" if there are no current Stage II, III or IV pressure ulcers OR if all current Stage II, III or IV pressure ulcers existed at the same numerical stage at most recent SOC/ROC)
a. Stage II	
b. Stage III	
c. Stage IV	
Instructions for d: For pressure ulcers that are Unstageable due to slough/eschar, report the number that are new or were a Stage I or II at the most recent SOC/ROC.	
	Enter Number (Enter "0" if there are no Unstageable pressure ulcers at discharge OR if all current Unstageable pressure ulcers were Stage III or IV or were Unstageable at most recent SOC/ROC)
d. Unstageable due to coverage of wound bed by slough or eschar	

M1308 and M1309 consist of tables that capture the length of time a patient had a pressure ulcer and the stage of the ulcer. Reviewing the specific instructions for these items, including the examples, increases the clinician's ease in completing this table, which provides much information about pressure ulcers with very few data entered.

Heart Failure Symptoms

To record process measures M1500 and M1510 in Section H of Chapter 3, the clinician must look back for two pieces of information: (1) whether the patient has been diagnosed with heart failure and (2) whether symptoms of heart failure were documented at the time of or at any time since the previous OASIS assessment.

(M1500) Symptoms in Heart Failure Patients: If patient has been diagnosed with heart failure, did the patient exhibit symptoms indicated by clinical heart failure guidelines (including dyspnea, orthopnea, edema, or weight gain) at the time of or at any time since the previous OASIS assessment?

　□ 0 - No *[Go to M2004 at (transfer); Go to M1600 at (discharge)]*
　□ 1 - Yes

☐ 2 - Not assessed *[Go to M2004 at (transfer); Go to M1600 at (discharge)]*

☐ NA - Patient does not have diagnosis of heart failure *[Go to M2004 at (transfer); Go to M1600 at (discharge)]*

(M1510) Heart Failure Follow-up: If patient has been diagnosed with heart failure and has exhibited symptoms indicative of heart failure at the time of or at any time since the previous OASIS assessment, what action(s) has (have) been taken to respond? **(Mark all that apply.)**

☐ 0 - No action taken

☐ 1 - Patient's physician (or other primary care practitioner) contacted the same day

☐ 2 - Patient advised to get emergency treatment (for example, call 911 or go to emergency room)

☐ 3 - Implemented physician-ordered patient-specific established parameters for treatment

☐ 4 - Patient education or other clinical interventions

☐ 5 - Obtained change in care plan orders (for example, increased monitoring by agency, change in visit frequency, telehealth)

M1500 is best answered by starting at the bottom response and working up. If there is no diagnosis of heart failure, the answer is "NA" (not applicable), and M1510 (heart failure follow-up) is skipped. If symptoms were documented, the actions taken is the last piece of information that requires looking back in the medical record. The likeliest scenario in which an occupational therapist would be collecting these data is at agency discharge after a nursing discharge earlier in the episode.

A caution not found in the item-specific guidance is in order: M1500 offers a response of "not assessed" (2), and M1510 offers an option of "no action taken" (0). If the clinician selects either of these responses without taking the time to look back for this information, the expectation is that the clinician will document the rationale for not completing these best practices. The "not assessed" and "no action taken" responses give the appearance of having opted out of performing these practices, which reflects poorly on the agency in the publicly reported outcomes. Again, finding out from the HHA the swiftest manner to look back in the medical record for this information increases efficiency in reporting this item.

Plan of Care Synopsis and Intervention Synopsis

Item M2250, Plan of Care Synopsis (Section N), asks whether the physician-ordered POC includes a series of elements, and M2400, Intervention Synopsis (Section P), asks whether a series of interventions were both included in the POC and implemented; each item is followed by a long list of elements or interventions for the clinician to check off. These items reflect best practices in care coordination with the physician. M2250 is completed at the beginning of an episode, and answering M2400 requires looking back to M2250.

Some of the interventions listed in these items reflect other process measures completed at SOC and ROC that CMS considers to be best practices, including falls risk screening (M1910, Section K), depression screening (M1730, Section J), and pain assessment (M1240, Section E). The item-specific guidance in the manual reminds us that the physician-ordered POC means that the clinician has engaged in both discussion and agreement with the physician before the end of the assessment window. Also, in the case of both M2250 (Section N) and M2400 (Section P), another rule of thumb is to read the tables from right to left. When selecting a response, the clinician should first consider whether a particular plan or intervention is not applicable to reduce the time spent looking for the presence of such a plan or intervention.

Medications

The medication process measures reflect industry expert guidance on safety and care coordination. Only two OASIS data items require the clinician to look back in the medical record for accurate completion: (1) medication intervention and (2) patient or caregiver drug education intervention (Section L).

> **(M2004) Medication Intervention:** If there were any clinically significant medication issues at the time of, or at any time since the previous OASIS assessment, was a physician or the physician-designee contacted within one calendar day to resolve any identified clinically significant medication issues, including reconciliation?
>
> ☐ 0 - No
> ☐ 1 - Yes
> ☐ NA - No clinically significant medication issues identified at the time of or at any time since the previous OASIS assessment

Selecting "yes" for M2004 means both that the HHA has notified the patient's physician's office and that the office responded to the HHA by the end of the next calendar day with the necessary information. Becoming familiar with the HHA's procedures for communicating with the physician's office may increase efficiency in selecting the correct response for M2004.

> **(M2015) Patient/Caregiver Drug Education Intervention:** At the time of, or at any time since the previous OASIS assessment, was the patient/caregiver instructed by agency staff or other health care provider to monitor the effectiveness of drug therapy, adverse drug reactions, and significant side effects, and how and when to report problems that may occur?
>
> ☐ 0 - No
> ☐ 1 - Yes
> ☐ NA - Patient not taking any drugs

When an occupational therapist is collecting data for M2015, it typically occurs on agency discharge after other skilled disciplines have completed their individual POCs. If skilled nursing was on the POC, information on drug education to the patient or caregiver is typically already completed. However, because a therapy-only episode is a possibility, the clinician should not assume that such education has not taken place. As Vance (2010) argued,

> Therapists do more education regarding medications than they realize. How many times does one or more of the following scenarios occur? The patient is advised to notify the physician that the pain medication does not appear to be working; to use strategies for reaching a bathroom in time when on a water pill, rather than not taking the water pill to avoid accidents; to tell the nurse that the new medication seems to cause dizziness; or to understand that nighttime pain relievers increase the risk for falls when getting up during the night to go to the bathroom. Consider that any scenario similar to these performed by yourself constitutes a "yes" response to [M2015] regardless of additional education by another clinician in a record review. (p. CE4)

References

American Occupational Therapy Association. (2014). Occupational therapy practice framework: Domain and process (3rd ed.). *American Journal of Occupational Therapy, 68*(Suppl. 1), S1–S48. http://dx.doi.org/10.5014/ajot.2014.682006

American Occupational Therapy Association. (2015). Standards of practice for occupational therapy. *American Journal of Occupational Therapy, 69*(Suppl. 3), 6913410057. http://dx.doi.org/10.5014/ajot.2015.696S06

Centers for Medicare & Medicaid Services. (2010a). *Outcome-Based Quality Improvement (OBQI) manual.* Baltimore: Author. Retrieved from https://www.cms.gov/HomeHealthQualityInits/Downloads/HHQIOBQIManual.pdf

Centers for Medicare & Medicaid Services. (2010b). *Outcome-Based Quality Monitoring (OBQM) manual: Agency patient-related characteristics reports and potentially avoidable event reports.* Baltimore: Author. Retrieved from http://www.cms.gov/HomeHealthQualityInits/Downloads/HHQIOBQMManual.pdf

Centers for Medicare & Medicaid Services. (2010c). *Process-Based Quality Improvement (PBQI) manual.* Baltimore: Author. Retrieved from http://www.cms.gov/HomeHealthQualityInits/Downloads/HHQIOASIS-PBQI.pdf

Centers for Medicare & Medicaid Services. (2011). *Part 484: Home health services.* Washington, DC: Author. Retrieved from http://www.gpo.gov/fdsys/pkg/CFR-2011-title42-vol5/pdf/CFR-2011-title42-vol5-part484.pdf

Centers for Medicare & Medicaid Services. (2012). Outcome and Assessment Information Set (OASIS): *Data set.* Retrieved from http://www.cms.gov/Medicare/Quality-Initiatives-Patient-Assessment-Instruments/OASIS/DataSet.html

Centers for Medicare & Medicaid Services. (2015). *OASIS–C1/ICD–10 version guidance manual.* Retrieved from http://www.cms.gov/Medicare/Quality-Initiatives-Patient-Assessment-Instruments/HomeHealthQualityInits/HHQIOASISUserManual.html

Centers for Medicare & Medicaid Services & National Center for Health Statistics. (2014). *ICD–10–CM official guidelines for coding and reporting.* Washington, DC: Authors.

Health Care Financing Administration. (1999). *OASIS implementation manual.* Baltimore: Author.

Health Insurance Portability and Accountability Act of 1996 (HIPAA), Pub. L. 104–191, 42 U.S.C. § 300gg, 29 U.S.C § 1181-1183, and 42 U.S.C. § 1320d-1320d9.

Institute of Medicine. (2000). *To err is human: Building a safer health system.* Washington, DC: National Academy Press.

Medicare Payment Advisory Commission. (2015). *Report to the Congress: Medicare and the Health Care Delivery System.* Washington DC: Author. Retrieved from http://medpac.gov/documents/reports/june-2015-report-to-the-congress-medicare-and-the-health-care-delivery-system.pdf?sfvrsn=0

Siebert, C. (2010, November). OASIS, scope of practice, and the therapies. *Caring Magazine,* pp. 28–33.

Vance, K. (2010). Occupational therapy and OASIS C. *OT Practice, 15*(13), CE1–CE8.

World Health Organization. (2011). *International statistical classification of diseases and related health problems, 10th revision.* Geneva: Author.

AOTA Fact Sheet: Occupational Therapy's Role in Home Health

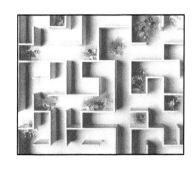

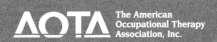 **Fact Sheet**

Occupational Therapy's Role in
Home Health

Occupational therapy practitioners are effective and important components of any home health agency's patient care and administrative teams. Occupational therapy practitioners can have many roles in improving efficiency, implementing new administrative requirements, and optimizing outcomes for patients.

Occupational therapy can perform admission visits.
Occupational therapists can conduct the initial assessment visit and the start of care comprehensive assessment on therapy-only patients for whom occupational therapy "establishes eligibility" (Conditions of Participation, 42 CFR 484.55). For many payers (e.g., Medicaid, private insurance), occupational therapy does establish the initial eligibility for home health, even though Medicare restricts occupational therapy as a qualifying service only to when

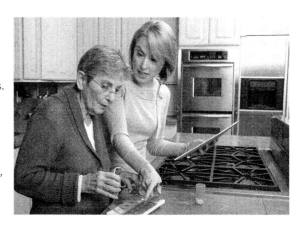

there is a "continuing need" (see below). But agencies and consumers should not restrict options for initial visits for non-Medicare beneficiaries. Occupational therapy can be a valuable resource to conduct the initial visits, increasing the number of available staff to conduct initial visits, addressing home safety issues earlier and identifying established routines to share with team members for improved participation by the patient in the plan of care.

Occupational therapy qualifies a Medicare patient for continued home health eligibility. A continued need for occupational therapy can extend eligibility under Medicare because the need for occupational therapy alone qualifies Medicare patients for continuation of the home health benefit and thus for any dependent aide and medical social work services the patient needs (*Medicare Benefit Policy Manual,* Chapter 7, Section 40.24). Occupational therapy may be the only continuing service needed by patients, but it is sufficient to qualify for continued coverage of Medicare home health services. "Subsequent to an initial covered occupational therapy service [visit], continuing occupational therapy services which meet the requirements of § 409.44(c) are considered to be qualifying services" ("Beneficiary qualifications for coverage of services," 42 CFR 409.42[c][4]).

Occupational therapy can collect OASIS data at any time point subsequent to the start of care. OASIS accuracy ensures that payment is appropriate and outcomes are accurate, benefiting the agency and the patient. Occupational therapy practitioners can contribute to this process. Once competency is established, occupational therapists are well prepared to perform assessments collecting OASIS data at resumption of care, other follow up, recertifications, and discharge time points (*OASIS Guidance Manual*). Furthermore, occupational therapists can help other agency staff understand the most effective techniques to assess patient needs, activities of daily living (ADLs), and instrumental ADLs to more correctly complete the OASIS and develop a plan of care. Occupational therapists can provide this guidance based on their unique training and perspective, which focuses on functional capabilities.

Occupational therapy can assist in aide supervision and in training of aides to maximize effectiveness and promote patient recovery. An occupational therapist may supervise the home health aide when nursing services are not on the plan of care, but occupational therapy is on the plan (Conditions of Participation, 42 CFR 484.36). (*Note:* Some states require nursing to always supervise aides; check your state regulations.) Whether supervising or not, occupational therapy can "fine tune" the aide care plan so that aide services help to move the patient toward independence in self-care, potentially speeding progress while reducing needed aide visits and the length of the home health episode.

Living Life To Its Fullest®
OCCUPATIONAL THERAPY

www.aota.org
4720 Montgomery Lane, Bethesda, MD 20814-3449
Phone: 301-652-2682 TDD: 800-377-8555 Fax: 301-652-7711

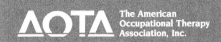 **The American Occupational Therapy Association, Inc.**

Occupational therapy contributes to stronger outcomes—for your patients and your agency.

Patients and their families are concerned about your patients' abilities to take care of themselves and to manage at home safely. Some patients have the potential to regain skills affected by their conditions. Other patients need strategies to prevent further loss of abilities. Regardless of specific diagnosis or condition, occupational therapy practitioners offer strategies for your patients to manage daily activities while reducing the risk of injury or further decline (Goldberg, 2009; Ryan, 2006). Occupational therapy practitioners find the right fit between patients' abilities, needed and desired activities, and their home environment so patients can manage safely and productively—*at home.*

You are also concerned about your patients' ability to *manage their conditions*. Management of chronic conditions is in large part management of daily activities. Occupational therapy brings expertise to help patients translate "doctor's orders" to manageable daily habits and routines (Bondoc & Siebert, 2010). Occupational therapy can strengthen outcomes related to:

- **Medication management:** Occupational therapy addresses strategies to enhance medication adherence and integrate medication management into patients' daily routines (Sanders & Van Oss, 2013; Touchard & Berthelot, 1999).

- **Daily management of conditions such as:**
    - *Diabetes:* Occupational therapy addresses the many aspects of diabetes management that must become daily routines: blood sugar monitoring, hygiene and foot care, meal planning and preparation, healthy coping strategies, and physical activity. Occupational therapy practitioners can also train patients with diabetes to use compensatory strategies for vision, sensory, or motor loss that may interfere with their daily activities (Sokol-McKay, 2011).
    - *Heart failure:* Occupational therapy addresses strategies to conserve energy and reduce the demands of activities, while integrating appropriate physical activity and self-monitoring. Occupational therapy practitioners can assist patients to master new activities—daily weights, modified diets—and incorporate these activities into regular routines (Branick, 2003; Norberg, Boman, & Lofgren, 2010).
    - *Chronic obstructive pulmonary disease:* Occupational therapy addresses strategies to conserve energy, reduce the demands of activities, and self-monitor to avoid exacerbations. Occupational therapy practitioners can assist patients to incorporate pacing, planning, and stress management into daily activities (Branick, 2003).
    - *Cognitive and behavioral health conditions:* Occupational therapy addresses daily routines, medication adherence, self-management, and stress management strategies. With a core knowledge base in psychosocial issues, occupational therapists can also address behavioral health conditions and train caregivers to provide appropriate cues and support to patients with cognitive limitations to optimize performance and reduce agitation or confusion.

References

Bondoc, S., & Siebert, C. (2010). *The role of occupational therapy in chronic disease management.* Retrieved from http://www.aota.org/Consumers/Professionals/WhatIsOT/HW/Facts/Chronic-Disease-Management.aspx

Branick, L. (2003). Integrating the principles of energy conservation during everyday activities. *Caring, 22*(1), 30–31.

Goldberg, A. (2009). Optimizing the skills of occupational therapy: An overview through a case study. *Home Healthcare Nurse, 27*(2), 120–123.

Norberg, E.-B., Boman, K., & Lofgren, B. (2010). Impact of fatigue on everyday life among older people with chronic heart failure. *Australian Occupational Therapy Journal, 57,* 34–41.

Ryan, J. M. (2006). Teamwork keeps the pressure off: The role of the occupational therapist in the prevention of pressure ulcers. *Home Healthcare Nurse, 26*(2), 97–103.

Sanders, M. J., & Van Oss, T. (2013). Using daily routines to promote medication adherence in older adults. *American Journal of Occupational Therapy, 67,* 91–99.

Sokol-McKay, D. A. (2011). *Occupational therapy's role in diabetes self-management.* Retrieved from http://www.aota.org/Consumers/Professionals/WhatIsOT/PA/Facts/Diabetes.aspx

Touchard, B. M., & Berthelot, K. (1999). Collaborative home practice: Nursing and occupational therapy ensure appropriate medication administration. *Home Healthcare Nurse, 17*(1), 45–51.

Living Life To Its Fullest®
OCCUPATIONAL THERAPY

Occupational therapy enables people of all ages to live life to its fullest by helping them to promote health, make lifestyle or environmental changes, and prevent—or live better with—injury, illness, or disability. By looking at the whole picture—a client's psychological, physical, emotional, and social makeup—occupational therapy assists people to achieve their goals, function at the highest possible level, maintain or rebuild their independence, and participate in the everyday activities of life.

Index

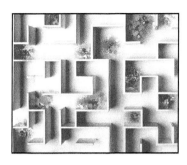

Boxes, case studies, exhibits, figures, and tables are indicated by "b," "cs," "e," "f," and "t," respectively, following page numbers.